DANVILLE PUBLIC LIBRARY
P9-CDA-259

REINVENTING AMERICAN HEALTH CARE

REINVENTING AMERICAN HEALTH CARE

How the Affordable Care Act Will Improve Our Terribly Complex, Blatantly Unjust, Outrageously Expensive, Grossly Inefficient, Error Prone System

EZEKIEL J. EMANUEL

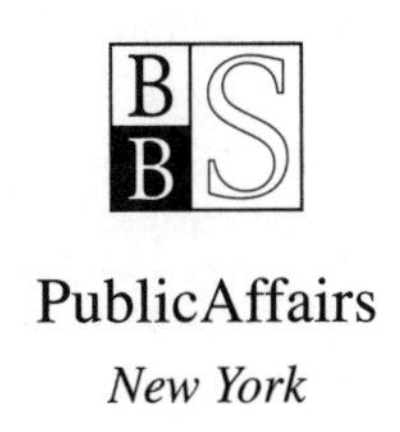

PublicAffairs
New York

Published in the United States by PublicAffairs™,
a Member of the Perseus Books Group

Printed in the United States of America.

PublicAffairs books are available at special discounts for bulk purchases in the U.S. by corporations, institutions, and other organizations. For more information, please contact the Special Markets Department at the Perseus Books Group, 2300 Chestnut Street, Suite 200, Philadelphia, PA 19103, call (800) 810-4145, ext. 5000, or e-mail special.markets@perseusbooks.com.

Editorial production by *Marra*thon Production Services. www.marrathon.net

Book design by Jane Raese
Set in 12-point Dante

Library of Congress Cataloging-in-Publication Data
Emanuel, Ezekiel J., 1957– author.
Reinventing American health care : how the Affordable Care Act will improve our terribly complex, blatantly unjust, outrageously expensive, grossly inefficient, error prone system / Ezekiel J. Emanuel. — First edition.
p. ; cm.
Includes bibliographical references and index.
ISBN 978-1-61039-345-4 (hardcover) ISBN 978-1-61039-346-1 (e-book)
I. Title. [DNLM: 1. United States. Patient Protection and Affordable Care Act. 2. Health Care Reform—United States. 3. Health Services—United States. 4. Health Services Administration—United States. 5. National Health Programs—economics—United States. WA 540 AA1]
RA413
362.1'0425—dc23
2013049343

FIRST EDITION
10 9 8 7 6 5 4 3 2

DISCLAIMER

Health care is dynamic. Though progress can seem maddeningly slow, the system is constantly reinventing itself. The cost estimates, enrollment numbers, and other data in this book were accurate as of December 1, 2013—when I stopped writing. Accurate is a matter of degree since different government agencies often report different numbers for the same data point and private organizations often have other numbers. We have done our best to comes as close as possible to reality. Complicating things even more is that health care is changing rapidly. The Supreme Court will agree to hear new cases related to health care, the Medicare actuary will issue new reports on cost growth in Medicare and Medicaid and the overall rate of health care inflation, the Congressional Budget Office will publish new estimates of long-term health care costs and their impact on the federal budget, and policymakers in Washington will craft new policy fixes and stake out new positions. It is possible that these or other changes could alter some of the trends, detailed numbers, and specific predictions discussed throughout this book. Nevertheless, the direction of change and what statisticians call the central tendencies are unlikely to be significantly altered.

To my many generous mentors
who supported, nurtured, and shaped
my ideas and intellectual drive

RAYMOND A. DWEK

RASHI FEIN

VICTOR R. FUCHS

GEORGE KATEB

MICHAEL J. SANDEL

JUDITH N. SHKLAR
(*in memorium*)

DENNIS F. THOMPSON

Contents

Acknowledgments

This book owes its existence to 2 journalists. Some time in 2011, the *New York Times* switched Sabrina Tavernise from writing on foreign policy matters to public health issues. Sabrina called me up and asked if I would meet her for coffee (or tea in my case) to get her up to speed on the American health care system. It was a joke of course. One hour is nowhere near enough to even begin to understand the insanely complex system. Nevertheless, we met at Union Station in Washington, D.C., and I did my best. But I wished I had a 300 page book explaining the system and the Affordable Care Act that I could give Sabrina for background reading. But no such book existed. So you can blame Sabrina for the fact that this book exists at all.

With the realization that there needed to be a primer on the American health care system I called Jonathan Cohn and asked him if he would be interested in co-authoring the book. Jonathan was hesitant. A book was a major undertaking, he said. He would have to talk to his family to see if they could sanction it. In reality, Jonathan was understandably reluctant to take on the task of writing another book. Not only did he have his own work, the prospect of writing with me was probably too much to bear. So you can blame Jonathan for the fact that this book is not better, and better written.

Many other people helped in bringing this book to fruition. Paul Begala offered recollections of both the Wofford Senate race and the Clinton health reform effort. Numerous experts read sections and the entire manuscript and gave insightful comments, including Henry Aaron, Ken Baer, Howard Bauchner, David Johnson, Bob Kocher, Farzad Mostashari, Peggy O'Kane, and Topher Spiro. They offered great advice, and saved me from many mistakes. Many of the remaining mistakes are because I did not adhere to their sage advice. I also managed to get Jonathan Cohn to read and critique parts of the text. In addition, several lay friends read the book to be sure it was clearly written and to catch errors, including Jen Homans, Corby Kummer, Michael D'Antonio, and Andy Oram. Paul Eberwine and Gabrielle Anderson did a tremendous amount of research, fact checking, and preparation of tables.

Special thanks goes to the very harshest but absolutely best—and fastest—editor I have, my youngest daughter Natalia Emanuel. She spent hours reading and "lovingly" attacking my words.

I greatly appreciate the willingness of Erin, Wayne, and Baltazar (not their real names, but they know who they are) to tell me their stories, and allow me to tell their stories. And to ensure they were factually accurate.

My agents, Suzanne Gluck and Jennifer Rudolph Walsh, and publisher Clive Priddle were enthusiastic from the start even about a book in a segment of the market that rarely sells and always loses money—health policy.

This book could not have occurred without the unbelievable hard work of my executive assistant Beth Walker Dunn, who jiggered my crazy schedule to create time to write and helped in so many other big and small ways.

Last but not least, Andrew Steinmetz, my academic chief of staff, was invaluable in making this book a reality. It would not exist were I not able to bounce ideas off Andrew, and rely on his help in delineating the chapters and organizing my thoughts. Andrew's thorough research and his careful reading saved me from many errors. He is a thoughtful and dedicated COS who makes me look much better than I really am.

REINVENTING AMERICAN HEALTH CARE

= INTRODUCTION =

Erin's Disease

Erin is unlucky.

Truly American, Erin says that despite her hardships, "she is the luckiest [woman] on the face of the earth"; that she "might have been given a bad break, but she has an awful lot to live for."

Erin, who comes from a large, East coast Irish family, arrived in Aspen, Colorado, one winter to visit her brother, who was taking some time off between college and graduate school. She fell in love with the place and remained for the next 23 years. She also fell in love with Justin, an accomplished mountaineer whom she married in 1999.

Justin and Erin made a good life together. He worked each winter as a ski patroller on Aspen Mountain. She started a marketing company and was self-employed. In 2000 Erin gave birth to their first daughter. Three years later they had their second.

Erin and Justin had the usual struggles of a young couple raising 2 children—finding affordable housing; expanding the hours in the day to accommodate the children, friends, work, themselves; keeping in touch with family out east.

But they also felt blessed. They lived healthy, active lives amid the beautiful scenery of Aspen. They hiked and biked and skied together as a family. And they formed close friendships.

They rarely needed to worry about their health or engage the health care system. Everyone ate a healthy diet. They were physically active. Neither Erin nor Justin smoked. Neither had any chronic condition nor took medications regularly. The girls did not have allergies, asthma, or any other childhood health problems. Besides 2 C-sections for the girls, no one had been admitted to the hospital.

Then tragedy struck. A few days before Christmas in 2008, Erin and Justin had an amazing morning skiing together. Two feet of fresh powder had fallen the previous night. Skiing conditions could not have been better. After lunch Erin left to meet their children, and Justin went back out to ski, alone this time, heading for his favorite, almost secret spot on the backside of Aspen Mountain. It was an area he had skied hundreds of times previously. Despite a promise to be home in a couple of hours, Justin never returned. A nighttime search of the mountain found his frozen body, buried in a freak avalanche 100 yards wide and 3 feet deep. The coroner's report concluded that Justin had died almost instantly of blunt force trauma, a result of hitting a tree and being buried under the snow.

With the support of her parents and her Aspen friends, Erin carried on as a single mother of 2 young daughters. Over the next few years she recovered from Justin's death. She began living her life again. Her daughters were recovering too. Her marketing business was thriving. They were still a healthy family.

In 2013 tragedy struck again. In March Erin and the girls went to Mexico with friends for a spring vacation. A few of the people on the trip got Montezuma's revenge that lasted for a day or 2. Erin did not experience any problems. But after being home 2 weeks she began to have severe abdominal cramping, followed by bloody diarrhea. Because of the blood, Erin went to her family physician. Once she heard Erin had been in Mexico, the physician thought it might be a bacterial infection. She ordered some stool cultures. Erin tested positive for a *Campylobacter* intestinal infection. She was treated with some antibiotics.

The cramps subsided and the diarrhea resolved. After she finished the treatment Erin did not feel great, but she seemed to be recovering. About 2 weeks later, however, the cramps returned. Erin's physician thought the medicine may not have gotten all the infection or that she may have developed a secondary infection. So they tried a combination of 2 additional antibiotics that would kill "90% of anything that was there."

It didn't work. Instead, Erin was getting worse. And then she felt a mass-like something in the lower part of her abdomen.

It was clear to Erin that something was wrong. On May 9 she went to the emergency room of the small Aspen Valley Hospital. The health care team was still focused on the possibility of an infection. They ordered a CT scan. While Erin was waiting for the CT results a nurse asked her whether there was anything she needed. Not having had anything to eat or drink all day, Erin asked for some water. After Erin had taken just 2 sips of the water, the nurse rushed back into the room and took the water away. "The doctor is coming to see you," she said.

Clearly something was wrong, seriously wrong. The ER physician said that Erin had a large section of "telescoping colon." Technically that is an intussusception in which one part of the colon swallows or overrides the other. Though regularly seen in younger children, this is very rare in adults. In the report the radiologist reading the CT wondered whether some fat bulge might be causing this telescoping. The ER physician said the intussusception could cause serious problems, strangulation of the colon and perforation, and that it had to be dealt with by emergency surgery in the next 20 minutes.

Trying to keep her head, Erin asked whether the surgery could be done laproscopically. Could the doctors wait to get a second opinion? Maybe send her to Denver for such a serious operation? But no other surgeon was available for a second opinion; indeed, the surgeon on call was not an Aspen hospital physician but rather a visiting surgeon from Maryland. The surgeon thought it was an emergency because they could not see what was wrong and a large stretch of colon was involved. He told Erin he felt it was imperative that he get in and operate immediately to investigate what was causing this telescoping and deal with the problem, hopefully before any serious damage was done to the colon tissue.

Erin, feeling that the situation was quite out of her control, had to "pretty much release myself to the medical team and trust that they were going to take good care of me." She went into surgery.

The next thing she remembers is groggily waking up in the recovery room. "I was later told that the surgeon had explained what he had found, but I don't remember any of that," she said. "I overheard someone saying something about cancer. I pulled over the surgical nurse. I looked at him and asked him, 'Are they saying I have cancer?' Poor guy. He was the one who had to tell me."

Erin was shocked. Neither the emergency room physician nor the surgeon had focused on cancer as a possibility. While dodging a perforation, Erin had suddenly become a cancer patient. "The surgeon thought

I would need 6 months of chemo and suggested that I should 'prepare' myself and my children. I had no idea where I would find the strength and what it was going to do to my children, who had already been through so much loss at just 12 and 9 years old. I was trying to process all this as a single mom."

Fortunately, Erin's support structure kicked into place again. Her mom was on a plane from New Jersey 24 hours later. Her friends took care of the children and lined up meals. "In these resort communities, where people live far from their relatives, they quickly find other people who become their circle of friends, their extended family," Erin observed. "It is a very supportive community, and I have a lot of close friends. I couldn't keep them out of my hospital room. I am not alone in Aspen."

Nevertheless, Erin says, "I never felt so all alone in all my life, including after my husband died. It was a really" she trails off for a long time, as though the moment is returning to her, then mumbles, "a very tough time."

A few days later the pathology report came back: "A 6.5 cm invasive adenocarcinoma of the right colon that is well-to-moderately differentiated. All margins uninvolved with tumor. Fifteen lymph nodes are negative for tumor." It meant that Erin had a very large colon cancer that did not look aggressive and did not appear to have spread.

The surgeon, however, did not believe the report because the lymph nodes he removed were too big and hard. He thought the cancer must have metastasized. So Aspen Valley Hospital sent the tumor and slides to the Mayo Clinic in Minnesota for another reading that confirmed the first report: no spread.

Erin followed up with a local Aspen oncologist whose view was positive that although her tumor was big and he could not say the surgery cured her, his review of all the recent studies indicated that chemotherapy was unnecessary, and that having the chemo would improve her survival prospects no more than 1% to 2%. In his view Erin would not need 6 months of debilitating chemotherapy or any other treatment.

For Erin it had been a wild ride. "On Thursday I had diarrhea. On Friday I had cancer and needed 6 months of chemotherapy. And on Monday I was cured," she said. "I had a lot to process and take in. It was really unbelievable that I was being told to forget I had cancer and get on with my life."

But Erin was not done yet. Given that she was only 48 years old, the oncologist wanted to get a genetic test to see whether she had Lynch Syndrome, an inherited disease characterized by colon and uterine cancers that present at a very young age. The oncologist said that the test would cost over $4,000, but given her situation, Erin's insurance company would probably cover the cost. Although cancer didn't run in her family—relatives had had heart disease and heart attacks, but no one had ever had cancer of any kind—the oncologist recommended it, so Erin agreed.

This was the first time anyone had ever mentioned the cost of anything. It was not the first bill Erin had seen. The bill for the initial stool culture test had come back in the weeks between the diarrhea and the visit to the Aspen emergency room. It was a whopping $1,200. Erin assumed her insurance would cover it.

Because she was self-employed, Erin had bought her own health insurance. In 2012 the monthly premium was about $800 for her and the 2 girls. She had chosen a high deductible plan, so every year she put $5,000 into a health savings account (HSA) to cover the deductible. If she did not spend it all, the remaining money would "roll over" to the next year. If she spent it all, the health insurance kicked in to cover the remaining bills. For the first few years Erin was able to roll over some money, but recently, because of higher health care costs, she knew she would be spending the full $5,000.

Many of her friends were urging that Erin get a second opinion from a colon cancer expert. "One of the nice things about living in Aspen is that everyone knows someone," she said. "A friend who grew up in the Houston area told me that her father has his name on a building at M.D. Anderson Cancer Center in Houston and could help open some doors there. She helped me get in contact with them." M.D. Anderson began the process to have Erin come for a second opinion, and she began filling out the paperwork. Three weeks later, however, as Erin was about to purchase her plane ticket to Houston, M.D Anderson called back. They told her that they contacted Erin's insurance company and that they were "out-of-network." This meant that to see an oncologist at M.D. Anderson, Erin would have to pay, in addition to her $5,000 deductible for in-network services, another $10,300 deductible for out-of-network services. The clerk said M.D. Anderson would be happy to see her, but she had to come to the appointment with a $10,300 check. For any services over that, her insurance would cover 70% of the cost, and she would be responsible for the remainder.

"If this had been life-and-death and I thought M.D. Anderson was going to have the magic bullet for me, I would have found a way to get the money," she said. "But given the circumstance—that I wasn't dying—I decided to see if there was a highly regarded colon cancer expert 'in-network.' I spent a lot of time on the phone with my health insurance company to see if they could help me find a Colorado colon cancer expert. The representatives I spoke with were based in Michigan and didn't have a lot of information about my network in Colorado. After several fruitless conversations with multiple representatives from the insurance company, I was directed to a website. The best I could come up with was a list of Colorado oncologists in-network with no hospital affiliation listed or designation of their specific cancer specialty. Basically the insurance company told me to call the doctors myself and ask if they were colon cancer experts."

Fortunately, Erin found that the colon cancer experts at the University of Colorado Cancer Center in Denver were considered in-network; it wouldn't cost her anything more to see them. "They were very accommodating and very helpful. They reviewed my case with their 'tumor board' and spent a good amount of time reviewing my pathology, my history, and my surgical reports. I was really pleased with the care and service there."

Ultimately, the University of Colorado colon cancer expert concurred with Erin's Aspen oncologist: "We would not recommend adjuvant therapy in this setting. We do recommend colonoscopy at 3 months out from surgery [and] CT imaging at 1 year."

But Erin was still not done. Even though the Lynch Syndrome test did not show evidence of an inherited cancer, the University of Colorado oncologists recommended Erin be seen at the Hereditary Cancer Clinic for further evaluation of other potential genetic changes.

About a month after her surgery Erin was feeling much better. Although her energy was not completely back to normal, she was able to resume biking, hiking, and a full work schedule. And she had started to recover emotionally as well. Of course, the episode left her and her daughters with a host of unanswered questions: Was she cured? How much should they worry about a recurrence? Should she change her diet or exercise or do anything differently? But Erin was grateful too—grateful that she had good care, grateful that her cancer was not as serious as it might have been, grateful for her life. "I am taking every day as a gift," she said. "I am not focusing on what could happen in a year or 5 years. No one knows better than me that we don't know what might happen tomorrow. Overall I feel really good—and lucky."

Then the bills began pouring in. The bill for the hospital stay for the CT and surgery, with the 6 days in postsurgical recovery, was a monster $71,397.91 (Figure I.1). The largest portion, nearly $30,000, was for the operating room services. Anesthesia added another $7,155, and sterile surgical supplies in the operating room added $8,655. Six days in a hospital room came to $9,031. The CT scan was $3,829, and the pathology for determining the cancer was $2,368. The surgeon's fee came separately at $4,174. The insurance company's negotiated rates with the hospital reduced that bill by about 8%, bringing it down to $66,382.11.

And there were other bills. The physician office visit and blood tests for the initial evaluation of the diarrhea came to $858. Another $287 was owed for the physician visit to change antibiotics after the cramping came back. Various antibiotics and other drugs added $96.71. For all the work they did reviewing the CT scans, medical records, and pathology, the consultation at the University of Colorado seemed reasonable—maybe even a bargain—at $480.42.

Altogether there was just about $73,000 in bills *after* the insurance company's savings. The total was nearly 140% of the median family income in the United States.

Then Erin 's insurance company initially denied the bill for the genetic test for Lynch Syndrome. Erin appealed, getting letters from her primary care physician, the University of Colorado Cancer Center physician, and the Aspen oncologist who ordered it. The company then reversed course and eventually approved the charge.

The follow-up colonoscopy was still to come, as was its bill.

Erin had not paid all of her deductible and she was responsible for $2,304 for the initial lab work surrounding the bacterial infection (stool samples and blood tests). Then there was $538.50 for the hospital stay and

FIGURE I.1 Erin's bill

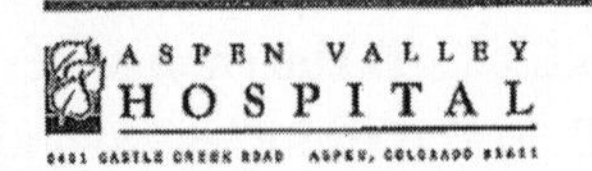

3401 CASTLE CREEK ROAD ASPEN, COLORADO 81611

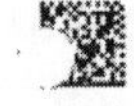

5396

000680 0202

PATIENT NAME: [redacted]
INSURANCE: [redacted]

CHECK CARD YOU ARE USING FOR PAYMENT

☐ MASTERCARD ☐ DISCOVER ☐ VISA ☐ AMERICAN EXPRESS

CARD NUMBER	AMOUNT
SIGNATURE	EXP. DATE

BILL DATE	PLEASE REMIT	ACCT. #
05/30/13	$ 0.00	[redacted]

SHOW AMOUNT PAID HERE $

PAGE: 1 of 2

ASPEN VALLEY HOSPITAL
P.O. Box 5244
Denver, CO 80217-5244

5/9/13 – ER + 6 days Recovery ft. Surgery

5396*SSP0M59T2000005

☐ Please check box if address is incorrect or insurance information has changed, and indicate change(s) on reverse. **SUMMARY BILL**

PLEASE DETACH AND RETURN TOP PORTION WITH YOUR PAYMENT

PATIENT ACCOUNT NUMBER: H008508004 ADMISSION SERVICE DATE: 05/09/13

DATE	DESCRIPTION	AMOUNT
	DRUGS W/ DETAIL (J) CODING	$ 1,536.08
	PRIVATE ROOM & BOARD	9031.00
	PHARMACY (IV)	1032.54
	IV SOLUTIONS	621.06
	OTHER PHARMACY (ORAL)	570.00
	MED/SURG NONSTERILE SUPPLY	702.00
	MED/SURG SUPPLY/DEVICE STERILE	8655.23
	LABORATORY	144.00
	LAB CHEMISTRY	1227.00
	LAB- IMMUNOLOGY	72.00
	LAB- HEMATOLOGY	395.00
	LAB/BACT/MICRO	371.00
	LAB-UROLOGY	27.00
	LAB PATHOLOGICAL-HISTOLOGY	2368.00
	CAT SCAN	3829.00
	OPERATING ROOM SERVICES	20005.00
	ANESTHESIA	7155.00
	ULTRASOUND	390.00
	EMERGENCY ROOM	128.00
	EMERGENCY ROOM EVAL/MANAGEMENT	1150.00
	EMERGENCY ROOM PROCEDURE	457.00
	RECOVERY ROOM	1366.00
	PROFESSIONAL FEES (CONT) ER	642.00
	PROFESSIONAL FEES- ONCOLOGY	644.00
	STATISTICS	0
	TOTAL CHARGES	$ 71,397.91
	ESTIMATED INSURANCE PORTION DUE --MC*COFINITY MIDWEST	$ 71,397.91
	PLEASE REMIT AT THIS TIME	$ 0.00

PATIENT NAME: [redacted]
INSURANCE: [redacted]

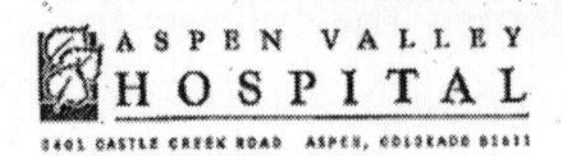

3401 CASTLE CREEK ROAD ASPEN, COLORADO 81611

PLEASE RETAIN THIS PORTION FOR YOUR RECORDS

3SP0M5TXU:1.2

an additional $1,505.87 for the surgeon. Paying just under $5,000 for a life saving surgery and cancer diagnosis seemed reasonable to Erin.

Erin's health insurance came up for renewal in the early fall, but this time she had a preexisting condition: colon cancer and a preexisting set of bills—about $73,000 even without any chemotherapy. Erin had heard stories of people with newly diagnosed cancer being denied coverage or charged exorbitant premiums when their insurance came up for renewal. Erin felt that because she had been paying health insurance premiums for many years, using very little most years because everyone in the family had been relatively healthy, she had been "saving up" for a time like this, when she would need the insurance coverage. But to the insurance company, she was a person who had had colon cancer and was at risk for really big bills if it came back.

October 2013 was her renewal date. Through the late summer she waited nervously for the insurance company's decision, which came in September. The good news was that the insurance company did not cancel her policy despite her preexisting condition. The bad news: they jacked up her premium 24%.

Luckily this was just as the Affordable Care Act began its coverage, when on October 1, 2013, the new online insurance exchanges opened for enrollment. People like Erin who do not get their health insurance through their employer can go online, view and compare different insurance policies, and choose the one they like best. In the exchanges, insurance companies are prohibited from considering preexisting conditions like colon cancer in setting the premiums, so people like Erin can go online and obtain insurance without preexisting condition exclusions and without cancer preexisting condition affecting the rates charged.

"I really didn't think that Obamacare applied to me," she said. "I thought it was health insurance for poor people who couldn't afford to purchase a policy. It never occurred to me that overnight I could become one of those people. I would read articles in the newspapers when the bill was passed, and frankly it all seemed very complicated and I could not follow it. And since I just didn't think it was relevant to my life, I would turn the page to another article."

Having an unexpected and unfortunate diagnosis and struggling with the current health care system is not limited to self-employed, relatively well-off people living in Aspen, Colorado. Wayne is a hairstylist in Philadelphia. He is a 40-year-old, divorced father of one child. For the last decade or so he has been going without health insurance and avoiding the doctor, almost at all cost. "The salon doesn't provide any health insurance—really any benefits at all," he said. "I haven't been to the dentist in . . . oh, I don't know the last time. I know I have a cavity, but I can't afford to get it taken care of. I just floss and brush my teeth really carefully twice a day."

A couple of years ago Wayne could not avoid the health care system. He smashed his elbow. Hoping it was just badly bruised, he carried on. After it became clear the injury was getting worse, not better, he went to the emergency room where, after an X-ray confirmed a broken bone, they put him in a cast and referred him to an orthopedic surgeon. The surgeon immediately took the cast off. "It was going to heal improperly and permanently restrict my range of motion." Wayne said. He hasn't been back to any doctor since.

In July of 2013 Wayne did not know anything about Obamacare and what it could do for him. When told there would be a health insurance exchange offering different health insurance plans and that he might be able to get a subsidy to buy coverage, Wayne became excited: "Do you think I could get coverage for $150 per month? $150 per month is probably the limit of what I can afford." After a long pause, during which he seemed to be pondering the possibility of health insurance, he continued, "Let's hope I can get insurance for $150 per month."

Baltazar is the quintessential immigrant. He came to Los Angeles from Mexico when he was 14 years old. He had few job prospects, few dollars in his pocket, and few English words in his vocabulary. He went to work as a gardener.

In his early 20s Baltazar took the risk of starting his own gardening company. "I started by myself 6 or 7 years ago. Now I employ a crew of 8 guys who work for me. I have 4 guys working for me [as well as] my little brother, my medium brother, and my cousin. It is better now." As Baltazar says, no one makes a lot. Working 8 hours a day, every day, his workers make only about $17,000 per year.

After a few years Baltazar looked into buying his workers health insurance. "We don't make a lot of money to have good health insurance. It is hard," he said. "Before Obamacare, all insurance is expensive, like $500 per month for each worker."

Over the years, however, his brothers and workers have needed some health care. A few years ago one worker cut his finger. He went to a general hospital in downtown Los Angeles and received 7 or 8 stitches. Baltazar paid cash for the $1,800 bill. About 5 years ago his younger brother developed appendicitis and went to the UCLA emergency room. The appendectomy cost $25,000. His brother has been repaying the hospital $400 in cash every month. He only recently sent in the last installment.

In July 2013 Baltazar was in Mexico on vacation with his girlfriend. They were driving along a highway when he suddenly felt a pain in his chest. "My heart started pumping real hard. Someone was crushing my heart," he said. He drove straight to a Mexican hospital.

Fortunately, Baltazar did not suffer a heart attack, but he did have a blocked coronary artery. The pain was just a warning. However, having a blocked coronary artery at age 30 is very serious, suggesting he has high cholesterol and/or high blood pressure. Who knows what else is causing his heart condition. "Since I came to this country I haven't been to the doctor," he said. "I haven't had a checkup. I felt healthy. I always worked fine. But I am sick. And now I have to take medicine and I have to see a doctor every 6 months. I now know all my workers have to have health insurance."

Throughout the summer and fall of 2013 Baltazar had been seeing commercials on TV for health insurance. He received a mailing and called the number to get more information. But he won't shop on the Internet. "The Internet is creepy," he said. "You never know if what you see is true or not." So he keeps calling to find out what he can. It is hard for him to understand. His English is not perfect, and he doesn't really understand about high deductibles, managed care, networks. What Baltazar knows is that he and his workers need to have health insurance on January 1, 2014, and that they can get subsidies. "I can't pay $500. No. No. Maybe $200 per worker," he says. "I am going to pay half price of the health insurance." And when he sees that a standard insurance plan at the silver level might be as low as $53 per month for a worker in California with the subsidies, he exclaims, "It's going to be fantastic. I have to get everyone health insurance."

Across the US there are tens of millions of people like Erin, Wayne, and Baltazar with their own stories of illness, struggles with health insurance, and bills that dwarf people's annual incomes.

Erin, Wayne, Baltazar, and millions of others remind us that illness and death can strike any of us unpredictably and that we all will need health care services—we just don't know when. They also remind us that we may not be able to control when we get sick and with what disease, but what happens next—the quality of care, the ability to get the best, how much it will cost, and who will pay—can be controlled. And it can be changed so that it does not oppress us with worries about whether we are getting the right care or will be stuck with endless bill payments or, even worse, the threat of bankruptcy.

This is a book about the United States' health care system. It tries to make sense of how the health care system affected Erin, Wayne, and Baltazar's care—and their lives. Its pages contain a complex web of facts, figures, statistics, and acronyms all presented in a way that, I hope, will allow you to understand how and why our system looks the way it does. It is an attempt to help you make sense of things that Erin, Wayne, and Baltazar confronted when they needed care—things like deductibles, in-network and out-of-network charges and policies, high deductible health plans, and hospital bills that total more than the average person earns in a year. It is an attempt to explain the problems with the health care system that prompted reform as well as all the changes that have already occurred and will continue to take place as part of the Affordable Care Act.

The American health care system is complex. Explaining how it works and doesn't work, its problems, attempts to reform it, and how Obamacare will transform it requires considering an unusual combination of topics. Consequently, this book will be an amalgam of history, health economics, sociology, contemporary politics, policy analysis, and forecasting that defies simple categorization.

The book is organized into 3 parts. In Part 1, The Current Health Care System, we review the American health care system—how we got here and our system's serious problems. Chapter 1 reviews the history of the American health care system to explain how we developed the system we have, with so many specialists, big hospitals, and hundreds of health insurance companies. Chapter 2 reviews the financing of the system: health insurance companies, Medicare and Medicaid, the role of employers, and who pays. Chapter 3 delineates how Americans such as Erin, Wayne, and Baltazar get care and how that care is paid for. It profiles other actors in health care, from drug and device companies to the government agencies that regulate them. Chapters 2 and 3 present the tremendously complex American health care system in a clear and comprehensible manner. Chapter 4 specifies 5 different problems with the American health care system, from the well-known problems of access and exorbitant costs to the less-discussed problems of lack of information about prices and quality and malpractice. It shows how these are not just problems about the health care system, rather they infect the rest of society, including education and the national debt. Part I makes the case for reform.

Given these complexities and problems, Part 2, Health Care Reform, then explores the efforts to reform the health care system, culminating in the Affordable Care Act (ACA). Chapter 5 reviews the 100-year history of failed attempts to reform the American health care system, including the many unexpected twists and turns, such as Democrats who killed reform and Republicans who championed it. Chapter 5 summarizes the hard lessons learned from the past failures to pass health care reform. Chapter 6 shows how President Obama was able to overcome the 100-year curse on comprehensive health care reform. It also reveals the vitally important but totally obscure practice essential to enacting any law—scoring by the Congressional Budget Office—and examines the fate of 3 key provisions of reform, thereby elucidating how politics intersects with policy in unexpected ways that defy simple political science theories. Chapter 7 analyzes the legal challenges to the ACA and the Supreme Court's decision. Chapter 8 analyzes what is in the nearly 1,000-page ACA. It delineates the law's provisions not by its titles, but according to 8 logical categories: (1) access, (2) cost control, (3) quality improvement, (4) prevention, (5) workforce, (6) revenue, (7) odds and ends, and (8) the CLASS Act that was eventually repealed. Chapter 9 makes the ACA more personal, showing how it will affect people like Erin, Wayne, and Baltazar, physicians and hospitals, as well as insurers.

In October 2013, the rollout of healthcare.gov was a disaster. While it was repaired within a matter of weeks, it has raised serious questions about health care reform. Part 3, The Future of American Health Care, opens with Chapter 10's dissection of the failure, indicating why it occurred and why it will not undermine the ACA's transformation of the health care system. The rest of Part 3 looks into the crystal ball. Chapter 11 delineates a dashboard to assess progress—or lack thereof—of reform. There are 4 dashboards with quantitative metrics: one for coverage, one for cost control, one for quality improvement, and one for overall health of society. Chapter 12 addresses healthcare reform 2.0 and additional reforms that need to be to be enacted over the next 5 years to further the transformation of the system.

Finally, in Chapter 13 I make bold—and risky—predictions about what will happen to the health care system over the next 20 years. Every actor in the health care system, from hospitals and physicians to insurers and government officials to pharmaceutical companies and venture capitalists, must make predictions—either implicitly or explicitly—about where they think the system is going. I am just being more candid and explicit—and precise, with dates and numbers—about my predictions. Given the ACA and how the various actors are responding and are likely to respond, I identify 6 megatrends that are likely to occur, from the end of health insurance companies as we know them to the end of health care inflation to the proliferation of VIP care for chronically ill patients. I know that the risk of making predictions, especially of writing them down and publishing them for posterity, is being shown a fool. But someone has to take up the challenge.

The American health care system is incredibly complex. At many points during the exploration of different facets of the health care system it is easy to get confused and forget what we are really talking about. If that happens, turn back to the Introduction and reread the stories. The reality is that the health care system is more than numbers and figures and acronyms. It is more than commissions or departments or febrile political rhetoric and slogans. Instead, it is about people and families and what happens to them when their health goes wrong and they need the health care system and their health insurance. It is about people like Erin and Wayne and Baltazar. And this is why the system needs fixing—and how it will surely be better by 2020.

Part I

THE AMERICAN HEALTH CARE SYSTEM

= CHAPTER ONE =

How Did We Get Here?

A Brief History of the American Health Care System

Why don't Wayne and Baltazar have health insurance? More profoundly, why is there health insurance at all? Sometimes it seems as though health insurance has always existed, but it has not. Where did it come from, and why do most Americans get it from their employer?

Why is medical care so expensive? Why did it cost Erin more than $70,000 for an operation and 6 days in the hospital? Or Baltazar's brother the price of a car for a pretty simple appendectomy? Or $1,800 for 8 stitches? And why are there so many separate charges on Erin's bill? Not just a charge for the operating room, but one for the sterile supplies, nonsterile supplies, IV solutions, anesthesia, and on? And why did her insurance company get that 8% discount when Baltazar's brother got none? Who sets the prices?

Why are physicians so super-specialized? Why did Erin have to go to a cancer physician who specialized in only one type of cancer and then another who specialized in the genetics of her cancer? Why is there not just a doctor for all cancers?

The American health care system was not created complex and ridiculously expensive from its origins. It evolved to become this way over a period of about 100 years. And there is nothing inherent in the way it evolved. It could have been different. But many decisions, often made for reasons having nothing to do with improving health care, shaped the health care system we have today.

Social scientists have a concept called *path dependence* that helps explain how decisions made in previous circumstances that may no longer be relevant today nonetheless shape and limit how current decisions are made. In other words, path dependence means that the institutions and arrangements created before—often created haphazardly or as an expedient—now constrain and shape the changes that are possible today. So the history of health care can help us understand why certain aspects of the health care system exist today, and this in turn helps us understand the constraints imposed on any health reform proposal.

Hospitals

Hospitals are dominant players in the US health care system and the overall economy. More money goes to the 4,985 acute-care hospitals ($970 billion in 2012) than all of Social Security ($730 billion) or national defense ($650 billion). In many cities hospitals are leading employers. For instance, in New York City 2 hospital systems, Long Island-Jewish Health System and Mt. Sinai, are the 4th and 5th largest private employers, by employees, in the metropolitan area.

Hospitals evolved in the United States in 3 historic phases. Phase 1 is the pre-1890 era. Benjamin Rush, a signer of the Declaration of Independence and attendee at the Continental Congress as well as a prominent Philadelphia physician who advocated for a clean environment and the abolition of slavery and also came to be known as the father of psychiatry, referred to hospitals during this period as "the sinks of human life." Early hospitals were mainly for the poor and offered very little in the way of therapy. They tended to treat patients more with moralistic and religious exhortations than with medical interventions. They offered lodging for the chronically ill in large, open, impersonal wards. Surgery was unsafe, often lethal. Infections regularly swept through the hospitals. Upper- and middle-class people avoided hospitals, preferring to receive their care at home.

Early American hospitals were largely funded and operated by leading citizens as part of their civic responsibilities. For 19th-century physicians these facilities mainly provided an educational function—doctors could learn by treating poor patients—and a way to enhance prestige. So valuable were these functions, in fact, that physicians volunteered their services. American physicians were not paid staff; hospital boards were composed of nonphysicians.

This organizational structure was very different from that in Europe, where there were permanent, hospital-based, and salaried physicians. Once patients were admitted to the hospital, their private practitioner no longer cared for them; the hospital physician managed all their care.

Between roughly 1890 and 1920 hospitals in the United States gained respectability and proliferated. Advances in medical science were largely responsible for this transformation. In 1846 the Massachusetts surgeon John C. Warren performed the first surgical procedure with anesthesia, and by the end of the century painless surgery had become common. Robert Koch in Germany and Louis Pasteur in France identified bacteria and propagated the germ theory of disease. Simultaneously, in 1867, Joseph Lister in England published his work on antiseptic procedures involving disinfectants. By the 1880s sterile and aseptic techniques supplanted those antiseptic procedures, and the incidence of hospital-acquired infections plummeted. Further, diagnostic tests were being developed, X-rays came into use in medicine in the mid-1890s, and ways of identifying bacteria were developed. The combination of radiology, anesthesia, and aseptic techniques transformed surgery and expanded the types of operations that were possible. And there were social changes too: urbanization meant that many people lacked families to provide nursing and other care for them at home when they were sick.

Beginning in the 1890s hospitals ceased providing just custodial care for the poor and chronically ill and began providing acute, mainly surgical care for a larger swath of society. Middle- and upper-class patients went to the hospital in larger numbers for safe, surgical operations, such as gall bladder removal. Hospitals, in turn, came to depend less on charity and more on payment from patients who could afford it and who valued the services the hospital offered.

By 1910 there were over 4,000 hospitals in the United States. The types of hospitals varied across the country. In the East, voluntary and municipal hospitals, funded by wealthy citizens, dominated, such as the Massachusetts General and Johns Hopkins Hospitals. In the Midwest, religious hospitals, such as Catholic, Methodist, and Baptist, arrived with immigrants. Hospitals were formed last in the West and South, and in those areas for-profit, physician-owned hospitals were an important segment of the market because of the paucity of wealthy donors or immigrant communities to found and fund them.

Importantly, hospitals were not organized in any formal way; there was no formal state oversight or master plan. Each hospital operated according to its own standards. The result was, as the Princeton sociologist Paul Starr puts it, a peculiar bureaucracy in which there was "very great uniformity [among the hospitals] and very little coordination. . . . [E]ach voluntary hospital had to raise its own funds for capital expenditures, set its own fees, do its own purchasing, recruit staff, determine patients' ability to pay, collect bills, and conduct public relations efforts." In addition, a voluntary physician staff who neither controlled nor operated hospitals meant that more authority rested with the hospital administrators, who quickly became professionalized.

The relationship between physicians and hospitals was tense, mainly because of money. Hospitals needed physicians to refer patients and to provide medical and surgical services. Yet hospitals did not pay physicians and had little control over how they practiced in the hospital. Simultaneously, physicians needed hospitals in which they could perform surgeries, obtain diagnostic tests, and admit their patients for care. Physicians also wanted the prestige of admitting privileges—that is, the permission to admit and treat their patients in a particular hospital. With the increasing use of hospitals, physicians often felt hospitals "stole" wealthier, paying patients. This tension between the voluntary physician staff and hospital administrators still persists today.

In the 1940s and 1950s the federal government fueled a huge expansion in the construction of hospitals. With the United States' entry into World War I, the federal government established veterans' benefits, including insurance and disability compensation. In 1930 various veterans' programs were consolidated into one federal agency. At that time the Veteran's Administration (VA) operated 54 hospitals, which were largely rural hospitals with low pay and poorly trained staff and were widely perceived to be of poor quality. After World War II the VA embarked on a major transformation, building urban hospitals affiliated with medical schools that became centers of medical research and training.

The *Hill-Burton Act of 1946* was the first major health care act that the federal government funded. It provided federal support for hospital construction in the United States. Over the next 25 years Hill-Burton contributed funds to approximately a third of all hospital construction programs. The formula allocated funds based on state population, with more money going to poorer states. It also required the communities to provide two-thirds of the construction costs. Consequently, because of political influence and the matching contribution requirement, poorer states were able to build hospitals, but within these individual states most of the federally funded hospital construction ended up in more prosperous communities. Access to hospitals in poorer communities remained limited.

Even as Hill-Burton disbursed billions of dollars, it significantly limited federal oversight and involvement in hospital policies and practices. For instance, although the act required hospitals receiving funds to provide a reasonable volume of services to people unable to pay; "reasonable volume" was not defined and this requirement was not enforced. Ultimately, however, Hill-Burton expanded the number and size of community hospitals and kept many viable when they would have otherwise failed financially.

Another postwar transformation in hospitals was the creation of Medicare in 1965. As Rashi Fein, one of the country's first health economists and the first employed by the government, has pointed out, many hospital administrators had plans for expansion and upgrades in technology but were waiting for donors. After the passage of Medicare in 1965 these hospitals now had the capital to realize these plans. Medicare obliterated the need for hospitals to provide free or subsidized care for poor elderly patients. In addition, to buy off hospitals and pre-empt any ideas of boycotting Medicare, the Medicare payments were generous. Essentially Medicare paid hospitals costs plus a percentage to compensate for capital expenditures related to expansion. This payment guaranteed all hospitals a profit. It incentivized both increasing costs to increase profits, and hospital expansion which would be paid for. This wildly inflationary payment system lasted until DRGs and prospective payment were introduced in the 1980s.

Advances in medical technology after the war, particularly in the 1950s and 1960s, reinforced the importance of the hospital as a place for health care miracles. In the late 1950s hospitals began establishing separate intensive care units as places where patients on breathing machines could be monitored intensively. In the 1960s monitoring of heart rhythms became routine, and cardiac catheterization to visualize blockages in the heart's arteries became possible. By the late 1970s techniques were developed not just to diagnose, but also to treat health problems through a cardiac catheter.

Dialysis for kidney failure and cancer treatment followed the same rough trajectory. It became possible to maintain a patient on long-term dialysis in the early 1960s with the discovery of a special shunt that could be maintained indefinitely. In 1972 dialysis proliferated when the federal government assumed payment for any patient who needed it. And beginning in 1955 cancer specialists began using combination chemotherapy. By the early 1960s they began curing previously fatal acute leukemia in children. By the late 1970s chemotherapy could cure several cancers, including testicular cancer and Hodgkin's disease, and it could extend survival in other cancers.

Scientific advances that occurred in the 1940s or 1950s had, by the 1960s, made possible surgical procedures and other treatments that allowed physicians to perform them, first at elite medical institutions and then, over the next decade or two, in almost all hospitals. Through the 1970s and 1980s high-technology medical care blossomed in US hospitals, enabling physicians to diagnose and treat most common conditions.

Beginning in the late 1990s, although hospitals still could perform amazing miracles, they increasingly became less desirable sites for care. Hospital-acquired infections became a major threat. With MRSA, methicillin-resistant *Staphylococcus aureus,* and other super bugs, hospitals returned to the "old days." According to the CDC, one out of every 20 hospitalized patients—about 1.7 million people—acquires an infection while in hospital care, and nearly 100,000 die from these hospital--acquired infections.

Alongside the increase in the number of conditions that physicians could and did treat came a disturbing growth in the frequency of medical errors. In 1999 the Institute of Medicine published a report entitled "To Err Is Human" that indicated at least 44,000 people and perhaps as many as 98,000 people die in hospitals each year as a result of preventable medical errors. Also, as hospitals grew in size and complexity they became increasingly impersonal. Patients' personal physicians stopped rounding in hospitals; instead, the European model expanded with a new breed of physician, the hospitalist, who is employed by the hospital to care for the patient. Usually the patient had no previous—or subsequent—relationship with the hospitalist.

And up went the costs. Hospitals, especially larger academic and central-city hospitals, have become exceedingly expensive places to deliver routine care. The costs of buildings, all the latest technology, and staff to provide these services exploded—as did the patients' portion of the bill.

Hospitals still perform miracles. And they remain invaluable for certain treatments, such as transplants and emergency opening of coronary arteries and other superspecialized interventions. But although they certainly are not Rush's "sinks of human life," they have lost some of their luster. Today many services they provide, such as treatment of serious infections with intravenous antibiotics, can be done better and more inexpensively in a patient's home. Hospitals seem to have devolved from the peak of their prestige as houses of hope to places to be entered reluctantly and only if absolutely necessary.

Physicians

The history of physicians mirrors the evolution of hospitals. Before 1900 the medical profession was disreputable. Doctors were viewed as quacks and snake oil salesman. Medicine had little to offer the sick. A symbol of their low status was the constant battles between different sects: homeopaths, eclectics, osteopaths, and allopaths (regular physicians). At the time most medical schools were proprietary institutions operated for the profit of their faculty. The standards were terrible. Students typically enrolled for 2 years—6 months per year—and simply repeated the same courses in each year.

The factors that converged at the turn of the 20th century to transform hospitals applied to physicians too: scientific advances made surgery safer, and the identification of germs made it possible to diagnose specific infections and control their spread. The improved efficacy increased use of physician services and allowed physicians to charge more.

In 1904, to marginalize and then eliminate poorly trained physicians, the American Medical Association established the Council on Medical

Education. It recommended 2 important changes in medical education: college training for admission to medical school and a standard 4-year medical education, to include 2 years of laboratory based preclinical work and 2 years of clinical instruction in hospitals. To support the AMA's new standards, the Carnegie Foundation for the Advancement of Teaching commissioned Abraham Flexner, who was neither a physician nor a scientist, to survey American and Canadian medical schools and recommend reforms. Over a 2-year period Flexner visited all 155 medical schools in the United States and Canada.

The 1910 Flexner Report was frank and harsh in its criticism of the vast majority of schools, describing them as "foul," "a disgrace," and worse. Ultimately he recommended that there be fewer schools and that the remaining ones be modeled on the most progressive medical schools such as the University of Michigan, Case Western Reserve, Harvard, and Johns Hopkins. His report urged that medical schools require admitted students to have college training in the sciences, require 2 years of laboratory-based preclinical training, and 2 years of clinical instruction based in hospital wards. The report also urged that medical schools be affiliated with universities and hire full-time faculty members to teach and engage in scientific research.

Simultaneously, physicians campaigned for licensing laws to purge their ranks of untrained or poorly trained physicians. Flexner supported this reform, and over the next few years many states required licensed physicians to have at least 1 year of college, diplomas from a reputable medical school, and then a passing grade on a licensing examination.

Over the next 25 years the Flexner Report prompted a significant drop in the number of medical schools, as the proprietary schools unable to support laboratories and standing faculty closed. This, in turn, decreased the number physicians but increased their quality—and income, due to demand and their much improved results.

The report also fostered 3 other enduring changes. Clinical training moved away from physicians' offices and patients' homes to hospital wards. The hospital became the site of training even though most medical care remained in the outpatient setting. This is still the case today. Second, by extending training to include both college and 4 years of medical school, thereby delaying the time when medical trainees earned an income, the report significantly reduced the number of students from poorer families who became physicians. This in turn reduced the number of physicians who would practice in poorer and rural communities. Finally, the Flexner Report catalyzed a change in medical school faculty. Private practitioners were eased out of their teaching roles at medical schools. Instead, medical students were taught by—and modeled themselves on—full-time university professors focused on the basic sciences and clinical specialties. Within medical schools the prestige shifted from generalists and primary care practitioners from the community to full-time research scientists and clinical specialists on faculty.

Two other peculiarities about American medicine, a lack of organization in the delivery of care and an emphasis on specialization, have deep historical origins. Neither corporations nor government structure physicians' delivery of care outside hospitals. Until recently, physicians worked in small groups and for themselves. For most of the 20th century physicians have strenuously resisted any large groups or other ways of organizing patient care.

Physicians have long defended their professional autonomy and, therefore, have been antagonistic to large, organized ways of delivering care, what physicians called corporate control of medicine. This resistance to any formal organization of the delivery of patient care was manifest in a vigorous defense of small practices and fee-for-service medicine. Because of their often remote geographic locations, railroad, mining, and lumber industries tended to employ physicians and directly control their workers' medical care. Other employers and organizations, such as fraternal lodges, tried to employ physicians to provide services for their workers or members, often at fixed prices. In response, workers and their unions were often leery of the company doctors' quality and commitment to patient care. Nor did physicians want to be treated like mere laborers, especially as the employers and organizations could drive hard bargains and force physicians to compete for the contracts, thereby lowering salaries, especially in an era of physician oversupply. So physicians came to distrust any intermediary between them and their patient because it could threaten the physicians' power and income. Intermediaries could drive hard bargains with physicians and take some of the profits that would otherwise go to physicians; engaging patients directly, however, left more of the money for physicians. As we shall see, this opposition to any intermediary even carried over to health insurance companies that might pay physicians.

Several factors allowed physicians to successfully oppose employers' control of health care and any other centralized purchaser of care. First, the decline in physician supply due to the decline in the number of medical schools and state licensing enhanced physician bargaining power. Second, state court cases prohibited employers from providing medicine because they were not licensed to practice. Third, organized medicine, namely the American Medical Association (AMA) and its state and local affiliates, became more powerful. They often excluded any physician who worked for a company, did contract work for fraternal lodges and other organizations, or advertised. Exclusion from the AMA made it hard for physicians to get malpractice insurance and gain admitting privileges at local hospitals, giving force to the AMA's policies. Finally, physicians had personal relationships with their patients, and because in the early part of the 20th-century care was relatively affordable, physicians could command loyalty of their patients without corporate intermediaries. Because setting up a practice was relatively inexpensive, with the cost of hospitals paid for by someone else, physicians could easily be their own bosses and not divide their patients' fees with others. All these measures encouraged small private practices with no organization of medical practice into larger groups.

Compared to other nations, the United States' health care system places great emphasis on medical specialization. In 2010 in the United States the number of generalists per 1 million population was 472, while the number of specialists was 636 per 1 million population. Comparatively, in 2009 49% of physicians in France and Australia were generalists. Five historical factors support this. First, specialty boards certifying physicians to practice certain types of medicine developed and proliferated, especially in the 1930s. Second, during World War II certified specialists were automatically given higher rank in the military to emphasize the value of being specialist. After the war the VA also required certification for physicians to be authorized to provide specialist care. Third, as medical schools developed their full-time clinical faculty, they eased—or forced—out generalists, instead encouraging specialists who were conducting research. NIH and VA funding for both research and training further fueled this emphasis on researchers. As more researchers were produced and funded, subspecialists proliferated and were hired by medical schools. Increasingly, the prestige of academia was associated with specialization. Finally, hospital-based specialists were paid more. This is because initially health insurance paid only for surgery and hospital-based care; insurance for office-based services came much later. Thus, surgeons and specialists primarily working in hospitals, such as cardiologists, had a more secure source of income. Furthermore, as Paul Starr emphasizes, with interns and residents in hospitals, hospital-based specialists could care for more patients, which also increased their income. Thus, the confluence of licensing, training and research grants, academic prestige, and higher incomes fueled the tremendous specialization now found in American medicine.

During the 20th century physicians went from being seen as disreputable quacks to highly regarded practitioners. They also remained fiercely independent and opposed to any organized body outside of medicine, whether it be a company or voluntary association, that would organize and potentially have authority over them. And the growth of licensure as well as expansion of biomedical research and the transformation of medical education strongly promoted specialization within the profession. By the end of the 20th century Americans were still favorably inclined to their personal physician but were beginning to be less favorably inclined to medicine and physicians in general. Simultaneously, objections to the overspecialization of the profession gained strength, and the need for a reorientation toward more primary care physicians became accepted as conventional wisdom.

Private, Employer-Based Health Insurance

Traditionally, the start of health insurance in the United States is fixed as 1929 in Dallas, Texas. Technically, however, this was not health insurance but rather prepaid hospital coverage. Baylor University Hospital provided Dallas schoolteachers up to 21 days of hospital care for $6 per teacher. This type of arrangement then spread to other Dallas hospitals.

With the rising cost of health care and the Great Depression that forced Americans to cut back on their health spending, hospitals found that fewer of their beds were occupied, and as a result, revenues declined. The Baylor-type of insurance became attractive. Indeed, to preempt interhospital competition, all the hospitals in particular cities began to offer joint hospitalization insurance. A significant advantage of such policies was that it gave patients free choice of which hospital to use. The American Hospital Association strongly supported this arrangement, and in 1939 it used the Blue Cross symbol for these types of hospitalization insurance plans.

At that time 25 states had laws permitting such Blue Cross plans to be tax-exempt charitable organizations. This offered the Blue Cross plans significant advantages, including waiving the normal requirement for insurance companies to have large financial reserves to meet their obligations to policy holders. Hospitals guaranteed that they would provide beds and health care services for insured patients. In return, these Blues plans offered community rating, charging the same premiums to all insured patients regardless of whether they were sick or healthy, old or young. These Blues plans were largely sold through employers, like that of the Dallas teachers.

However, this version of history that locates the development of health insurance at Baylor University Hospital is only partially right. Before 1929 there were a variety of efforts to cover health care costs. Commercial insurance companies largely avoided health insurance, worrying that voluntary insurance was untenable for 4 reasons. First, sick people would preferentially buy insurance, leading to adverse selection and high premiums. Second, the insurer would have to assess the risk of each individual and set the premium based on that risk; doing this for each individual would be very expensive and again increase the premiums.

Third, they worried that "health and sickness are vague terms open to endless construction," opening up avenues for uncontrollable abuse and fraud. Finally, in the early part of the 20th century demand for health insurance was low. Hospital costs were relatively low, and people used hospitals so rarely that few people perceived a need for insurance; they simply paid cash.

Nevertheless, there were some pre-1929 efforts to provide health cost coverage. One effort focused on companies that were in remote locations where there were no physicians. In 1877 the Granite Cutter Union established the first sickness fund in the United States. And by 1917 in California, 41% of union members had benefits through union-based sickness funds. In 1910 Montgomery Ward offered its workers group health insurance, although it was structured more like disability insurance. In addition, there were early prepaid group practice arrangements, especially in rural regions such as Oklahoma and Iowa. These efforts at providing health coverage were isolated and never proliferated widely. It was the Baylor arrangement that caught on.

The success of Blue Cross plans encouraged commercial insurers to jump into the hospitalization market. By insuring all the workers at a company, the Blues showed how the problem of adverse selection and high underwriting costs could be overcome. If the pool—the number of people insured—was big enough, the risk could be shared. As a result, commercial insurers started competing with the Blue Cross plans and, by 1951, surpassed them in the number of people they covered with health insurance.

Physicians, still wary of any financial intermediary between them and patients, were hostile to any form of health insurance that covered physician services. In addition, physicians often price discriminated; they tended to charge their wealthier patients more than they did poor patients. Insurance, however, would eliminate the option to price discriminate. But 3 factors made physicians and, in particular, the AMA soften their opposition to health insurance for physician services. As with hospitals, the Great Depression depressed the utilization of physician services, and physicians' income fell. Furthermore, there were increasing calls for compulsory, government-sponsored national health insurance, but the AMA viewed private voluntary health insurance as preferable to government insurance. Finally, physicians were worried that Blue Cross plans might include payment for physician services performed in the hospital, thereby cutting them out of the market entirely.

In 1934, as a prelude to the battle over compulsory health insurance that they suspected would be in Roosevelt's Social Security legislation, the AMA specified 10 principles that should govern any insurance for physician services, including patients' freedom to choose any physician, no third party should come between physician and patients, and the medical profession should control medical practice. The principles also stated that patients should pay the physician at the time of service, implying that insurance companies should then pay or indemnify patients for what patients paid rather than involving physicians in the insurance-patient transaction.

Then, beginning in 1939, first in California and then in Michigan, state medical societies began offering coverage for office visits, house calls, and in-hospital physician services. These plans came to be known as Blue Shield plans. State medical society Blue Shield plans covering physician services proliferated, often with Blue Cross assistance, to combat commercial insurers that were packaging physician coverage with hospital coverage. What was important to physicians was that physicians controlled the Blue Shield plans. Physicians insisted that physicians serve on the Blue Shield boards.

By 1940 20 million Americans had some form of health insurance. But World War II changed all that. With millions of men in the military fighting overseas, labor was in short supply. Workers wanted higher wages, and employers, needing to attract workers, wanted to pay those higher wages. However, the Stabilization Act of 1942 required that the president stabilize prices and wages at September 15, 1942, levels. The day after its passage President Roosevelt issued an executive order that included the following paragraph:

> No increases in wage rates, granted as a result of voluntary agreement, collective bargaining, conciliation, arbitration, or otherwise, and no decreases in wage rates, shall be authorized unless notice of such increases or decreases shall have been filed with the National War Labor Board, and unless the National War Labor Board has approved such increases or decreases.

Importantly, the executive order excluded insurance benefits from controls:

> Salaries and wages under this Order shall include all forms of direct or indirect remuneration to an employee or officer for work or personal services performed for an employer or corporation, including but not limited to, bonuses, additional compensation, gifts, commissions, fees,

> and any other remuneration in any form or medium whatsoever *(excluding insurance and pension benefits in a reasonable amount as determined by the director)*. (italics added)

To satisfy both employers searching for workers and workers hoping for higher wages, the National War Labor Board ruled that health insurance did not constitute wages or salaries limited by the Stabilization Act. Furthermore, establishing what constituted "insurance . . . in a reasonable amount," the board ruled that the insurance could be provided if it did not exceed 5% of the value of the worker's wage. As a consequence, by 1950 nearly two-thirds of working Americans had health insurance coverage for hospital stays.

After 1942, 3 rulings by government boards and courts entrenched the employer-based health insurance structure in the United States. First, in 1945 the War Labor Board ruled that employers were bound by a contract not just for wages but also for the insurance plans that were part of the negotiations; in other words, they could not cancel the health insurance after the war when there was no longer a severe labor shortage. Second, in 1949 the National Labor Relations Board ruled in the famous Inland Steel Company case that unions, as part of their negotiations for wages, could negotiate for fringe benefits like health insurance. The US Supreme Court affirmed this ruling, thereby encouraging unions to demand employer-sponsored health insurance. As a result, in 1946 only 600,000 union workers had employer-sponsored health insurance, but by 1954 nearly 30 million workers and their dependents had employer-sponsored health insurance.

Most importantly, in 1954 the IRS issued the so-called tax exclusion. This policy explicitly declared that the monetary value of the health insurance employers sponsored was not part of the worker's income; consequently, it was not included in determining a worker's income or payroll taxes. This made the value of a dollar in health insurance benefits worth more than a dollar in wage increases because the latter are taxable. Thus, the combination of exempting health insurance from the World War II wage controls and then giving health insurance a significant tax break firmly institutionalized employer-sponsored health insurance in the United States.

Then, beginning in the 1950s, 2 trends propelled health insurance coverage to expand beyond voluntary employer-based programs. The first was the growing costs of health care, especially hospital care. The second was the increasing realization that an employer-based health insurance arrangement would necessarily leave certain groups out, with one conspicuous group in particular: the elderly who were no longer working. They were more likely to be sick, and rising costs for health care were imposing serious financial strain on them.

In 1957 Aime Forand, a congressman on the House Ways and Means Committee, sponsored a bill to cover hospital costs for seniors. His plan, which linked health insurance for the elderly with Social Security, was called Medicare. After Forand introduced his bill, numerous congressional hearings on the issue demonstrated significant problems in health coverage for the elderly. In 1960, for instance, health care costs were one of the main reasons that 35% of the elderly were living in poverty, causing health coverage for the elderly to become a major issue in the 1960 presidential election. In response, the Eisenhower administration denounced Forand's bill and introduced its own legislation to cover the older Americans. However, southern Democrats led by Senator Robert Kerr of Oklahoma and Representative Wilbur Mills of Arkansas, chair of the House Ways and Means Committee, offered a compromise: Eldercare. Enacted in 1960, Eldercare was a means-tested program for the aged poor. States could voluntarily opt into the program to get federal funds, while the states administered the program. But after just 3 years the program was widely viewed as a failure. A 1963 report by the Senate's Special Committee on Aging began by stating, "After 3 years of operation, the Kerr-Mills Medical Assistance for the Aged (MAA) program has proved to be at best an ineffective and piecemeal approach to the health problems of the Nation's 18 million older citizens."

The history of hospitals and physicians shows the transformation that advances in science have catalyzed. Anesthesia, germ theory of disease and sterile techniques, and safe surgery made hospitals and physician services at the turn of the century much more effective and valuable. These scientific advances brought about a process of transformation that expanded the number of hospitals and enforced the requirement of more rigorous physician training, which in turn increased physician power, prestige, and income.

These changes were then reinforced and amplified by policies that were often exigent responses to immediate circumstances, not well vetted courses of action. For instance, the need to fill the expanded number of hospital beds during an economic downturn spawned employment-based health insurance, and the need to appease workers during World War II tremendously expanded employment-based health insurance. Then the IRS ruling on the tax treatment of health insurance added even more drive to expanding employment-based coverage.

Simultaneously, other policies also enhanced the role of hospitals and the physicians who practiced in them. Government funds expanded the number of hospitals nationwide and, in the 1950s and 1960s, financed the discovery of new tests and treatments along with their increased availability in community hospitals in the 1970s and 1980s. The focus of health insurance for hospital payments reinforced the importance of hospitals and hospital-based specialist care, and the way Medicare was then structured further amplified this emphasis on hospital-based care. It also encouraged surgeons and specialist physicians working in the hospitals.

This is the structure of the American health care system we have inherited. The next chapter delves more deeply into how we pay for it.

= CHAPTER TWO =

Financing Health Care

Insurance Companies, Medicare, Medicaid, and the Rest

There is an old joke in health policy: there are 2 people who actually understand the American health system, and both Vic Fuchs and Alain Enthoven are 90 and 83, respectively.

When opponents were campaigning against the Clinton health care reform ideas in 1993 they adopted a graphic originally developed by Senator Arlen Specter's (R-Pennsylvania) staff to explain the American health care system and the proposed reform to him. The diagram showed all the different parts of the health care system and drew the interconnections between each of the actors in the system. The result was so complex that it looked more like a computer circuit board with tangles of connections than an organizational chart or any other logical structure (see Figure 2.1). And this was before a host of new elements, such as the Children's Health Insurance Program (CHIP) and Medicare Part D, even existed. The chart became famous when Senator Bob Dole (R-Kansas) used it to attack the Clinton health care reform effort. The irony, of course, was that it represented the *existing* health care system, not the Clinton reforms.

Unless we understand at least the main parts of the system, it will be impossible to intelligently identify the sources of problems and assess how the system can be improved. So we must dissect Specter's chart, which is still the best representation of the whole system before the Affordable Care Act, and understand its various elements and actors. While we are doing this we must keep 3 things in mind. First, all the elements of the health care system are interrelated and symbiotic. How Erin's care is organized, where it gets done, how insurance pays for it, and which parts

FIGURE 2.1 Arlen Specter showing the diagram developed by his staff to explain the American health care system. © John Mottern/AFP/Getty Images

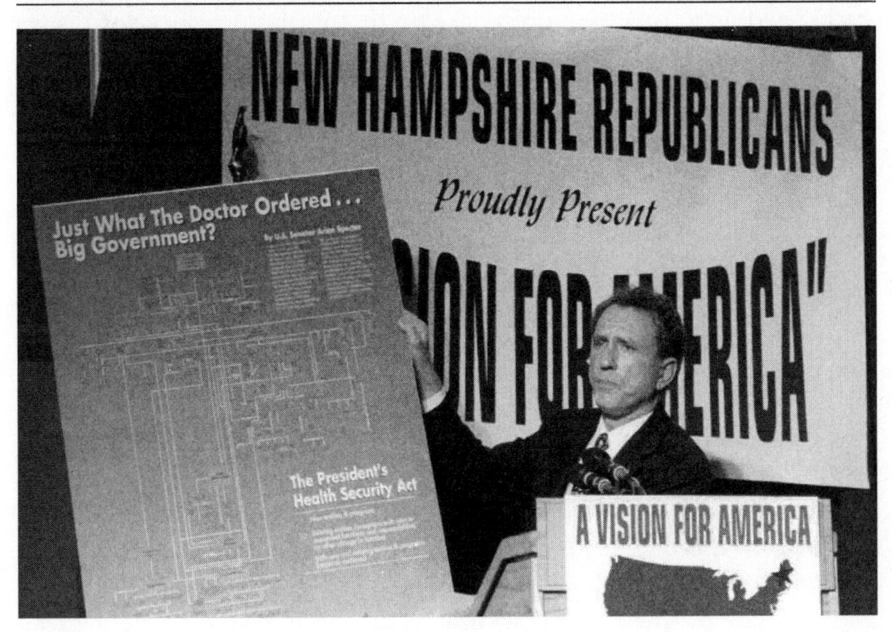

of the government and private sector are involved are intimately related. This complexity and system of interconnections make it hard to explain any single part of the system, such as payment, without explaining other parts. This can be confusing until we have a broader grasp of the entire system. So it is important to keep reading until the full picture emerges, as many elements of the picture will come into focus at the same time.

Second, the complexity of the system guarantees that every change or reform will have both positive and negative consequences and also unforeseen consequences. Even dramatic improvements are inevitably going to cause serious dislocation to many other parts of the system. Because of the huge complexity, even conscientious and thoughtful policy makers who thoroughly game out what might happen can easily fail to anticipate how various actors will respond. Things will happen that no one predicted—and often do.

Third, this complexity means there is no "ideal" system and no final reform. There are always myriad compromises and trade-offs in any reform. Just as one set of policies are expounded and becoming settled, other problems, evasions, and flaws will become clearer, thus necessitating further reforms. Efforts to improve the health care system are inherently Sisyphean. However, unlike the myth, the boulder does not always roll all the way back down the hill; many changes do measurably and decidedly improve the health care system.

The only way to get beyond slogans and actually be rational and thoughtful about how to improve the system and how policies like the Affordable Care Act will affect the system is to truly understand it in all its interconnected weirdness.

Health Insurance

There are 3 primary reasons for health insurance to: (1) protect individuals and families from large financial losses, (2) reduce financial barriers to using necessary medical services, and (3) make utilization predictable and costs lower through pooling.

The main purpose of any insurance product, such as home owner's or car insurance, is to protect people against large random—that is, unpredictable—financial losses. The idea is that people pay a predictable, comparatively small amount of money up front—the premium—and in exchange the insurance company promises to pay a large amount if a specified event randomly happens. For example, with home owner's insurance, people pay a premium, and their insurance company pays them if, unfortunately, their house burns down in an unexpected fire. They are thus financially protected against the large loss of having to rebuild their house. Similarly, health insurance protected Erin from paying over $70,000 for her unexpected colon cancer operation. Because Baltazar's brother did not have insurance, he had to pay the hospital $25,000 over 4 years for his appendectomy.

For the most part this function of insurance works. In 2008 Oregon wanted to assess its Medicaid program's efficacy. Medicaid is the joint federal-state government-sponsored program that pays for health services for poor children, pregnant women, and mothers of young children as well as mentally and physically disabled and very poor elderly individuals. Because of a shortage of funds, there were 90,000 uninsured people on the state's Medicaid waiting list. Oregon only had funds to expand coverage to one-third of the uninsured. The state conducted a lottery to enroll 30,000 people in Medicaid; the rest were left uncovered. Researchers found that Medicaid coverage "nearly eliminated . . . catastrophic expenditures, defined as out-of-pocket medical expenses exceeding 30% of income." Health insurance, in this case Medicaid, did protect people from large random financial losses.

A second important function of insurance is that it reduces the financial and psychological barrier to utilizing health care services. Insurance frees people from weighing the costs of health care against pain relief, getting an operation, or other tests and treatments. As Erin's operation or Baltazar's worker's stitches show, even simple health care services are very expensive, so high costs could inhibit people from using these important services. Indeed, even paying a small amount can deter people from seeking out life-saving tests and treatments. For instance, Medicare used to require people to pay 20% of the cost of a mammogram. When they eliminated this payment and essentially made mammograms free, the proportion of women who had mammograms increased 25%. A similar scenario occurs for vaccinations, well-baby visits, and many other beneficial services. Health insurance reduces the effective price people see for health care services, leading more people to utilize those services. In the language of economists, this increasing demand for services is termed insurance-induced demand.

A third reason for health insurance is pooling and spreading risk across a large number of people. Even if Erin's cancer is unpredictable, the need for health services of a large group of people is predictable. Aggregating people allows more predictability in how much health care they will use and, therefore, what the overall costs will be.

One of the most important facts about health care is that people's health is not random. In any particular year half the American population hardly uses any health care services (the small bar in Figure 2.2). Indeed, about one-third of people who have private insurance never submit a claim in a year. Conversely, 10% of Americans use nearly two-thirds of all health care services (see Figure 2.2).

When individuals buy health insurance the companies need to estimate which group the person will fall into: the low-user or high-user group. *Actuarial science* involves the calculations that insurance companies use to determine how likely individuals are to become sick and how

FIGURE 2.2 Concentration of health care spending in the US population, 2010

Percent of Population, Ranked by Health Care Spending	Percent of Total Health Care Spending
Top 1% (≥$53,238)	21.0%
Top 5% (≥$18,086)	49.5%
Top 10% (≥$10,044)	65.2%
Top 15% (≥$6,696)	75.0%
Top 20% (≥$4,639)	81.7%
Top 50% (≥$829)	97.3%
Bottom 50% (<$829)	2.7%

A small proportion of the US population accounts for half of all US health care spending. The 5% of the population with higher health care expenses (>$18,086 annually) was responsible for half (49.5%) of total health care spending, whereas the 50% of the population with the lowest expenses (<$829) accounted for only 2.7% of total spending.

Dollar amounts in parentheses are the annual expenses per person in each percentile. Population is the civilian noninstitutionalized population, including those without any health care spending. Health care spending is total payments from all sources (including direct payments from individuals and families, private insurance, Medicare, Medicaid, and miscellaneous other sources) to hospitals, physicians, other providers (including dental care), and pharmacies; health insurance premiums are not included.

Source: Kaiser Slides, The Henry J. Kaiser Family Foundation, March 13, 2013. *US Data Sources:* Department of Health and Human Services, Agency for Healthcare Research and Quality, Medical Expenditure Panel Survey (MEPS), Household Component, 2010.

severe that sickness will be. Then, given the risk that the person will fall sick, the insurers *underwrite* how much to charge for a premium. For instance, they know that, on average, younger people are healthier and are less likely to use health care services than older people. Similarly, the typical employed person is working and, therefore, is less likely to be chronically ill and use health care services than are the unemployed. Conversely, someone with a chronic illness such as asthma is likely to need medications, physician office visits, pulmonary function tests, visits to the emergency room, and hospitalizations. Insurance companies can use this kind of information to set premiums.

Pooling people and providing insurance to a big group of people allows the law of large numbers to kick in. Based on the law of large numbers, the average cost of care for a large group is easier to predict and subject to fewer fluctuations year to year than it is for small groups. Purely by chance, a small group may contain a large proportion of very sick people, but the larger the group, the lower that chance is. That is, the larger the group, the proportion of sick people is likely to be more consistent. To compensate for the lower predictability—or what is also called greater risk—insurers increase their prices for smaller groups and individuals.

Providing insurance to larger groups can lead to lower prices in part because it increases predictability and reduces the risk that the insurance company will itself experience a large unpredictable loss. This is one of the reasons why insuring big businesses is cheaper than insuring small businesses.

Two Problems Inherent in Health Insurance

Providing health insurance causes 2 problems. One problem is *moral hazard*. When insurance induces demand for necessary medical services it is a good thing; however, by lowering prices, insurance can also induce demand for services that might not be necessary. It can also allow people to choose a more expensive test or treatment when they are faced with choices between different interventions for the same medical condition. Moral hazard leads to overconsumption of health care services.

To counter moral hazard or insurance-induced demand, insurance companies employ several strategies. One is to make people pay part of the cost of health care before their insurance begins to pay. This portion is called the *deductible*. Deductibles come in wide ranges, from zero-deductible plans to what is now a moderate deductible of $250 or $500 per person. Erin had a *high-deductible* plan that required her to pay $5,000 before the insurance company covered any health care costs.

In addition to the deductible, insurers typically require individuals to pay a portion of the cost each time they use a service. This can be a *co-payment* (or co-pay), in which people pay a set amount of money, such

FIGURE 2.3 Key Insurance Terms

CONCEPT	DEFINITION
Premium	The amount paid for a health insurance policy. The average premium for a family in 2012 was $15,745 and for a single person was $5,615.
Deductible	The amount insured people pay out of their own pocket before the insurance company begins to pay medical bills, such as $500 per year.
High-deductible health plan	In these plans the amount people pay before the insurance company pays medical bills is very high, such as $5,000 per year. This really is catastrophic health insurance. It keeps premiums low and is thought to make people more prudent in their use of health care services.
Co-payment (co-pay)	A flat amount insured people pay when they use a medical service before the insurance company pays, such as $40 for a physician office visit or $10 for a prescription drug.
Co-insurance	A percentage of the total bill insured people pay when they use a medical service, such as 20% of the bill for a hospitalization.
Out-of-pocket payments (also "skin in the game")	All the costs covered by an insurance policy that insured people pay themselves. People pay for these out of their own pocket. This typically includes 4 payments: premium, deductibles, co-pays, and services not provided by insurance. There is an out-of-pocket maximum per year that an individual can pay, and then the insurance company must assume all further costs for that year.
Health savings account	A savings account used to pay for health care bills usually linked to a high-deductible health plan. If there is money left over in the health savings account at the end of the year, it can be rolled over to the next year. The money deposited into these accounts is not subject to federal income tax when deposited.
Consumer-driven health care	The combination of a health savings account with a high-deductible health plan places greater control over spending in the hands of consumers but also exposes them to potentially higher health care costs.
Beneficiary	An individual who is covered by a health insurance policy or by a government program, such as a person 65 years or older who is a Medicare beneficiary.

FIGURE 2.3 (*continued*)

CONCEPT	DEFINITION
Risk	The chance that people will need health care services and incur health care costs. High-risk people have a high chance of using health care services usually because they already have a serious illness that is likely to mean they will see a physician or require hospital care.
Claim	Bill presented to a health insurer by a health care provider for giving services to a beneficiary, such as a physician sending a claim into Medicare for seeing a Medicare beneficiary in the office.
Reimbursement	Payment by a health insurer to a health care provider such as a hospital or physician for providing a health care service to a beneficiary, such as Medicare paying $100 to the physician when a Medicare beneficiary had an office visit.
Self-funded plans	Large businesses do not really buy health insurance; instead, they pay the medical bills for their employees themselves—they self-fund the insurance. Typically, a commercial insurance company, such as Aetna, processes the medical bills.
Stop-loss coverage	This is insurance bought by a business that self-funds its worker's health care to limit how much it might pay. The insurance covers bills beyond a threshold.

as $20 per physician office visit or $10 per generic prescription. Alternatively, it can be a *co-insurance*, in which people pay a set percentage of the costs, such as 20% of the hospital bill. For instance, Medicare charges people 20% co-insurance for hospitalizations. Striking the right balance between facilitating the appropriate use of medical services while not increasing overuse is one of the complexities of health insurance.

A second problem is *adverse selection*. This is the tendency for sicker people or those disposed to use health care services such as the worried well to want to purchase health insurance and for healthier people to forego buying coverage. Individuals have some—albeit imprecise—ways of estimating how much health care they are likely to use in the next year. People who are likely to use a lot of services because they already have an illness, such as heart disease or diabetes, or engage in riskier activities, such as construction, are more likely to buy health insurance and buy policies that cover more medical services. Conversely, people who are healthy and have no history of chronic illness may think they do not need to buy health insurance.

One consequence of adverse selection is to increase the price of health insurance for all policyholders. If there are more sick people buying insurance, there will be greater use of health care services, thereby generating higher costs. Insurance companies then need to charge more in order to cover their costs. This can lead to a reinforcing downward spiral. As health care costs go up, the cost of health insurance increases, inducing more and more healthy people to forego insurance because it costs too much. This, in turn, concentrates sicker people in the group buying insurance and forcing costs up even further. And as costs continue to go up, even more healthy people stop buying insurance. Voilà: a downward spiral.

Insurance companies counter adverse selection in several ways. One approach is to exclude or charge very high prices for people with preexisting medical conditions. For example, Erin's insurance company increased her premiums 24% after her cancer diagnosis. Another approach is to exclude coverage for certain health care services associated with the preexisting condition either permanently or for a period of time. Erin's company might have written her policy to avoid paying for any future colon cancer–related care.

A third way is compulsion. This involves creating a very large pool of people who have no choice of whether to buy health insurance. This can be done by making a whole country one pool, by making a large geographic region a pool, or by making a large company or other large organization a pool. Enrollment of a large group—or everyone—eliminates adverse selection within that group. This is what occurs in Medicare. Similarly, a mandate or requirement that everyone have health insurance reduces adverse selection.

Private Health Insurance

One way of dividing up the American health care system is to identify 2 types of people: those who have coverage—the insured—and those who do not—the uninsured. Before implementation of the Affordable Care Act (ACA) roughly 85% of Americans were covered and 15% were uninsured (see Figure 2.4). However, the breadth and depth of coverage among the insured varied enormously.

In 2012 private health insurance covered approximately 165 million Americans, or 54% of the population. Among Americans who have private insurance, 150 million people get their health insurance through their employer or are on the insurance plan of a spouse or family member who gets coverage through an employer. They have *employer-sponsored insurance (ESI)*. This is why the American health care system is called an *employer-based system*. Another term for the employer-based coverage is the *group market*, because workers at a company are pooled into one "group" for buying insurance. Another 5% of the American population—15 million—buy private health insurance as individuals. This is called the *nongroup or individual market*. Erin is in the individual market.

In the employer-based system larger employers are much more likely to offer health insurance than are smaller employers. About 98% of employers with 200 or more workers provide insurance, whereas just 50% of businesses with fewer than 10 workers do. There are 3 reasons for this difference. First, for the same plan larger employers can get lower rates, not so much because they have better bargaining power—although they do—but because having more employees makes health care costs more predictable. Predictability reduces the amount of money that insurers must keep in reserve to cover uncertainty over the demand for health care services. In addition, the fixed administrative costs associated with insurance can be spread over a larger number of workers, reducing premiums for larger employers.

Second, workers at large employers tend to have higher wages, so the cost of health insurance is a smaller fraction of their total compensation. For Baltazar's low-wage gardeners, for instance, a health insurance plan that is $500 per month is a very large part of their income. For many low-wage workers in smaller companies it is much more important to have higher wages than health insurance.

Finally, there is just practicality. Unlike small employers, large employers have human relations departments that can more easily navigate the complexities of health insurance to offer their workers policies.

FIGURE 2.4 Health insurance coverage of the American population (310.2 million, 2012)

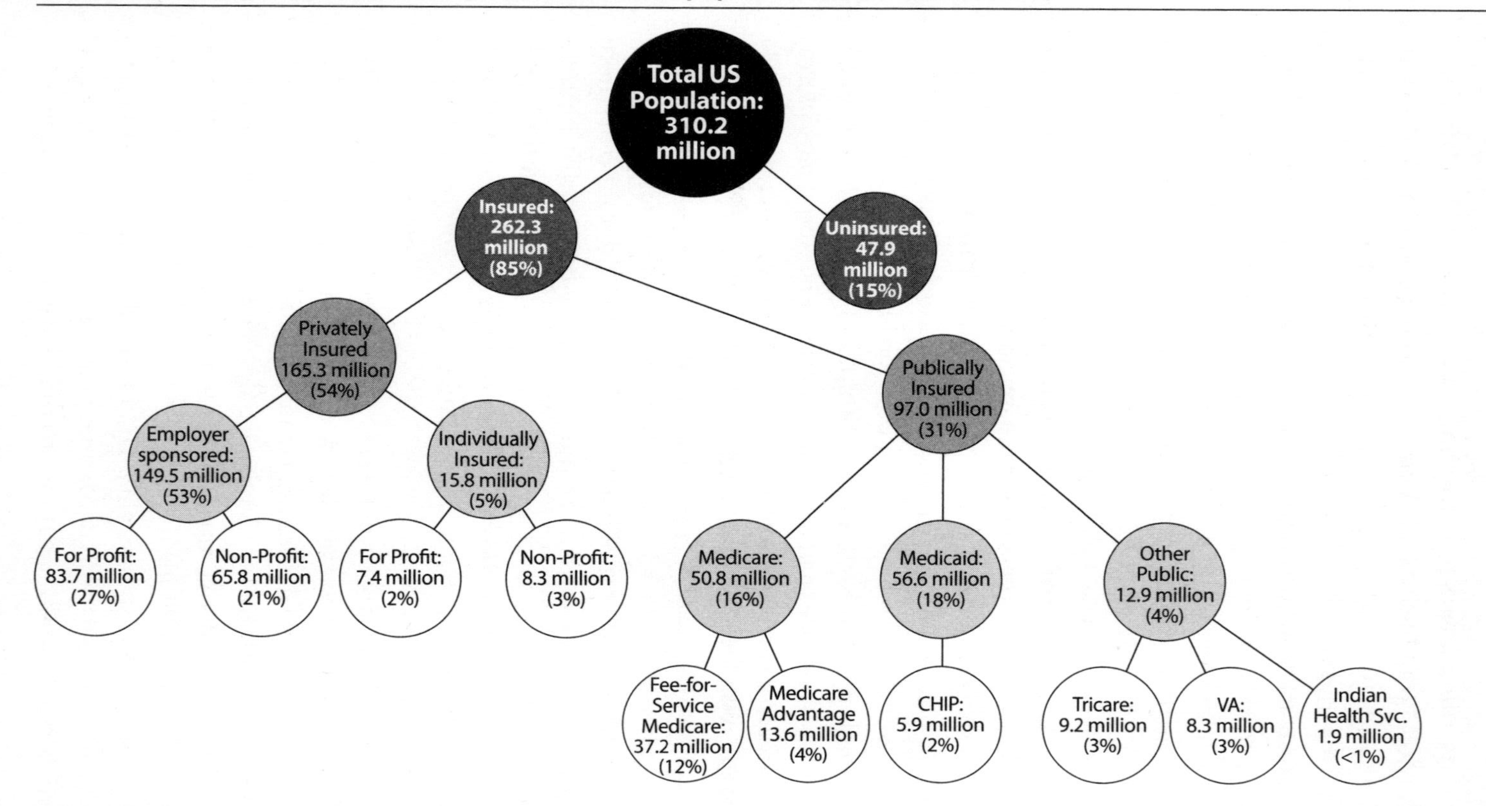

Note: Numbers reflect totals from 2010–2011. Numbers may not add up due to rounding and individuals who are covered by multiple insurers, and conflicting data from different government and private sources.

Sources: The Kaiser Family Foundation's State Health Facts. *Data Sources:* Centers for Medicare & Medicaid Services, US Census Bureau, Current Population Survey, Indian Health Service, Department of Defense, Veterans Administration, *AIS's Directory of Health Plans: 2013,* ©2013 by Atlantic Information Services, Inc., www.AISHealth.com.

There are other important characteristics of Americans who have employer-sponsored health insurance. Importantly, they are richer. For instance, of nonelderly people in households where the income is 400% or more of the poverty line (in 2013, $94,200 for a family of 4), 90% had private health insurance. Conversely, only 39% of nonelderly Americans making between 100% and 200% of the poverty line ($23,550 to $47,100) were insured. Because whites and Asian Americans tend to be better off than African Americans and Hispanics, these privileged groups are more likely to have employer-sponsored health insurance.

One peculiarity of the American health care system is that employers offer insurance at all. Until the Affordable Care Act there was no law requiring any employer to offer health insurance. Why did General Electric, General Motors, Intel, IBM, or your local law firm sponsor health insurance for their workers?

The primary reason is that many people, especially highly skilled people, would not consider working for a company that did not offer health insurance. Further, employers have economies of scale; they offer insurance companies a ready-made group, thereby getting lower rates than workers could get if they were to buy it for themselves. Similarly, health insurance also helps retain high-quality workers; it serves as a kind of "golden handcuffs," in which workers with a good policy, especially those with a preexisting condition, do not want to leave if they won't get an equally good policy from another employer.

There are 2 other reasons companies offer health insurance. First, many people believe their employer pays for health insurance. On average, in 2012, employers paid 72% of the insurance premium for family coverage and 82% of the premium for individual coverage. Yet this belief is misleading. It is really workers who pay for their health insurance by taking lower cash wages. Many studies have shown that if employers were to stop providing health insurance, workers' salaries would go up, not necessarily instantly but instead after a transition period. Similarly, if an employer-sponsored insurance plan includes more benefits and its premiums rise, then workers' other forms of compensation, especially cash wages, will grow less rapidly or fall to offset the added premium. In this sense employers who offer health insurance do not really pay for health insurance; they merely substitute one form of compensation, health insurance, for another, cash wages or vacation time. By appearing to pay the vast majority of health insurance premiums, employers win their workers' appreciation and loyalty.

The second incentive for employers to provide their workers' health insurance is the *tax exclusion*. In 1954 the IRS formally ruled that employer contributions to their workers' health insurance were excluded from the workers' taxable income. This ruling meant that workers who receive health insurance do not have to pay income or payroll taxes on the employers' financial contributions and, thus, employers do not have to pay their share of payroll taxes on the health insurance premiums. This is a huge financial incentive for workers to want more employer-sponsored health insurance: it is paid before taxes, and therefore, a dollar in health insurance is worth more to them than a dollar in cash wages. Employers also prefer compensating workers in health insurance.

The tax exclusion is the single largest tax break in the entire US tax code, worth about $250 billion in 2013. In comparison, the mortgage interest deduction is worth just $70 billion.

The tax exclusion is highly regressive; it gives much more benefit to the rich than to the poor. This is because, first of all, many lower-wage workers, like Wayne and Baltazar's, do not receive employer-sponsored insurance and, therefore, cannot take advantage of the tax exclusion at all. Secondly, wealthier workers are in a higher tax bracket, so the benefit of excluding money spent on health insurance saves them more money than it does lower-wage workers who get the same insurance policy. If an employer pays $10,000 in health insurance, the executive in the 39% tax bracket gets $3,900 in savings from the tax exclusion, but the janitor who is in the 15% tax bracket gets only $1,500.

Public Health Insurance

About 97.0 million, or 31% of the American population, has health coverage through a wide variety of public programs (see Figures 2.4 and 2.5). *Medicare* and *Medicaid* are far and away the largest and were created in 1965. Medicare covers 51 million Americans in 4 groups at a total cost in 2012 of $552 billion. Medicaid covers about 57 million Americans at any one point in time. However, over the course of a year about 72 million Americans will receive Medicaid benefits. For instance, over the course of a year a woman with children on Medicaid might find a job that provides health insurance and would leave Medicaid. Conversely, a worker with a wife and a 2-year-old might lose his job, and the mother and child could become eligible for Medicaid. In 2012 Medicaid's total cost was $414 billion, with $238 billion coming from the federal government.

Surprisingly, even though Medicare and Medicaid were enacted and signed into law at the exact same time, their structure, governance, financing, eligibility, and the services they pay for are very different (see Chapter 5). Medicare is *social insurance*. It requires that people pay taxes for a large part of their lives in order to earn eligibility for services when they become old or disabled. It protects a whole class of people—65 years and older and the disabled, regardless of income or need—from the financial risks of ill health through a compulsory program the government organizes and finances.

Conversely, before the ACA Medicaid has been a *means-tested, needs-based* program. People are eligible if they have low income *and* fit into other categories, which are (1) children, (2) blind or physically disabled, (3) elderly, (4) mentally ill, (5) pregnant women, and (6) mothers, but only when their children are young. It is almost impossible for young, healthy, but poor males or females without children to be on Medicaid. Being poor is necessary to qualify for Medicaid, but it is not sufficient.

Medicare and Medicaid also differ by how they are operated and funded. Medicare is paid for and administered exclusively by the federal government; Medicaid is paid for by a combination of the federal and state governments and is administered by the states. States are not required to participate, although since 1982, when Arizona finally joined after 17 years, all do. (As will be discussed in Chapters 8 and 9, not all states are joining the expansion of Medicaid under the Affordable Care Act.) On average before the ACA the federal government paid 57% of Medicaid's costs, but the amount varied by state, depending on the state's per capita income. Poorer states receive more federal support.

Many Americans who are eligible for Medicaid do not enroll. For instance, it is estimated that there are 8 million uninsured children in the United States, but 5 million are eligible for Medicaid or CHIP (see

FIGURE 2.5 Three main government health programs

PROGRAM	ADMINISTERED BY	NUMBER OF ENROLLEES	COST (2012)	
			FEDERAL	STATE
Medicare	Federal government only	50.8 million Americans, composed of: • 42.2 million Americans who are 65 years of age or older, • 8.6 million younger people with disabilities, • 500,000 people with end-stage renal disease who need dialysis or a kidney transplant, and A small but unknown number have Amyotrophic Lateral Sclerosis (Lou Gehrig's disease).	$552 billion	$0
Medicaid	Jointly by states and federal government	50.7 million Americans including CHIP (eligibility varies by state), including: • 22.0 million children; • 12.9 million adults, mainly pregnant women and mothers of eligible children; • 9.8 million people who are blind or have disabilities; and • 5.0 million very poor elderly—these are *dual eligibles:* eligible for both Medicare and Medicaid.	$238 billion	$176 billion
CHIP—Children's Health Insurance Program	Jointly by states and federal government	5.9 million children (eligibility varies by state)	$9 billion	$4 billion

below). This lack of enrollment is partly because many states discourage enrollment by requiring many forms and documentation as well as frequent re-enrollment with all the required paperwork. In addition, many Americans abhor the idea of taking government aid; doing so does not fit with their self-image or ideology. Even when they are eligible for Medicaid they do not enroll. Finally, many believe they will soon be "on their feet again" and do not think they need the help.

After the failure of his health care reform initiative in 1993, President Clinton allied with Senator Edward Kennedy (D-Massachusetts) to enact the *Children's Health Insurance Program (CHIP)* in 1997. CHIP was meant to provide insurance for US and immigrant children up to age 19 who were uninsured but did not qualify for Medicaid. Eligibility varies from state to state. In New Jersey children are eligible if their parents' monthly income is under 350% of the federal poverty level, while in Wyoming parents' income must be under 200% of the federal poverty level.

In addition to Medicare, Medicaid, and CHIP, there are many other public health programs, which are described later in the chapter.

The Uninsured

Before implementation of the ACA about 15% of the population at any given time were uninsured, representing just under 50 million Americans. Approximately 12 million are undocumented aliens. The image many people have of the other 38 million are unemployed, maybe even lazy people who are taking advantage of the system by showing up at the emergency room for routine care.

This image is totally wrong (see Figure 2.6). Like Wayne and Baltazar, the vast majority of uninsured Americans are the working poor. Approximately three-quarters, about 36.5 million, are either workers or in households with a full- or part-time worker. Indeed, 10% of the uninsured have 2 full-time workers in the family. The problem is that even if they are working, they are poor: 40% of all uninsured have incomes under 100% of the poverty line and, like Baltazar, cannot afford the premiums. For many of these workers, like Wayne, their employers do not offer insurance. For instance, 55% of those earning under 100% of the

FIGURE 2.6 Characteristics of the nonelderly uninsured population, 2012

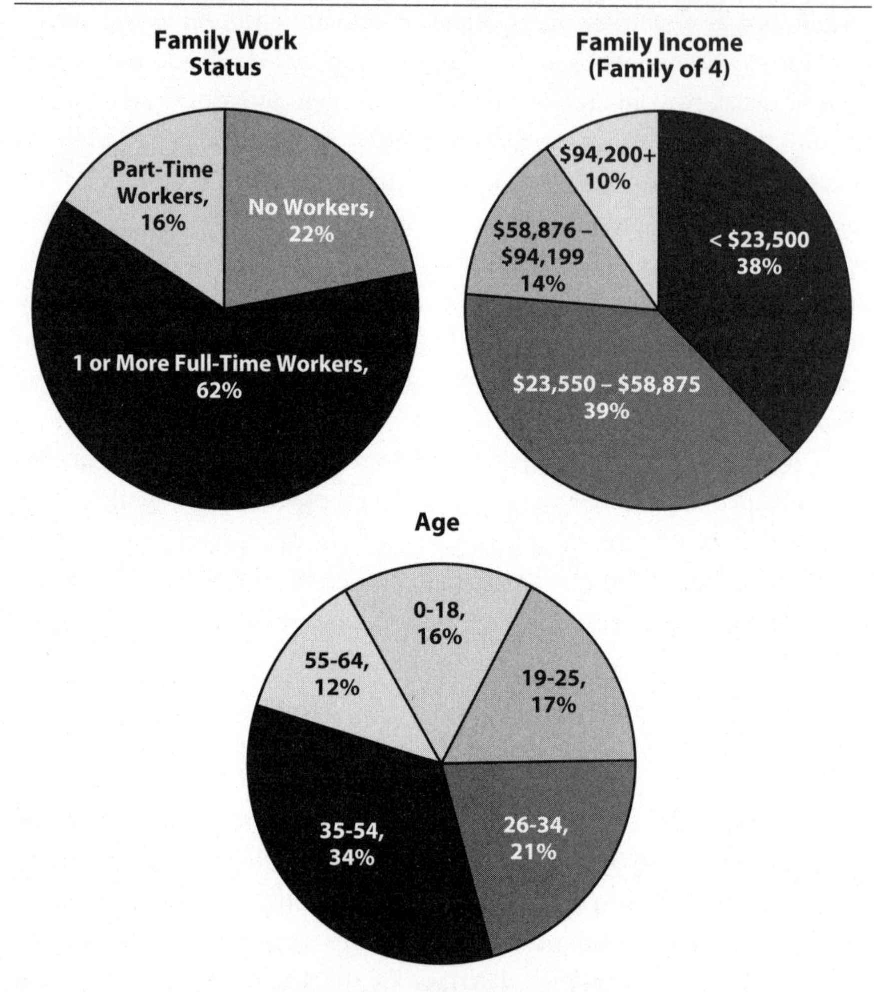

Note: Data may not total 100% due to rounding.

Source: Kaiser Slides, The Henry J. Kaiser Family Foundation, March 13, 2013. *Data Source:* KCMU/ Urban Institute analysis of 2012 ASEC Supplement to the CPS.

federal poverty line are not offered health insurance from their employers. About 8 million are children, of which 5 million qualify for Medicaid or CHIP but are not enrolled for one reason or another. Importantly, these 2 groups—the working poor and children—are relatively healthy and, therefore, are relatively cheap to insure.

Surprisingly, about 10% of the uninsured, nearly 5 million Americans, are in families who actually earn a good income, more than $94,200 per year for a family of 4 in 2013. Insurance companies may reject these relatively well-off people because they have a pre-existing condition, such as a nonfatal type of skin cancer, and be denied coverage or charged an exorbitant amount for coverage.

Lacking health insurance is not a transitory issue for most people. Fully 51% of the uninsured have been uninsured for 3 years or more. For only 17% does being uninsured last 6 months or less. This is probably the case because, like Wayne, many of the uninsured are long term employees of businesses that just cannot afford to purchase insurance, and this is not transitory.

Private Payers and Insurers

Private Insurers

One way to divide private payers for health coverage is into health insurance companies and employee health plans (see Figure 2.7). Health insurance companies are regulated at the state level, and there are 3 types: (1) for-profit commercial insurers, (2) Blue Cross and Blue Shield Plans, and (3) health maintenance organizations (HMOs), also known as integrated delivery systems.

Altogether there are over 1,000 for-profit commercial insurance companies, yet only a handful of companies dominate the industry. The top 11 for-profit insurers are in the Fortune 500; the 5 largest and most well-known are United, Aetna, Wellpoint, Cigna, and Humana. Together these 11 companies insure well over 100 million Americans. In 2012 the top 11 health insurance companies had revenues of $301.8 billion and profits of $13.7 billion, with the big 5 for-profit health insurers dominating with revenues of $255.2 billion and $12.5 billion in profits.

A second type of private health insurance company is the "Blues"—the Blue Cross and Blue Shield plans. Historically these were not-for-profit, state-based plans, and many, such as Blue Cross and Blue Shield of Tennessee and of Illinois, still are. But over the last few decades many

FIGURE 2.7 Private insurance hierarchy

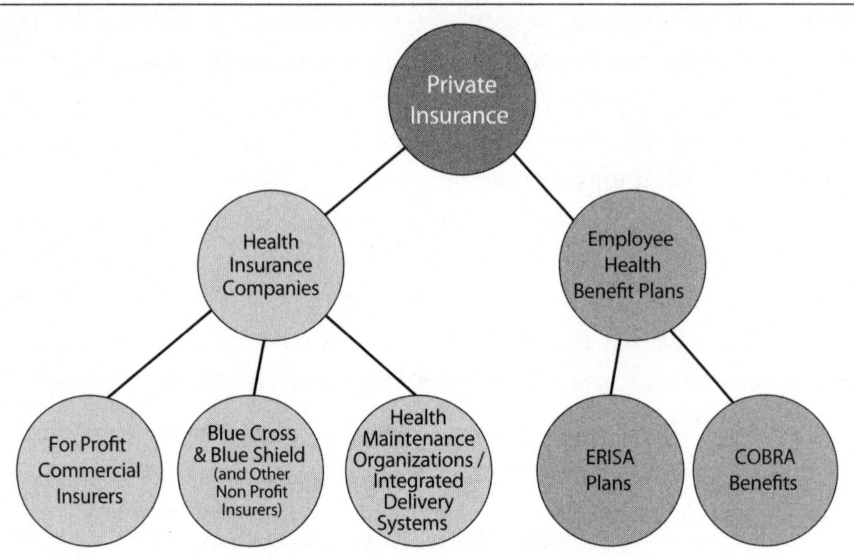

have become for-profit commercial insurers. Wellpoint, for instance, was originally formed from a California Blues plan.

Traditional Blues plans often view themselves as having special missions and have to fulfill special state requirements such as insuring all applicants or using community rating—that is, charging a similar premium to all enrollees, regardless of age or health status—and in return they often get special consideration such as special tax benefits. Overall, the 38 independently operated not-for-profit Blues plans insure around 40 million Americans, with revenues of over $179 billion and margin—"profit" without the profit—of $5.5 billion.

Finally, among private health insurance plans are *health maintenance organizations (HMOs)*, such as Kaiser and Group Health of Puget Sound. These are better thought of as *integrated delivery systems* because the insurance function is integrated with the health delivery function in one organization. Thus, integrated systems typically operate hospitals and offices, and they employ physicians, nurses, pharmacists, and other health care personnel directly. Often, for legal and liability reasons, the insurance function is in a separate subsidiary from the health care providers and is separately regulated by state officials. Thus, Kaiser Permanente Medical Group is the physician side and exclusively contracts with the Kaiser health plan. Conversely, commercial insurers and Blues plans pay private hospitals, physicians, and others for health care services but do not directly provide the health care services, own hospitals, or employ physicians.

Kaiser is by far the biggest integrated system, providing insurance to 9.1 million people, employing nearly 15,000 physicians, operating 37 hospitals, and showing revenues of $50.6 billion. Group Health of Puget Sound provides insurance to 616,000 people largely in Washington State, with revenues of $3.3 billion.

Commercial insurers and Blues plans offer different insurance policies. The most expensive and generous cover any hospital and physician. These *indemnity* or *conventional plans* were common through the 1980s; since the 1990s, however, they have become almost extinct. During the 1990s both HMOs (integrated systems) and *preferred provider organizations (PPOs)* became more common. In PPOs, insurers create special networks of hospitals and physicians, sometimes called *preferred provider networks*. One reason to establish these networks is that the insurer negotiates with these providers lower prices that they will pay for services. As a result, the insured patient will pay less to see these preferred physicians. Physicians accept these lower prices to see more patients than if they were not in the network. During the 2000s the HMOs decreased in popularity while the PPOs expanded.

High-deductible health plans, like the one Erin has, require the insured to pay the first several thousand dollars of medical bills, and then the insurer pays the rest. (Legally the limit is $6,250 in out-of-pocket expenses for an individual and $12,500 in for a family.) Recently these high-deductible plans have greatly expanded. Their appeal to employers is that they keep costs down by having the insured pay more of the medical bill. High-deductible health plans are designed to counter moral hazard, but it also discourages people from using health care services.

With such high-deductible plans, individuals whose medical bills will be small and do not use a lot of health care services will be affected, whereas the 10% of Americans who use a great deal of services are less likely to change their use of health care services. These high health care users quickly spend all of their deductible with one hospitalization or even a small surgical procedure, and then the rest of their care is essentially free because insurance covers it all.

Another category of health insurance plans is *employee health plans, or ERISA plans*. Employers or, to a lesser extent, employee organizations sponsor the plan and are self-funded: the employers pay the health care costs directly. The federal government regulates these plans under *ERISA, the Employee Retirement Income Security Act* of 1974. This is an extremely complex law that regulates employee benefit plans, such as health insurance, and was meant to protect workers when employers provide benefits. Large employers that operate across state lines prefer ERISA health plans because the law largely exempts them from specific requirements of state law and allows them to provide uniform benefits to their employees throughout the country. In ERISA plans employers pay and determine the benefits that they will provide to their workers.

Typically an employer with an ERISA plan will hire a health insurance company to process and pay the bills from hospitals, physicians, and other providers. Frequently, these companies are for-profit insurers, such as Aetna, providing *administrative services only (ASO)*. Importantly, in ERISA plans the employer or business is really paying the health bill; the administrator is just processing payments. An employee may think they have health insurance through Aetna, but that is just the "nameplate"; the employer is the one that is actually assuming the financial risk and telling the administrator what services should be paid for and what should not be paid for.

Finally there is *COBRA (Consolidated Omnibus Budget Reconciliation Act)* health benefits. This was enacted in 1986, and it allows workers whose employment has been terminated or whose work hours have been reduced, as well as retirees and workers' spouses and dependent children, to purchase the company's health insurance at group rates. This lowers the cost compared to what the individual would pay were they buying health insurance on their own. Typically the employer does not pay any part of the premium, so it is more expensive than what active workers would pay. COBRA coverage can last a maximum of 18 months.

One hotly debated aspect of commercial insurers, such as United, Wellpoint, and Aetna, is their administrative costs and the related *medical-loss ratio (MLR)*. The MLR is a way of determining what percentage of a person's insurance premium goes to paying for health services they use and what goes toward administrative costs and profits.

An MLR of 90%, for example, means that 90 cents of every dollar of a premium goes toward paying for medical bills and 10% goes toward administration, sales, and profit. (The reason the MLR is characterized as a "loss"—how much the insurance company loses on its payments for services—is because this is viewed from the perspective of the business and shareholders, not the insured patient.)

The MLR should be higher for larger groups because fixed administrative costs, such as creating a network of physicians and actuarial estimates of total costs over the years, can be allocated to the large number of employees. For instance, IBM can spread its fixed health insurance administrative costs over its 400,000 full-time workers, raising the premium of each worker a tiny amount. Conversely, a small company might have only 25 workers to spread its fixed costs over, meaning that a larger share of the premium will go toward administrative costs, generating a lower MLR.

What is the right MLR? There are 3 activities insurers engage in that require administrative expenses. One relates to clerical activities such as credentialing physicians, processing claims, combating fraud, and the IT infrastructure to support these efforts. A second relates to developing networks and monitoring as well as enhancing quality of care and developing new payment methods. A third relates to marketing, risk selection, and other competitive practices. And then there is profit (see Figure 2.8).

There is no doubt that many of the administrative costs, especially those related to the first 2 categories, are vital but could be reduced. For instance, there could be administrative simplification with greater use of use of standardized electronic claims transactions. Similarly, brokers are paid a percentage and thus have an incentive to sell higher-cost plans; savings might be found if they were paid a flat fee. The costs related to the third category, especially risk selection, seem inappropriate and unjustified. And, of course, there is the issue of what constitutes the right level of profit.

The MLR can be high for bad reasons. Spending more money on higher-cost services that may not be necessary constitutes overtreatment. This would raise the MLR but would not represent a good use of money. A rule of thumb that has been put into the Affordable Care Act

FIGURE 2.8 2012 Insurer operating expenses (in millions)

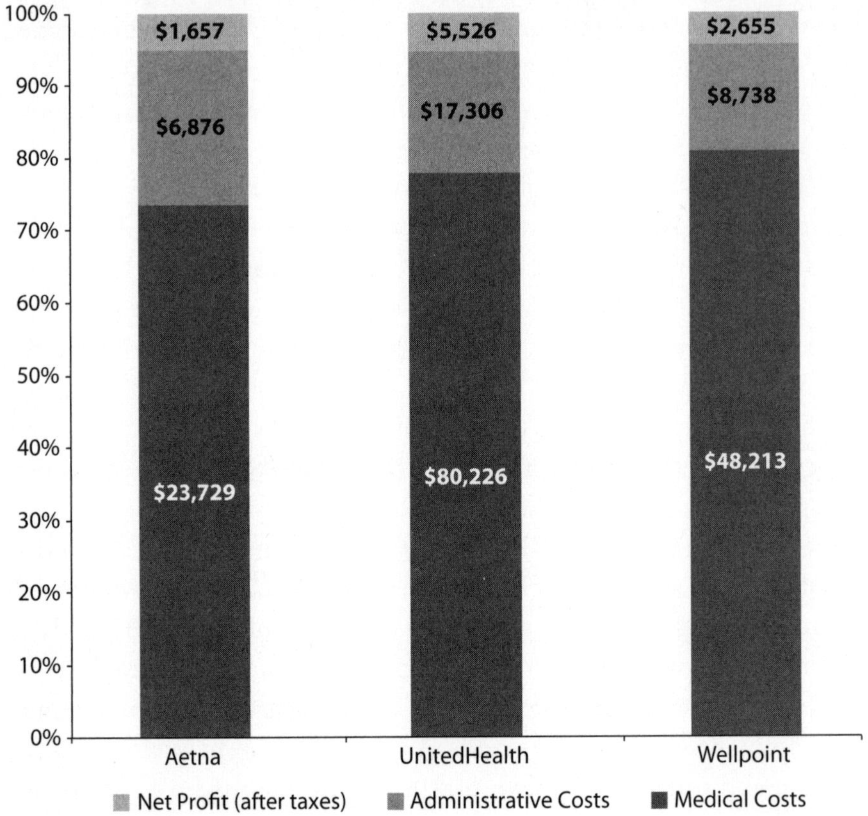

100%
90%
80%
70%
60%
50%
40%
30%
20%
10%
0%

Aetna: $1,657; $6,876; $23,729
UnitedHealth: $5,526; $17,306; $80,226
Wellpoint: $2,655; $8,738; $48,213

Net Profit (after taxes) Administrative Costs Medical Costs

(see Chapter 8) is that for larger groups the MLR should not be lower than 85%, and for individual and small groups it should not be lower than 80%. These thresholds are also controversial.

Public Insurers

Medicare. Medicare is organized in a different manner from a private insurer. Medicare is divided into 4 parts (see Figure 2.9). Parts A and B were established in the initial 1965 legislation. Part A covers hospital costs, and a payroll tax pays for it. Workers and their employers each pay 1.45% of total wages to support Part A.

Part B covers physician visits, other nonhospital services like physical therapy and rehabilitation, and X-rays, laboratory tests, injectable chemotherapy provided by oncologists, walkers, wheelchairs, and other

FIGURE 2.9 Medicare's Parts

	YEAR ESTABLISHED	NUMBER OF PEOPLE ENROLLED	PURPOSE	FINANCED
Part A	1965	50.8 million	Pays for hospital care	Payroll tax: 1.45% from workers and 1.45% from employer (2.9% from self-employed individuals).
Part B	1965	47.6 million	Pays for physician visits, nonhospital services, X-rays, lab tests, walkers, wheelchairs, other medical equipment, physical therapy, rehabilitation, and emergency room visits	Income-linked premiums from enrollees and general federal revenue. Premiums cover only 25% of costs.
Part C	1997	13.6 million	Managed care that must cover services in Parts A and B and usually covers prescription drugs	Not separately financed. Plans receive capitated payments from Medicare. Additional premiums and cost-sharing obligations vary by plan.
Part D	2006	31.9 million	Pays for prescription drugs	Income-linked premiums from enrollees and general federal revenue. Premiums cover only 25% of costs.
Medigap	Revised in 1992 by National Association of Insurance Commissioners into 10 standard packages that were expanded to 12 in 2006	10.2 million	Pays for costs that enrollees would have to cover, such as deductibles, co-payments, and co-insurance	Premiums exclusively from enrollees or their employers.

Source: Edgar Online.

medical equipment. Part B also covers hospital outpatient and ambulatory surgery services.

Two sources of revenue pay for Part B: general federal revenue and income-linked premiums from enrollees. The beneficiary premiums cover only 25% of the cost of the Part B program, so general federal revenue heavily subsidizes these services.

Not all Medicare enrollees use Medicare services every year; only about 20% of all Medicare beneficiaries end up in the hospital each year and use Part A services. After a beneficiary pays a deductible—the cost of one average hospital day—Medicare covers all the cost of the first 60 days of each hospitalization and three-quarters of the cost of the next 30 days.

In addition to traditional hospital and physician visits, Medicare also pays for stays of up to 100 days in skilled nursing facilities, home health care services, and hospice services for patients who are expected to die in the next 6 months.

Most Medicare patients have supplemental insurance to cover medical expenses that are not paid for by Medicare such as the co-payment and co-insurance costs. About 34% of Medicare beneficiaries have coverage for these costs from their employer, usually as retiree benefits. Another 17% of Americans with traditional Medicare also buy *Medigap* supplemental insurance plans from private insurance companies and others such as AARP. Many Medigap plans offer *first dollar coverage*, meaning that they eliminate deductibles. This exacerbates insurance-induced demand because the financial barrier to seeing a doctor or getting a test is eliminated.

Medicare Part C, Medicare Advantage, provides private managed care or preferred provider plans to Medicare beneficiaries. Initially promoted by Republicans, it allows insurance companies to expand their business by offering Medicare patients private insurance plans. The federal government pays these plans a fixed premium for each beneficiary, determined by a complex competitive bidding process. Many of these private plans offer additional benefits beyond the Medicare Parts A, B, and D coverage, such as vision care and gym memberships. Historically, Medicare Advantage plans have appealed to healthier seniors who were less likely to use many health care services and liked the added benefits such as free gym memberships. Their benefits are structured more like traditional managed-care or preferred-provider insurance, with, for instance, a $20 co-pay to see the in-network physician and a $5 co-pay for generic drugs. The Medicare Advantage Plan Star Rating system rates these plans based on quality and customer service standards.

Enacted in 2003 and implemented on January 1, 2006, Medicare Part D covers prescription drugs. It is a voluntary program in which Medicare beneficiaries can select to enroll in a plan run by an insurance company or other private company approved by Medicare. (Seniors who enroll in Part C usually get drug coverage through those plans.) About 60% of seniors have Part D coverage (or drug coverage in a Part C plan), about 30% get drug coverage from another source, such as retiree benefits, while 10% of seniors lack drug coverage. In 2014 there are 1,169 Part D plans across the United States; each plan decides what drugs it will pay for, the amount of the deductible and co-pays, and the premiums. Some plans have restricted formularies, meaning they only cover a limited number of drugs in each drug category, emphasize generics, and charge low or no deductibles and co-pays, whereas other plans may provide extensive choice of drugs but with higher premiums, deductibles, and co-pays.

One of the peculiarities of Part D is the so-called donut hole. To keep the total costs of the program down, Congress permitted no coverage when a beneficiary spent $2,850 in drug expenses (in 2014 dollars), and then coverage resumed, with seniors paying just 5% of drug costs when the senior had more than $4,550 in drug expenses. Beginning in 2011 the ACA progressively closes the donut hole.

Part D is paid for like Part B. Beneficiaries pay an income-linked premium that covers about 25% of the cost of the insurance, and, using general tax revenues, the federal government pays the other 75% of costs.

Parts A and B constitute fee-for-service or traditional Medicare. About 75% of all seniors in Medicare, 37.2 million, are enrolled in traditional Medicare. Medicare Advantage or Part C enrolls the other 25%.

Medicare is administered at the federal level by the *Centers for Medicare and Medicaid Services (CMS)*, an agency within the Department of Health and Human Services. (CMS also administers the federal portion of Medicaid and the CHIP programs.) CMS employs just over 4,000 people and is overseen by a Senate-confirmed administrator. CMS receives over 1 billion claims from hospital, physicians, and other health care providers a year, but it does not itself pay the bills. CMS pays private contractors, typically insurance companies, to receive claims and process payments, operate call centers, and combat fraud, all under government-specified rules.

Probably CMS's most important functions include issuing regulations establishing the rules for each part of Medicare and Medicaid, determining the annual payment rates for various providers each year, granting waivers to federal rules for states to try new approaches to delivering care, and operating demonstration projects to test new ways of delivering and paying for services that might improve quality and/or reduce costs.

It is worth noting that in some circumstances Medicare sets prices and in others it pays whatever it is charged. In its payments to hospitals, for instance, Medicare sets the formula and rates for hospitals. CMS tells hospitals how much they will be paid for specific services provided to all Medicare beneficiaries receiving Parts A and B services. (Each private insurance company determines how much it will pay hospitals participating in its Medicare Advantage plan.)

Conversely, there are other services in which Medicare is required to pay whatever it is charged. For instance, Medicare Part B pays oncologists for intravenous cancer chemotherapy drugs administered in the office. The price Medicare pays is determined by the *average sales price (ASP)*—that is, the average of the actual prices paid in the previous quarter. Congress has prohibited CMS from bargaining with pharmaceutical companies to lower the price of the chemotherapy drugs. Legally, Medicare must pay whatever the pharmaceutical companies charge oncologists for the drugs. In this case, Medicare is a price taker: the price is set by the drug companies, and Medicare has no flexibility or negotiating power to pay a lower price.

Medicare is filled with "extra" payments, or payments that are added on to base payments to encourage certain activities (Figure 2.10). For instance, Congress decided it wanted to assist hospitals that take care of a large number of uninsured or poorly reimbursed Medicaid patients. Rather than directly paying these hospitals based on how many patients they provide care to and the types of services they provide, Congress created the Disproportionate Share Hospital (DSH, pronounced "dish") payment. Similarly, Congress wanted to keep very small rural hospitals open, so it pays higher Medicare rates to these hospitals than the

FIGURE 2.10 Other Medicare payments

OTHER MEDICARE PAYMENTS	PURPOSE OR TARGET	DESCRIPTION OF THE PROGRAM	COST
Graduate medical education (GME)	To support training of interns and residents in hospitals	DME: direct medical education, pays salaries and supervision of interns and residents IME: indirect medical education, pays for extra tests and longer hospital stays that arise because interns and residents care for patients	$10 billion
Disproportionate share hospital (DSH, pronounced *dish*)	To compensate hospitals for the care they provide to the uninsured and a high proportion of Medicaid patients	Primary method: designated for hospitals that serve a disproportionate percentage of low-income patients as determined by the disproportionate patient percentage	$11 billion (65% of these funds go to academic teaching hospitals)
Critical access hospitals	To keep small rural hospitals open by providing higher payments	For hospitals with 25 or fewer beds located at least 35 miles from another facility that offer 24 hour emergency services. Medicare pays for 101% of inpatient and outpatient costs, as well as ambulance expenses.	$8.5 billion
Health professional shortage areas (HPSAs)	To identify a medically underserved geographic area, population group or health care facility, physician scarcity areas	There are 3 types of HPSA designations with individual requirements: primary medical care, dental, and mental health HPSAs. The requirements for each designation depend on geographic area, population groups, and facilities, and they include criteria such as population and full-time primary care physician ratio.	$274 million

hospitals would normally receive based on the price they actually pay for rent, wages, electricity, and other expenses related to providing care in their rural communities.

Medicaid. Whereas Medicare is entirely a federally financed and administered program, Medicaid is jointly financed and administered by the federal and state governments. The federal government sets minimum standards of service delivery for Medicaid, eligibility, and quality of care, while the states have significant flexibility in determining eligibility standards, services actually paid for, and the payment rates for hospitals and physicians. Some states pay for many services above the federal minimum and have generous eligibility requirements. Consequently, rather than having one benefit package for the whole country, there is a common core set of benefits that the federal government mandates, while actual Medicaid benefits differ from state to state.

Interestingly, Medicaid has more extensive benefits than Medicare. Whereas both cover the usual hospitalizations, office visits, emergency department visits, and most diagnostic tests, Medicaid also covers dental care, eyeglasses, nurse midwives, and nursing home care. For children, Medicaid operates an *early and periodic screening, diagnostic and treatment (EPSDT)* program to prevent and diagnose medical conditions early before they become major issues.

Over half of the states have opted to provide their Medicaid program through managed care, paying insurance companies to administer the program, whereas others continue basically a conventional insurance program where the state directly pays hospitals and physicians for their services. This managed care program applies mainly to mothers and children. Typically the disabled, mentally ill, and others remain on a traditional fee-for-service program.

The numbers of Medicaid enrollees is not closely linked to the cost of the program. For instance, 49% of Medicaid recipients are children, but they use about 20% of Medicaid dollars (see Figure 2.11). Conversely, some people are eligible for both Medicare and Medicaid. These are called *dual eligibles*. They are the elderly or disabled whose income is below 100% of the federal poverty line (which in 2013 was $11,490 for an individual). For these duals, Medicaid pays for the premiums as well as the co-payments and co-insurance of Medicare along with long-term

FIGURE 2.11 Medicaid enrollees and expenditures, FFY 2009

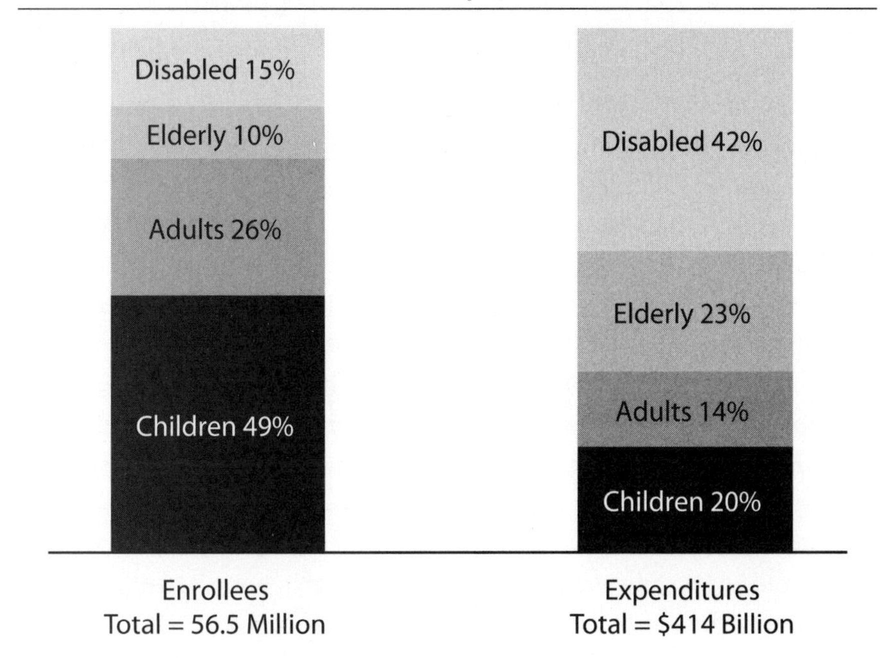

Note: Percentages may not add up to 100 due to rounding.

Source: KCMU/Urban Institute estimates based on data from FFY 2009 MSIS and CMS-64, 2012. MSIS FFY 2008 data were used for PA, UT, and WI, but adjusted to 2009 CMS-64.

care costs. There are about 9 million duals representing 15% of Medicaid enrollees. The duals are very expensive; they use about 40% of all Medicaid dollars and 36% of all Medicare dollars. Most of the Medicaid money funds long-term care. Thus, although most people think of Medicaid as a program for poor mothers and children, its big expenditures support the poor elderly and disabled.

Although Medicaid offers generous benefits, few people actually get the benefits. In theory almost all hospitals take Medicaid, but due to geographic location, many care for few Medicaid patients. For instance, the Aspen hospital where Erin was treated is not likely to admit many Medicaid patients. More importantly, fewer than half of all physicians actually take Medicaid patients, and even fewer dentists do. The lack of physician participation in Medicaid is partly because of very low payment amounts and partly because of excessive paperwork and other bureaucratic requirements. This is particularly problematic for Medicaid beneficiaries who need specialists. Consequently, it is often said that

Medicaid offers the most comprehensive health insurance benefits on paper but the worst in reality.

The Veterans Administration. Medicare and Medicaid are government-financed programs, but their beneficiaries receive their care in hospitals that are typically privately owned and from physicians who are not employed by the government. Conversely, the Veterans Administration (VA) is a true socialized health care system. The government pays the bills; owns the hospitals; and employs physicians, respiratory and physical therapists, pharmacists, and other providers. In this sense, the VA is akin to an integrated health system in which the federal government, not a private organization, is both the insurer and the provider of care. This also means it has a real interest in providing high-quality, cost-effective care.

The VA used to be criticized for the poor care it provided. Beginning in the mid-1990s, however, the VA embarked on a coordinated effort to measure performance and improve quality. Ironically, the VA also had an older, sicker, and poorer patient population. A 2010 independent assessment by RAND, a nonprofit policy think tank, concluded that, especially on the standards the VA measured, it outperformed regular medical care. For instance, among patients with chronic diseases VA patients received about 70% of recommended care, compared with about 60% in the national sample. For preventive care VA patients received about 65% of recommended care, whereas patients in the national sample received 20% less.

There are many other public health care programs (see Figure 2.12). For instance, the *Federal Employee Health Benefits Program (FEHBP)* covers nearly 9 million federal employees, their families, and retirees at an annual cost of $40 billion in 2012.

Conclusion

The US health care system really is a circuit board with a huge number of different components. There are private for-profit and not-for profit insurance companies, integrated delivery systems, and a whole variety

FIGURE 2.12 Other government health coverage programs

PROGRAM	TARGET POPULATION	TYPE OF HEALTH COVERAGE	COST
Veterans Administration	8.3 million veterans	Health care services through 153 hospitals, 788 out-patient clinics, and 232 veterans centers	$53 billion
Tricare	9.2 million active-duty military personnel, retirees, dependents, and survivors	Health insurance covering the costs of receiving care from private, non-military physicians and hospitals	$33 billion
Indian Health Service	1.9 million Native Americans and Alaskan Natives	Health care services through 33 hospitals and 59 health centers and health stations	$4.3 billion
Federally qualified health clinics (FHQCs)	20 million Americans: 39% uninsured, 36% Medicaid, 8% Medicare	Health care services	$1.2 billion
Public Hospitals	Insured and uninsured Americans	Inpatient and outpatient hospital services	$72 billion

Source: Kaiser Slides, The Henry J. Kaiser Family Foundation, March 14, 2013.

of public programs, from Medicare and Medicaid to the VA. Each component is itself incredibly complex; for instance, Medicare alone has 4 parts along with supplemental insurance. It would be great if there were a single graphic that integrated all of it. But there is not. What we have helps but cannot easily capture the complexity without becoming incomprehensible (see Figure 2.13 on next page).

The challenge—or depressing fact—is that this is just the financing part, the part that pays for health care. The next chapter details the delivery side of health care—the physicians, hospitals, home health care agencies, drug and device companies, and regulators—and it may well be even more complex. This is why they say that only 2 old and wise people really understand the American health care system.

FIGURE 2.13 Health coverage map

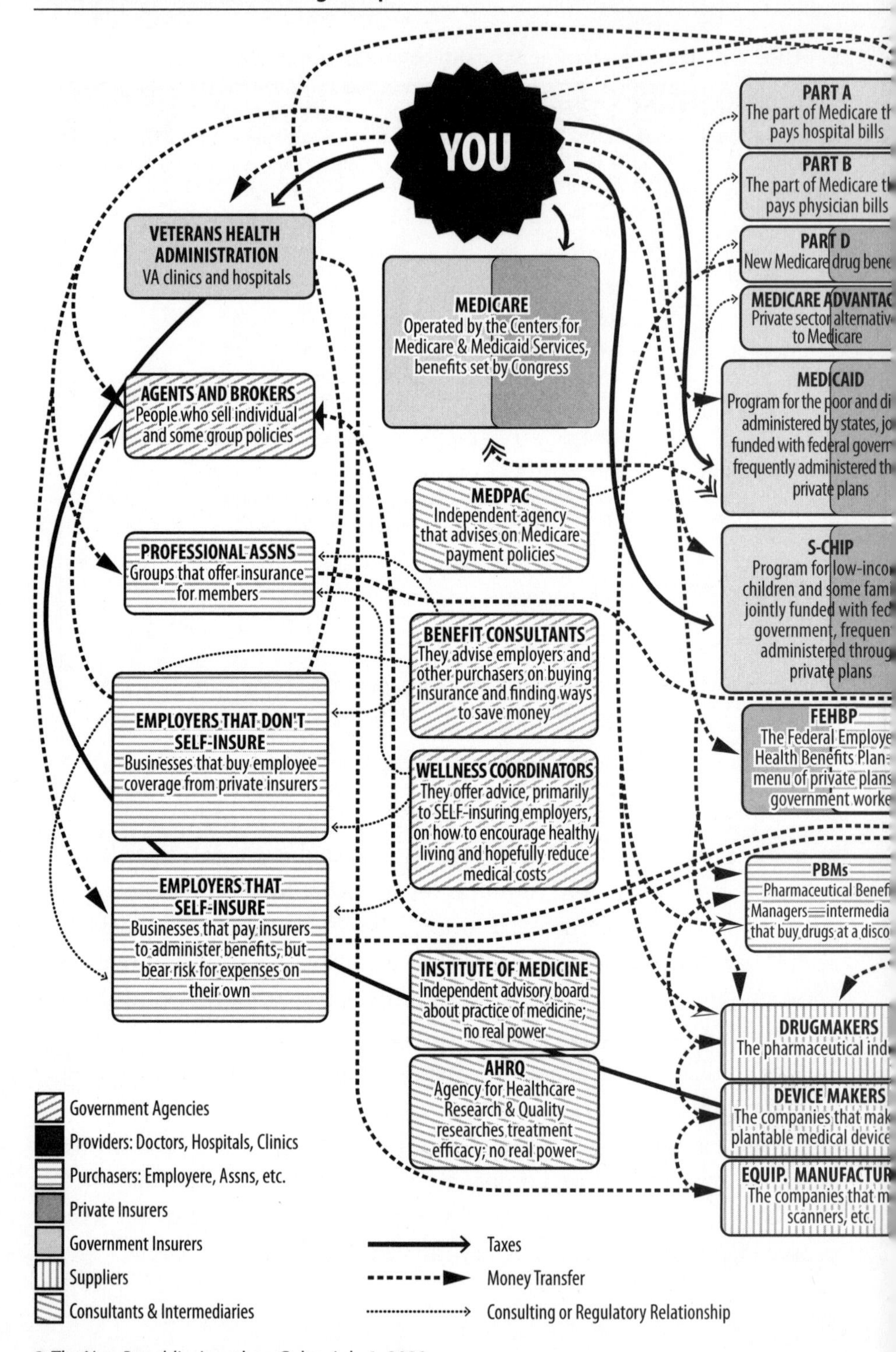

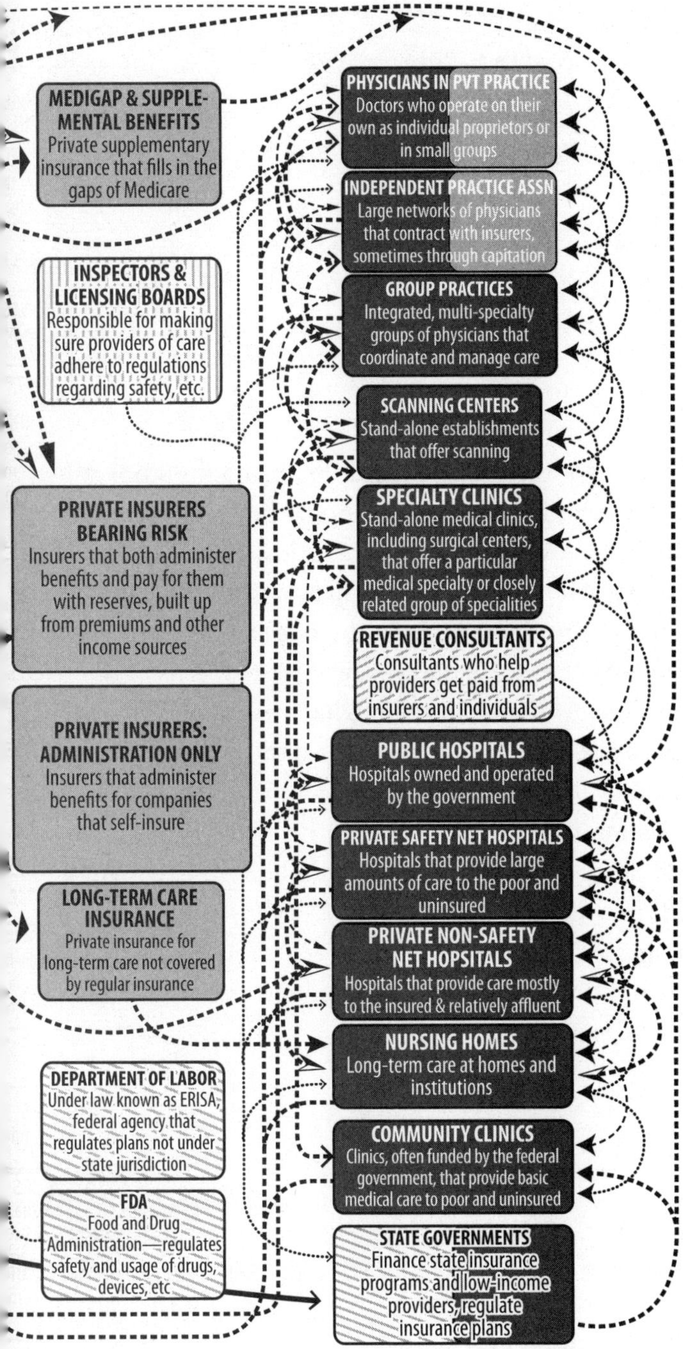

MEDIGAP & SUPPLEMENTAL BENEFITS
Private supplementary insurance that fills in the gaps of Medicare

INSPECTORS & LICENSING BOARDS
Responsible for making sure providers of care adhere to regulations regarding safety, etc.

PRIVATE INSURERS BEARING RISK
Insurers that both administer benefits and pay for them with reserves, built up from premiums and other income sources

PRIVATE INSURERS: ADMINISTRATION ONLY
Insurers that administer benefits for companies that self-insure

LONG-TERM CARE INSURANCE
Private insurance for long-term care not covered by regular insurance

DEPARTMENT OF LABOR
Under law known as ERISA, federal agency that regulates plans not under state jurisdiction

FDA
Food and Drug Administration—regulates safety and usage of drugs, devices, etc

PHYSICIANS IN PVT PRACTICE
Doctors who operate on their own as individual proprietors or in small groups

INDEPENDENT PRACTICE ASSN
Large networks of physicians that contract with insurers, sometimes through capitation

GROUP PRACTICES
Integrated, multi-specialty groups of physicians that coordinate and manage care

SCANNING CENTERS
Stand-alone establishments that offer scanning

SPECIALTY CLINICS
Stand-alone medical clinics, including surgical centers, that offer a particular medical specialty or closely related group of specialities

REVENUE CONSULTANTS
Consultants who help providers get paid from insurers and individuals

PUBLIC HOSPITALS
Hospitals owned and operated by the government

PRIVATE SAFETY NET HOSPITALS
Hospitals that provide large amounts of care to the poor and uninsured

PRIVATE NON-SAFETY NET HOPSITALS
Hospitals that provide care mostly to the insured & relatively affluent

NURSING HOMES
Long-term care at homes and institutions

COMMUNITY CLINICS
Clinics, often funded by the federal government, that provide basic medical care to poor and uninsured

STATE GOVERNMENTS
Finance state insurance programs and low-income providers, regulate insurance plans

= CHAPTER THREE =

How Americans Get Their Health Care

Why did Erin's surgery cost over $70,000? And the $1,200 for stool cultures? And who determined that her surgeon should be paid $4,174, but the cancer doctors at the University of Colorado just $500? And why would she have had to pay over $10,000 of her own money to see oncologists at M.D. Anderson but nothing to go to the ones at the University of Colorado? Why did 8 stitches for Baltazar's brother cost $1,800?

Insurers, employers, government, and individuals pay for health care services. They are the *payers.* Those who deliver health care services are the *providers.* Of the total *national health care expenditures (NHE)* of $2.87 trillion in 2012, $921 billion (about 32%) went to hospitals, $555 billion (20%) to physician and other clinical services, $280 billion (10%) to drugs, and the rest went "in the weeds" (see Figure 3.1). For instance, just 4% of health care spending goes to dental care and 3% to public health measures. So hospitals and physicians are the big components accounting for over half of all health care spending.

Hospitals

According to the American Hospital Association, in 2010 there were 4,985 acute-care hospitals in the United States, with just over 800,000 beds and 4.6 million employees. These hospitals admitted just over 35 million patients in 2010, a number that has been fairly stable for the last 5 years. They also had 127 million emergency room visits.

There is a wide distribution of hospital sizes (see Figure 3.2).

FIGURE 3.1 Components of national health care expenditures, 2010

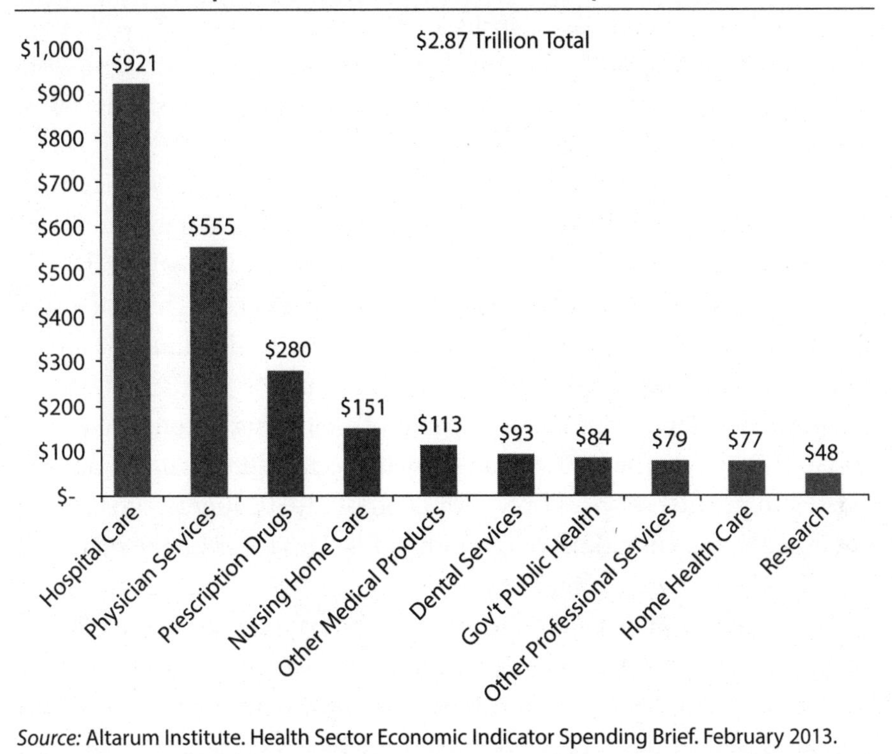

Source: Altarum Institute. Health Sector Economic Indicator Spending Brief. February 2013.

FIGURE 3.2 Hospital size and type, 2010

HOSPITAL SIZE	NUMBER (PERCENT OF TOTAL)	% NOT-FOR-PROFIT	% IN RURAL AREAS
Less than 100 beds	2,561 (51.4%)	48.4%	60.8%
100 to 199 beds	1,029 (20.6%)	61.5%	31.3%
200 to 499 beds	1,122 (22.5%)	73.3%	9.4%
More than 500 beds	273 (5.5%)	76.9%	0.7%
TOTAL	4,985	58.3%	39.9%

Source: AHA Hospital Statistics, 2012.

Of the acute-care hospitals, 18% were for-profit hospitals. The large for-profit hospital companies include HCA, founded in 1968, which operates 162 hospitals and 113 surgical centers, and Tenet, established in 1967, which operates 49 hospitals and 125 outpatient centers. Their hospitals are mainly located in the South.

Increasingly, physicians are opening specialty hospitals that they themselves own in order to provide particular services. For instance, cardiologists created the Arkansas Heart Hospital in Little Rock, and there is the Arizona Spine and Joint Hospital with just 23 beds. There are now about 240 physician-owned specialty hospitals devoted mainly to cardiac and orthopedics services that are high-profit types of practices. Because these are not general hospitals capable of delivering a comprehensive range of services, these physician-owned specialty hospitals tend to be created to provide services only for uncomplicated patients, those without other health conditions or comorbidities. This focus on the relatively healthy adds to their profitability.

How are hospitals paid? They used to be paid fee-for-service based on the cost they expended in providing a service. If a patient with a hip replacement stayed 7 days, hospitals were paid for 7 days; if the patient stayed 10 days, they were paid for 10 days. Beginning in 1983, however, Medicare shifted to paying hospitals for a particular diagnosis, so called *diagnosis-related groups (DRG)*. The DRG system was developed to identify discrete conditions or products that hospitals provided, such as hip replacements or care for acute heart attacks, and then provide a uniform price for providing the package of services. The prices were modified based on patient characteristics such as age and other health problems. Thus, the system is known as the *medical-severity adjusted diagnostic related groups system (MS-DRG)*. There are 335 DRGs and 746 distinct MS-DRGs.

DRGs are prospective payments; that is, "rather than simply reimbursing hospitals for whatever costs they charged to treat Medicare patients, the new model paid hospitals a predetermined, set rate based on the patient's diagnosis" or treatment. Under DRGs, patients with a medical problem—say, a stroke—that falls under a particular case grouping should have similar costs in hospitals with average efficiency. The objective is to encourage hospitals to be more efficient and to bear the financial risk for slow delivery of care or mistakes.

The consequence of introducing DRGs was revolutionary: the average length of stay (LOS) in hospitals declined. As a result, many other insurers adopted DRGs for hospital stays.

How does Medicare determine the actual MS-DRG payment? As with everything in health care, it is complicated, but Uwe Reinhardt, a professor of health economics at Princeton, has developed an excellent diagram to explain it (see Figure 3.3). There are 4 critical steps:

1) Medicare determines a "base case." This is an imagined, hypothetical single medical patient. The cost of the base case incorporates 2 factors: operating expenses, such as medical labor and supplies, and capital expenses, such as rent of hospital space and depreciation. Because labor constitutes nearly two-thirds of the cost of the base, Medicare adjusts the base case's labor costs for regional variations in wages. Adding up the geographically adjusted operating costs and the capital costs generates the base case.
2) Then Medicare adjusts the base case by the 746 different MS-DRG weightings that are supposed to reflect patients' clinical condition and treatment strategies. In other words, this weighting is supposed to capture the relative costliness of the particular patient's condition. For instance, does the patient with a heart attack have other medical problems, such as diabetes and emphysema, and does a stent need to be placed? If so, the patient would be more costly than an otherwise healthy patient admitted for an uncomplicated heart attack without stent placement. The base case times the MS-DRG weighting gives the adjusted payment rate.
3) Now the add-ons start (see Chapter 2, page 61). If the patient is treated in a teaching hospital, a factor for graduate medical education is added. The hospital might also receive disproportionate share (DSH) payments that are add-ons for taking care of the uninsured or a large number of Medicaid patients.
4) If the patient stays unusually long because of a complication or some other reason, the hospital might receive an additional "outlier" payment.

There are at least 5 important characteristics of Medicare's approach. First, as has been noted, it is prospective; it pays based on a predeter-

FIGURE 3.3 Algorithm for calculating Medicare's acute-care inpatient payment

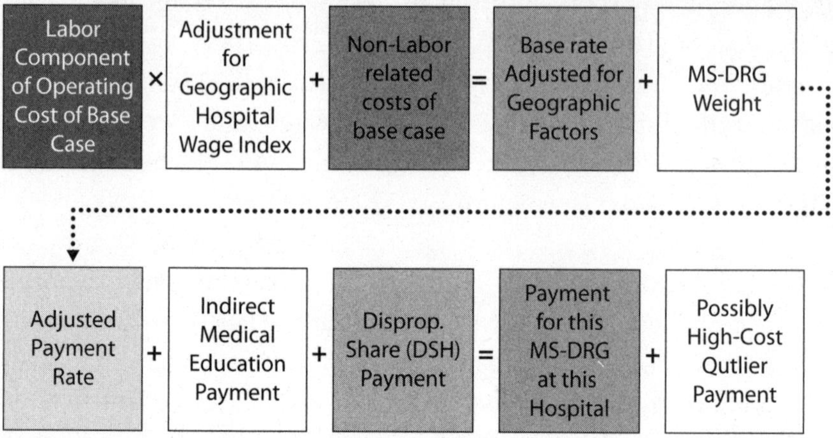

Labor Component of Operating Cost of Base Case × Adjustment for Geographic Hospital Wage Index + Non-Labor related costs of base case = Base rate Adjusted for Geographic Factors + MS-DRG Weight

Adjusted Payment Rate + Indirect Medical Education Payment + Disprop. Share (DSH) Payment = Payment for this MS-DRG at this Hospital + Possibly High-Cost Qutlier Payment

Source: Uwe Reinhardt, "How Medicare Sets Hospital Prices: A Primer," *New York Times*, November 26, 2010, http://economix.blogs.nytimes.com/2010/11/26/how-medicare-sets-hospital-prices-a-primer/. See also "Hospital Acute Inpatient Services Payment System," Medpac, October 2010, www.medpac.gov/documents/MedPAC_Payment_Basics_10_hospital.pdf.

mined price that Medicare sets rather than a price the hospital charges. This promotes efficiency but also may promote stinting on care. Second, it is based on average costs, not the costs actually incurred in a particular hospital. Third, it is cost based not value based; there is no modification based on the quality of the service delivered. Fourth, it has add-ons that allow Medicare to encourage certain behaviors deemed desirable, such as training residents and caring for the poor. Finally, it is very complicated, which, unfortunately, allows for the gaming of the system. Nevertheless, it has some key virtues, especially compared to the previous payment system, and these are recognized, in part, because many other countries have adopted the DRG system of payment.

How does this payment system influence how others, such as Erin's insurance company or Wayne, pay for their hospital care? There really are 6 different payment rates for hospitals (see Figure 3.4). The first is what hospitals list as their price, often called charges. This list price is the *charge master rate*, which is akin to the list price. The charge master rate is a comprehensive listing of billable items such as medical procedures, laboratory tests, X-rays, drugs, supplies, and the like. This is the derivation of the $10 aspirin or the $7,000 MRI scan the hospital in Aspen

FIGURE 3.4 Six Different Payment Rates for Hospitals

PAYMENT RATE	DESCRIPTION
Charge Master Rate	The list price determined by the hospital for billable items such as lab tests, medical procedures, drugs, and supplies—everything from an x-ray to an aspirin to a pad of gauze. Very few patients or insurance companies actually pay the charge master rate.
Medicare Rate	The rate at which Medicare reimburses hospitals and physicians for various services. Medicare sets this rate on its own—it is not a negotiated rate. The rate is typically much lower than the charge master rate and it can vary from provider to provider.
Commercial Insurer and Blues Rate	The price that is ultimately paid by a private insurer to hospitals and physicians for the delivery of medical services. Each insurer negotiates rates for various services with each hospital and physician. Rates for private insurers are higher than the Medicare rate and they vary widely among insurers.
Usual, Customary, and Reasonable Rate	Rate used by insurers to determine what they will pay providers who are out-of-network. It is supposed to reflect "reasonable" costs for providing services within a particular geographic area, but this is highly subjective and how it is determined is largely unclear. It is usually less than the charge master rate.
Medicaid Rate	The rate at which Medicaid reimburses hospitals and physicians for various services. Often quoted as a percent of the Medicare rate. This is typically the lowest rate of reimbursement for providers.
Actual Cost	The actual cost of rendering a service for a hospital or physician. This includes the actual cost of supplies, technology, time, and labor. This is very difficult to calculate definitively. As a result, nobody really knows the actual cost of delivering most health care services.

Source: Andrew Ziskind, Kristin Ficery, and Richard Fu, "Adapting to a New Model of Physician Employment," *Accenture, Outlook Point of View*, No. 2, August 2011.

charged Erin. Every hospital system maintains its own charge master rates. As has been shown by Steve Brill in his 2013 article "Bitter Pill: Why Medical Prices Are Killing Us" and the release of the list of service prices for which hospitals billed Medicare (but not what Medicare paid), these charges vary widely from hospital to hospital. Typically, only a few people pay list prices, such as Arab sheiks flying in for a service, who are asked to pay cash. Tragically, however, they are often collected from the uninsured, who have no leverage to negotiate lower prices. Wayne paid the charge master rate for his emergency room visit, and Baltazar's brother paid it for his appendectomy.

The second is the *Medicare rate*. This is not negotiated but rather is the rate that Medicare says it will pay for an office visit or the surgeon's time for a hip replacement or a hospital stay for the hip replacement based on diagnosis-related groups (DRGs). The Medicare rate is much lower than the charge master rate or list price.

The third is the price paid by commercial insurers and Blues plans. This commercial rate is usually higher than the Medicare rate but lower than the charge master rate. Each insurer actually negotiates its particular rate with each hospital; therefore, different insurers will obtain different rates and discounts. In this sense, there is no single commercial rate but instead multiple commercial rates. These commercial rates are usually denominated as a percentage of the Medicare rate. For instance, the Mayo Clinic's Medicare rate for a hip replacement is $16,109, but its rate for commercial payer A may, for example, be 180% of the Medicare rate, while Mayo's rate for commercial payer B might be 140% of the Medicare rate and, for commercial payer C, 220%. Because individual negotiations determine these commercial rates, the rate with any one insurer will depend on a hospital's bargaining power, how many patients the insurer covers, whether the hospital wants those patients, and whether the insurer perceives it *needs* to have the hospital in their network of hospitals. Also because these rates are determined one on one between insurers and each hospital, there are significant administrative costs to these negotiations. Erin's insurance company paid its commercial rate to the Aspen Hospital and received the 8% discount off the charges.

The fourth rate is the *usual, customary, and reasonable price (UCR)*. This rate was written into the original Medicare legislation to determine what the government would pay. Historically, it has heavily overpaid for doing and underpaid for diagnosing—that is, paying more for procedures, such as surgery, and skimping on office visits. Today, insurers use it primarily to determine what they will pay physicians and hospitals with whom they do not have a signed contract. For instance, if one of their insured patients needs emergency services at a hospital in another state, the insurance company will pay the UCR. The UCR rate is almost always less than a hospital's charge master rate, but how insurers determine the UCR price is largely shrouded in secrecy. It is supposed to reflect the reasonable costs in a geographic area of providing a service, such as an electrocardiogram (ECG). But what constitutes "reasonable" is highly debatable, as charges vary widely even within local areas.

The fifth is the *Medicaid rate*. This is typically the lowest rate paid. It might be quoted as 17 cents on the $1 billed, where the billed rate is the list price.

Finally, there is the *actual cost* of providing a service. It is fair to say no one really knows this rate. Hospital administrators cannot even tell you what a day in the hospital actually costs, as so many different people interact with a patient and for such varied amounts of time, and hospitals have rarely conducted time-motion studies to determine the actual interactions and their actual costs. This creates a problem: when hospitals say Medicare rates are lower than the cost of delivering services, this is hard to validate because we can't know the actual cost of care.

These various rates explain the current merger mania among hospitals. Within the last few years larger hospitals have been buying up neighboring hospitals to form large hospital systems. A primary rationale is to increase the hospitals' bargaining power with the commercial insurers in order to be able to raise their rates. If many of the hospitals in a geographic region are part of a single hospital system, then the insurer must include them in a network and the hospital system can demand higher rates. This consolidation of hospitals also allows one hospital with high rates to get those same rates applied to the other hospitals in its system; however, this raises hospital prices with no change in actual practices or quality.

Importantly, the Medicare payment is transparent—everyone can look up the rates. Conversely, the payments from commercial insurers are not transparent. The prices are not known to other insurers, other hospitals, or average Americans. Insurers view their negotiated rates as proprietary information.

These different rates also highlight a common practice at hospitals and other health care providers: *cross-subsidization*, in which high payments in one area subsidize low payments in another area. There are 2 types of cross-subsidization, one based on the type of insurance patients have and another based on the types of services provided. Typically the rates hospitals receive from commercial insurers and Blues plans are where they make profit that, in turn, subsidizes the lower payments they receive from Medicaid and, to some degree, Medicare. Therefore, to boost their profits, hospitals are always trying to get more privately insured individuals and reduce the number of Medicaid patients they admit. This so-called *payer mix*—what percentage of patients are Medicaid versus Medicare versus privately insured—is critical to determining a hospital's profitability, even its financial viability. It also helps explain why new hospitals or a hospital's satellite facilities are often located in relatively prosperous areas where most people are likely to have high-paying private insurance.

In addition, fees for some services typically exceed costs, whereas fees for other medical services do not cover costs. For that reason hospitals and other providers manage their *case mix* as much as their payer mix. Hospitals tend to make a profit on organ transplants and neurosurgery, and those profits subsidize other services for which payments may not cover costs, such as talking to diabetic patients about improving their diet. Typically, hospitals will make money only on a limited range of services, such as transplants, cardiac surgery, cancer treatments, and CT, MRI, and other imaging, and lose money on other services, such as care for patients with arthritis and psychiatric conditions. The profit on the MRIs will subsidize the psychiatric department or the care for the uninsured.

Finally, nothing necessitated the development of 6 different payment rates. There could be one single rate that all payers, whether government or private insurers, pay all hospitals. This is an *all-payer rate* system. The state of Maryland has such a system. In 1971 Maryland enacted a law establishing the Health Services Cost Review Commission, which had the power to set hospital rates. By 1977 this commission was setting rates for all private payers as well as Medicare and Medicaid. Over time this has moderated hospital cost increases. In 1974 Maryland's hospital rates were significantly above the national average, but between 1975 and 2005 Maryland became the state with the lowest rate of increase of cost per admission. Furthermore, this has eliminated the patient cross-subsidization. Because private payers, Medicare, and Medicaid all pay the same price, there is no need for one group of patients to subsidize the other group. Maryland no longer has any public government-operated acute-care hospitals, and the indigent and uninsured have access to all hospitals. And hospitals have no reason to adjust their payer mix—that is, to prefer patients with private insurance to those with Medicaid.

Physicians

Physician services account for about 20% of total national health expenditures. According to the American Medical Association's *Physician Characteristics and Distribution in the US*, in 2010 there were 985,375 physicians in the United States, or 3.19 physicians for every 1,000 Americans (see Figure 3.5). Currently about 70% of physicians are male and 25% were trained outside of the United States as international medical graduates. But these ratios are changing with women occupying half of medical school classes.

FIGURE 3.5 Types of physicians, 2010

TYPE OF PHYSICIANS	NUMBER	PERCENT OF TOTAL (985,375)
Office-based practice	565,024	57.3%
Hospital-based practice	187,548	19.0%
Researchers	13,755	1.4%
Training (interns and residents)	109,065	11.1%

The mix and distribution of physicians in the United States is far from ideal. There are too many specialists compared to primary care physicians, while the large majority of patients' contacts with physicians are for services that do not require specialty training. Of the 643,000 physicians who provide direct patient care, excluding interns and residents, just 48% could generously be classified as primary care physicians, working in general medicine, family medicine, internal medicine, pediatrics, and obstetrics and gynecology. Further, this percentage has been falling. Between 1975 and 2010 the number of physicians more than doubled, but the number of primary care physicians increased only 10%. This distribution of specialists and primary care physicians is very different from other countries; for instance, more than 62% of Australian physicians do primary care. One piece of potential good news is that more women go into primary care; therefore, as the percentage of women in medicine increases, there may be more primary care physicians.

The main reason physicians specialize is not hard to fathom: specialists are paid more—often vastly more—than primary care physicians. The historical bias remains strong toward paying physicians who do hospital-based interventions. According to a survey conducted by Profiles Database in 2011, the average pay for a family medicine physician was $199,850 and a pediatrician $202,500, whereas for cardiac surgeons it was $522,875, and orthopedic surgeons who specialize in spine surgery make $625,000 per year.

Physicians deserve to be paid well. They tend to work long hours, typically over 50 hours per week. They have had at least 7 years of post-college training. But the differential between primary care physicians and specialists makes a significant difference in career choice even if money is not a physician's primary motivator. The difference between a pediatrician and a spinal orthopedist is $400,000 per year. Over a 35 year career, that amounts to a $14 million pay difference. It is no wonder more physicians become specialists.

There is also a geographic maldistribution of physicians, with few working in rural areas. For instance, in the northeast there are 4.63 physicians per 1,000 Americans, whereas in the mountain states it is 2.60 physicians, and in Texas, Oklahoma, Arkansas, and Louisiana it is just 2.45 physicians per 1,000 Americans. Although some of this is related to the fact that there are more interns and residents in the northeast, the fact is physicians, like other well-educated and higher-income individuals, prefer to live in urban areas that provide social, cultural, and other amenities. Despite numerous efforts and incentive programs, getting physicians to locate in smaller, more rural communities has been very difficult, and this is particularly true of specialists. The whole state of Alaska has just 18 neurologists and 28 cardiologists (2.5 per 100,000 people and 3.8 per 100,000 people, respectively), Idaho has 34 neurologists and 49 cardiologists (2.3 per 100,000 people and 3.3 per 100,000, respectively), and Wyoming has just 13 neurologists and 13 cardiologists (2.3 per 100,000 people). Conversely, Massachusetts has 477 neurologists and 743 cardiologists for 6.5 million people, or 7.2 per 100,000 people and 11.4 per 100,000 people, respectively.

Historically, physicians have been fiercely independent or, as some might say, poor at working with others. The consequence has been the dominance of small physician practices. In 2008 just under half of all physicians worked in groups of 5 or fewer physicians, while only 19% worked in groups of 6 to 50 physicians. In addition, physicians have largely been self-employed private practitioners, refusing to work for a boss, whether that is a hospital, company, or other entity. Small physician groups are not inherently bad, but it does create problems of coordination. Having a slew of small independent groups increases the fragmentation of care, especially for patients with chronic conditions who typically receive care from 5 to 7 different physicians. Furthermore, small physician groups do not have the size and capital to install electronic records and include services such as care coordinators or wound care specialists that would help prevent problems necessitating additional medical care.

The number of small practices is declining, however, as hospitals buy up physician practices. Hospitals foresee a drop in the number of patients, so they want to secure physicians who will admit those patients. In addition, the hospitals are looking to compensate for declining revenues from fewer patients in hospital beds by increasing revenues from outpatient services. Physicians are willing to be bought because they recently have experienced lower payments both from Medicare and commercial insurers. Hospitals can also assume many of the administrative chores of running a private practice, such as rent and maintenance on a facility, HR policies, billings, and malpractice payments. More importantly, hospitals have greater bargaining power and can increase the payments commercial insurers make to their physicians. The consequence is that, in 2014, more physicians will be employed by hospitals than will be self-employed (see Figure 3.6).

How are fee-for-service physicians, like the ones Erin saw, paid? Again, physician payment is exceedingly complex but can be distilled into 3 steps. The first step is *medical coding*. This takes medical services that physicians, nurses, or other health care providers render and converts them into codes.

FIGURE 3.6 Physician employment, 2000–2013 (thousands)

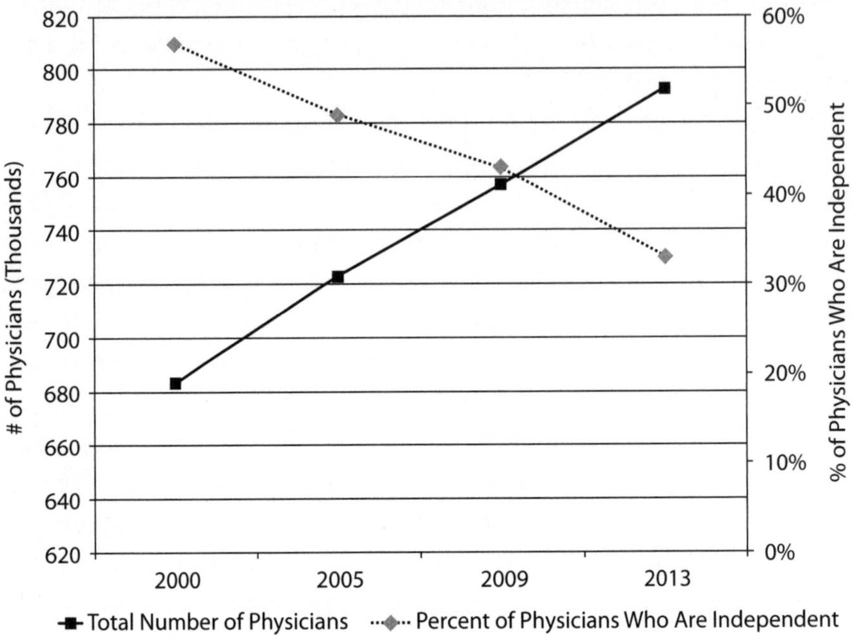

Mechanistically, the physician distills the services provided to the patient during the office visit. These services can be divided into several types:

- Physician taking a patient's history of illness, conducting a physical examination, and decision making
- Physician procedures, such as skin biopsy
- Nonphysician procedures, such as immunizations
- Other tests, such as rapid strep tests
- Office work, such as reception

These services are then converted into *current procedural terminology (CPT)* codes. The AMA created and copyrighted CPT codes to create a uniform system for cataloging medical, surgical, and diagnostic services. It provides a single code for each physician visit and the other procedures. There are 6 sections of codes: (1) evaluation and management (E&M) codes, covering office visits, emergency room visits, or preventive services, including a physicians' history, physical, and decision making; (2) anesthesia codes; (3) surgical codes; (4) radiology codes, including ultrasound, nuclear medicine, or radiation oncology; (5) pathology and laboratory codes, including urinalysis, chemistry, and microbiology; and (6) medicine codes, such as dialysis and pulmonary care.

The CPT codes must then be aggregated and linked to a specific diagnosis, such as strep throat, skin lesion, or chest pain, in order to document that the services provided, as specified in the CPT code, are appropriate for the medical diagnosis. This is to prevent fraud—that is, billing for a service unrelated to the diagnosis. The diagnoses are specified by the *International Classification of Diseases* ICD-9 (or, more recently, the ICD-10) produced by the World Health Organization to classify diseases systematically.

The second step is *medical billing*. The codes and diagnoses are converted into a bill by figuring out the financial cost of each CPT code. A physician thus submits the CPT codes with their ICD-9 diagnosis and the charges to the insurer, Medicare, or some other payer.

The third step is for the payer to take the codes and bill and determine what will be paid. Decades ago payers would just pay whatever the physician charged. In the 1980s, however, when Medicare was introducing DRGs for hospitals, they also changed how physicians were paid. A team of Harvard researchers developed the *relative value unit (RVU)* system that was supposed to be a common metric to compare the human and other resources needed to provide physician services. Basically, the RVU system gives each CPT code a "value" that is supposed to reflect the amount of resources needed to deliver that service. There are 4 steps when using the RVU system.

1) The RVU for a particular service is based on 3 components (see Figure 3.7):
    - *Physician work: RVU* reflects the relative amount of time, skill, training, and intensity required of a physician to provide a specific service.
    - *Practice expense: RVU* reflects the nonphysician labor, the building, equipment, and other practice's expenses.
    - *Malpractice: RVU* reflects the cost of malpractice premiums for a specialty.

2) These different RVUs are adjusted to reflect the cost of living variations in different geographies.
3) The 3 adjusted RVUs are then added up to determine the RVU for a particular service.
4) The RVU is then turned into dollars paid when it is multiplied by a conversion factor. Medicare and each private insurer set their own conversion factors.

There are many subtleties to calculating RVUs. Practice expenses vary by whether the service is provided in a facility—that is, hospital or ambulatory surgical center—or a nonfacility, such as a physician's office. The same exact service—a skin biopsy, for instance—will be paid more if performed in a hospital. Thus, service providers have an incentive to make sure activities occur in hospital-owned facilities.

Assessing the physician work in each of the CPT codes is obviously complex and controversial. Historically, office visits to discuss Erin's cancer and whether she should get chemotherapy or other cognitive activities have been given low RVUs, whereas surgical procedures, such as Erin's colon cancer operation, have been given higher RVUs (see Figure 3.7). Health policy experts as well as primary care physicians strongly object to the bias favoring procedures and specialist care. It minimizes the skill and intensity of, for example, discussions of end-of-life care and preventive measures such as dieting.

FIGURE 3.7 RVUs for medical procedures

SERVICE	PHYSICIAN WORK	PRACTICE EXPENSE	MALPRACTICE	TOTAL
Office visit	1.50	1.54	0.1	3.05
Colonoscopy	3.69	2.20	0.59	6.48
Cardiac bypass surgery, one vessel	34.98	14.90	8.41	58.29

Medicare defines the RVU per service. This means it is responsible for determining the RVU value of physician work, practice expenses, and malpractice for each particular service—that is, each component of the 58.29 for cardiac bypass surgery. Commercial insurers and the Blues do not alter that number—they just take Medicare's number. Physicians get paid a different amount from Medicare and commercial insurers and the Blues because each of them uses a different conversion factor that translates the RVU number into dollars paid to the physician. In 2001 the conversion factor Medicare used was $38.251 per RVU, and in 2012 it was actually lower, at $34.0376. In 2012 that meant a physician made $1,984 ($34.0376 × 58.28) for the cardiac bypass surgery. Commercial insurers and the Blues have a higher conversion factor, closer to $55 per RVU for evaluation and management of patients and over $70 per RVU for surgical and other procedures. They would pay about $4,080 for the same cardiac bypass ($70 × 58.29). And you can see the bias toward higher payment for surgery and other procedures is built right into the payment conversion factor.

The RVUs are supposed to be updated every five years because the complexity of the physician work might have increased or decreased or the practice expenses associated with a particular service might have declined. The American Medical Association's Relative Value Scale Update Committee (RUC) has given recommendations on how to change the RVUs for each service. Historically, CMS has adopted over 80% of the RUC's recommendations. This practice has been criticized, however, because the RUC is heavily biased in favor of surgeons and specialists who want to preserve their higher RVUs at the expense of primary care physicians. Furthermore, there appears to be a conflict of interest: CMS, a government agency, should not take such a high proportion of recommendations on how much to pay for certain services from the very constituency who will be paid.

In this complex payment system there are ways to game the system. *Upcoding* is putting in a CPT code for more extensive and costly services than the services that were actually delivered. For instance, you see your physician for a quick checkup, but she might bill for an expanded checkup that is paid at a higher rate. That is upcoding, and it is fraud. The extent to which upcoding occurs is controversial. However, studies have shown that over the last decade physicians have steadily submitted a higher number of the more complex codes even when there is no evidence that American patients are getting much sicker. The generous interpretation of this trend is that even with very specific rules there are still judgment calls about how to classify various actions, and these are often based on how complicated it is to manage the patient.

Importantly, Medicare's *Sustainable Growth Rate formula (SGR)* has shaped physician pay. SGR was part of the Balanced Budget Act of 1997 to control the yearly increase in spending on physician services. Basically the act set an SGR target for how much physician services should increase. The rate of increase depends on the growth of 3 factors: physicians' costs, Medicare enrollment, and the GDP. If spending for all physicians in Medicare in a year exceeds the SGR target, then the amount paid to physicians in the next year is to be reduced in order to hit the SGR target.

Unfortunately, the SGR applies to the cost of physician services for the whole country; it provides no incentive to individual physicians to control their costs. For the first few years after the SGR was implemented the cost of physician services kept within the target. But since 2002 the cost has consistently exceeded the SGR target for a variety of reasons, in particular an increase in the number of services provided and in the complexity of the procedures and services. Exceeding the SGR target should have necessitated a cut in per service payments to physicians, but beginning in 2003 Congress has enacted a series of temporary "SGR fixes" that prevent the legally required cuts to physician pay from being implemented but has not changed the SGR target or formula for calculating it. Consequently, using the SGR formula now requires cuts in physician payments of about 24%. To change the formula and permanently eliminate the threatened cuts to physician payment would increase Medicare spending by about $117 billion over a decade, depending on the details. There are active Congressional discussions to finally replace the SGR.

Nurses

Altogether, there are about 3.6 million nurses working in the United States. Nurses can be divided into 3 groups:

- Registered nurses (RNs)—2.8 million
- Licensed practical nurses (LPNs)—690,000
- Advanced practice nurses, requiring a master's or doctorate, which include nurse practitioners (NPs), anesthetists, and nurse midwives—180,000.

Although there are great worries about nursing shortages, the number of nurses grew during the 2000s. The number of RNs grew by 500,000 and LPNs by 90,000, outpacing growth in the US population. Indeed, in 2011 alone more than 142,000 RNs passed the licensure exam. Similarly, between 2001 and 2011 there was a 69% increase in the number of nurse practitioners.

There are a substantial number of nurses from foreign countries. The largest pool is from the Philippines, and then from South Korea, India, and Nigeria. Consequently, 25% of RNs are nonwhite, but nursing remains largely a female profession—only 9% are men.

Nearly two-thirds of RNs and one-third of LPNs work in hospitals, and another one-third of LPNs work in nursing homes. Few nurses work in physician offices. About 16% of RNs and 25% of LPNs work in rural areas with some rural states, such as South Dakota, Nebraska, and Maine, being at the top of the list of nurses per person in the state. The salary level of nurses ranges from the average of $39,361 for LPNs to $63,944 for RNs.

One of the most important issues facing the nursing profession is the *scope of practice laws* that determines what services health professionals, such as nurses, can provide, in what setting, and under what supervision. State governments set these laws, and not surprisingly, they vary widely. For instance, about 16 states allow NPs to practice as independent primary care providers, including allowing them to evaluate patients, order diagnostic tests, make diagnoses, write prescriptions, and refer patients to specialists without physician supervision. Another 22 states reduce what NPs can do and require physician collaboration. The other 12 states require physician supervision for the NP to provide patient care. Greater easing of restrictions on NPs is likely to occur in order to meet the need for primary care services as well as care in rural settings.

Home Health Care

Over the last 25 or so years a large and growing part of health care has been migrating out of the hospital. Home health care agencies have expanded to provide medical services in homes. The services now include intravenous medications, respirator treatments, nutritional supplements, and physical therapy. In 2012 there were approximately 12,000 home health care agencies, with over 75% operating as for-profit agencies.

There is great focus on home health care agencies. On the one hand, they have been very profitable and the federal government has sought ways to limit these expenditures. On the other hand, they are essential to migrating care out of the more expensive hospital setting. Recently the Institute of Medicine showed that 73% of variation in costs among and even within regions arises from differences in the care after a hospital stay, the so-called post-acute care. Care in institutions, such as rehabilitation facilities, increases costs, whereas utilization of home health care agencies can reduce these post-acute-care costs. Thus, there is tension in wanting to expand use of home care while not incurring high costs per service from the agencies.

Federally Qualified Health Clinics (FQHCs)

Beginning in the 1960s community health centers began to provide care to indigent and underserved people. In 1975 the federal government began providing grants to these clinics, and in 1996 they were brought under the supervision of the US Department of Health and Human Services (HHS).

Federally qualified health clinics (FQHCs) provide comprehensive primary care as well as preventive services, such as dental and mental health services, to underserved urban and rural communities, including migrant workers and non-US citizens. They are supposed to charge fees on a sliding income scale and provide services regardless of the person's ability to pay. They receive grant support from the federal government as well as reimbursement for Medicaid patients and free malpractice coverage from the federal government. They also receive special pricing on pharmaceuticals.

In 2011 there were 1,124 FQHCs in the United States, delivering care at over 7,800 different sites caring for over 20 million people. In 2009 FQHCs had $11.5 billion in revenue, an average of $10 million per FHQC. The average federal grant was $1.7 million per FQHC.

Other Providers

There are a variety of other providers of health care services (see Figure 3.8), most of whom are for-profit.

FIGURE 3.8 Other health care providers

TYPE OF PROVIDER	NUMBER
End-stage renal facilities for dialysis	5,800
Ambulatory surgical centers	5,300
Outpatient physical therapy facilities	2,350
Hospices	3,600

Manufacturers

There are many different types of manufacturers of supplies needed in health care. These range from drug companies to manufacturers of medical equipment such as wheelchairs and hospital beds, to manufacturers of gauze pads and other surgical supplies. Probably the most important are drug and device manufacturers, as they create new technologies that simultaneously improve care and drive up drive up health care costs.

Drug Manufacturers

Drugs account for at least 10% of total health care spending. Drug companies develop, produce, and market drugs. Drug development occurs through preclinical testing of molecules or biological compounds on cells and animals to establish dosing, formulation, and an initial safety profile. For drugs that seem to have a therapeutic benefit without serious side effects, companies submit to the FDA an *Investigational New Drug (IND)* filing to proceed to human or clinical testing. Clinical trials typically involve 3 phases of progressively larger trials used to establish initially the safety and then the effectiveness of a new compound. If the drug passes the 3 phases of research and the FDA grants marketing approval, a drug company then has the exclusive right to make, market, and sell the drug. It is then a branded drug.

This process of drug development is both long and financially risky. It takes about 7 to 10 years to get FDA approval. Few drugs make it through the process. The FDA actually approves roughly 1 out of 10,000 discovered compounds and roughly 3 to 5 drugs of every 100 that enter human clinical trials. Only 3 of out of every 20 approved drugs ever manages to recover their development costs.

The drug industry claims it costs more than $1 billion to develop every drug. This figure includes the cost of laboratory research, clinical trials, and regulatory filings, but it also includes costs associated with the development process of drugs that fail either in the laboratory or in clinical trials. More controversially it also includes interest on the money invested in drug development. Others claim the proper cost of drug development may be less than $100 million per marketed drug. These critics also note that much of the basic science research drug companies use to develop their drugs is generated through publicly funded, mainly National Institutes of Health (NIH), basic science research and some clinical trials. They also argue there is a lag between investment and research in new products and financial returns for all companies—telecommunications, computer, and manufacturing companies—and that the "cost of money" should not be counted as part of the cost of drug development.

Although there may be high financial risk in developing new drugs, the profit margins are substantial. The largest pharmaceutical company is Pfizer, and its revenue in 2011 was $67.9 billion and its profits were 14.7%. The most profitable large drug company, Gilead, had profit margins in excess of 33%. Historically, the high prices for brand-name drugs in the United States meant that in excess of 60% of drug company worldwide profits came from sales in the United States. This percentage, however, has been declining over time. Nonetheless, approximately 45% of drug company profits are from US sales.

The future for pharmaceutical companies is clouded. Use of drugs in the United States is predicted to increase with the aging of the population, the increase in chronic illnesses, and the insurance expansion from the ACA. Conversely, revenue growth is expected to slow down to under 4% per year. More importantly, many well-selling brand-name drugs, such as the cholesterol-lowering statin Lipitor, the antipsychotic drugs Zyprexa and Serquel, the antiplatelet drug Plavix, and Enbrel for arthritis, have come off patent, reducing drug companies' profits.

Once a drug loses its patent protection and exclusivity, other drug makers can manufacture the drug, making it "generic." The FDA requires that generic drugs have the same active ingredient as their brand-name counterparts. They also must meet FDA standards for quality, purity, and potency. But they do not have to go through the clinical trials to prove the drug works.

Typically, when a drug becomes generic the price drops by 80 to 95%. Importantly, as one drug in a class becomes generic, patients should be able to change specific drugs to generic versions in the same class. For example, there are 7 statins, cholesterol lowering drugs. Many, such as simvastatin, are now generic and sell for just a few dollars for a month's supply. Patients taking the brand-name statins, such as Crestor, can switch to simvastatin and save money. Only a few patients might need the special characteristics the brand-name drugs offer.

Over the past decade use of generics among American patients has dramatically increased. There are about 4 billion prescriptions a year. The percentage of all prescriptions that were generic increased from 47% in 2002 to nearly 80% in 2012. A big factor in this shift is probably the introduction in 2006 of Medicare Part D (Chapter 2, page 59). Seniors began getting their medications from pharmaceutical benefit managers who shifted seniors from brand-name drugs to equivalent generics.

There has been significant consolidation among generic drug manufacturers, leaving only several large ones. The largest is Mylan, with $6.1 billion in sales and profit margins of 8.7%, and Teva, an Israeli company, with worldwide sales in excess of $20 billion.

Finally, over the past few years there has been a rise in so-called specialty pharmaceuticals. These are high-cost prescription medications, often biologic agents, and they have 3 defining characteristics: (1) they may need special handling, like refrigeration; (2) they treat chronic conditions like cancer, rheumatoid arthritis, pulmonary hypertension, and multiple sclerosis; and (3) they are expensive, with average prices in the range of $35,000 to $75,000 per patient per year. Typically one manufacturer with no competition makes these drugs, allowing for monopoly pricing. Examples include Avonex for multiple sclerosis, Avastin and Provenge for cancer, and Enbrel for rheumatoid arthritis.

In 2011 these specialty pharmaceuticals accounted for 24% of all drug costs. There are over 900 specialty drugs in development, and Wall Street analysts anticipate that by 2018 half of the best-selling drugs will be these high-cost specialty drugs. This sector is attracting the attention of private equity firms, pharmacies wanting to distribute these drugs, and others who will fuel growth in this market to compensate for declines in the profits from brand-name drugs.

Traditionally, drug companies marketed to physicians through detailing—that is, sending sales representative to hospitals and physicians' offices. This has been heavily criticized, and various institutions have begun restricting the practice. Beginning in 1981 Merck ran the first *direct-to-consumer (DTC)* advertisement. In 1997 the FDA finally issued regulations permitting drug companies to market their drugs directly to the public through broadcast and other advertisements. The United States and New Zealand are the only 2 developed countries that allow DTC marketing. Although DTC has expanded, current projections estimate that drug companies will reduce their use of DTC marketing.

Device Manufacturers

There are myriad medical devices, ranging from cardiac stents and pacemakers to artificial hips and knees, from insulin pumps to tear duct plugs, from surgical robots and radiation machines to sutures. Although the usual measures of health care expenditures do not delineate the costs associated with devices, an international comparative study showed that the United States was second in the greatest percentage of total health care costs going to medical devices. Switzerland was first. In 2011 4.3% of US total health care expenditures, approximately $116 billion, went to medical devices.

In 2012 Advanced Medical Technology Association (Advamed), the trade organization for the device industry, claimed that there were 7,000 device manufacturers in the United States. According to Advamed, the majority were small, with fewer than 100 employees each. However, the biggest device companies in the area are large corporations that do more than manufacture medical devices, such as Johnson & Johnson, General Electric, and Siemens. Medtronics describes itself as the world's leading manufacturer, with sole focus on devices and revenues of $16.2 billion. Like drug companies, device companies are also highly profitable; Medtronics's profits are very high, above 60%.

Health Care Regulators and Health Care Providers

There are scores if not hundreds of different regulators involved in the health care system. Some regulate providers, setting standards and assessing hospitals, physicians, nurses, pharmacists, and other providers. Others regulate insurers. Others regulate drug and device manufacturers. These regulators can also be divided into public and private regulators. We will explore the roles of just a few of them.

Public Regulators

At the federal level the Food and Drug Administration (FDA) has significant oversight authority for drugs, devices, and the food supply. The FDA's 2012 budget was $3.83 billion, less than the revenue of many best-selling drugs, and it employs over 13,000 people.

For drugs the FDA is responsible for determining whether a drug is safe and effective as assessed by clinical trials. The FDA does not have authority for determining whether a new drug is better than an existing agent, whether it is an important addition to medical care, or whether its proposed cost is worth its benefits.

In 2012 the FDA approved 95 drugs, but few are new compounds; many are new manufacturers of already approved drugs. It also approved 6 biological compounds, such as antibodies.

The FDA also monitors drugs when they are marketed for any unexpected adverse effects that might arise. Historically, this has been described as a passive monitoring process, collecting information voluntarily reported by physicians and other providers rather than proactively and systematically collecting information as drugs are being prescribed.

The FDA also regulates devices. FDA classifies medical devices into 3 categories: Class 1: low-risk devices such as dental floss and tongue depressors; Class 2: moderate-risk devices that need to be safe and effective, such as sutures and intravenous-infusion pumps; and Class 3: devices that tend to be technologically complicated and high risk, such as heart valves, stents, pacemakers, HIV testing kits, and surgical robots.

The FDA provides 2 types of reviews for medical devices: approval and clearance. The most rigorous is a *premarket approval (PMA)*. This approval is meant to assess whether the device is safe and effective for its intended use and whether there have been any adverse reactions and complications, device failures, and replacements. The other is 510(k) approval. In this process the device must show that it is "substantially equivalent" to an existing device that was previously approved. The 510(k) process is mainly for Class 2–type devices but can be used for Class 3 devices.

The *Dietary Supplement Health and Education Act (DSHEA)* of 1994 prohibits the FDA from regulating dietary supplements, such as vitamins, amino acids, herbs, and other botanicals, even though some of these supplements, such as ephedra (which has now been removed from the market after it caused several deaths), have been shown to have adverse health effects and even cause deaths.

The FDA is not the only public regulator in the health system. Another set of public regulators license physicians. Every state operates a board of medical licensure, evaluating whether physicians are "in good standing" and requiring them to reapply every few years for licensure.

Going forward a major issue for these state boards will be creating an efficient way for physicians to be licensed in multiple states without going through the paperwork of each state so as to enable telemedicine and other forms of practice across state lines.

Another set of important public regulators is state insurance commissioners, who oversee the health insurance industry. The state requirements as well as the powers of the insurance commissioners vary. Most state insurance commissioners make certain that insurers selling in the state have sufficient reserves. In many but not all states the insurance commissioner has the power to review rates proposed by insurers especially in the individual and small-group market.

Private Regulators

One important private regulator is the *Joint Commission*. Begun in 1951, it is an independent, not-for-profit organization that establishes standards and accredits mainly hospitals, nursing homes, home health care agencies, and clinical laboratories. Accreditation is focused on meeting defined standards that cover a wide range of issues so as to ensure the facility is providing quality care. For the last decade or so, a major focus of the Joint Commission review and accreditation process has been patient safety, such as medication safety and infection control, as well as improved and standardized clinical processes.

Although the Joint Commission is a private entity, most states require its accreditation for hospital licensure and participation in Medicaid. From 1965 to 2010 Joint Commission accreditation was necessary for hospitals to participate in Medicare. Congress changed this, however, and allows severed organizations to accredit hospitals for Medicare payments.

Another important private regulator is the *National Committee for Quality Assurance (NCQA)*. Founded in 1990 as a not-for-profit entity, NCQA was initially focused on assessing the quality of health plans and managed-care organizations. Since then it has branched out to accrediting accountable care organizations and medical homes.

The *National Quality Forum (NQF)* is a membership organization that endorses national consensus standards for measuring and publicly reporting on health care quality. The NQF has endorsed quality standards and has also defined 28 so-called "never events"—that is, events that should never happen. Examples include operating on the wrong leg or administering incompatible blood. In 2009 HHS contracted with NQF to help establish a portfolio of quality and efficiency measures for use in reporting on and improving health care quality. NQF has been criticized because its consensus process is overly cautious and slow; approving a quality standard can take over 2 years.

Just as the Joint Commission largely accredits hospitals and NCQA health plans, there are numerous private regulators that certify physicians. The *National Board of Medical Examiners*, for instance, administers the "boards"—the medical equivalent of the bar exam for lawyers—except that the medical boards have 3 parts. Part 1 is given to medical students after their first 2 years of medical school, part 2 at the end of medical school, and part 3 after their internship year. Passing the boards is necessary in order to apply for a state license to practice medicine.

All of this information only begins to describe the full complexity of the health care system. There are more components and interconnections than there are even on Senator Specter's chart. And as we have seen, calculating payment to hospitals and physicians is a multistep and incredibly complex system that is heavily biased in favor of specialists who perform surgery or other hospital-based procedures rather than primary care.

It is also clear that although at one time there may have been good rationales for many of the components, the system has really become incomprehensible and largely unjustifiable. Why should there be 6 different rates for the same procedure, with the uninsured people like Wayne and Baltazar paying the highest rates while insured patients, like Erin, receiving lower bills? Further, this system has created perverse incentives that create problems not just for the health care system but well beyond it. The next chapter will examine 5 of the most serious adverse consequences of the utterly crazy, complex health care system.

= CHAPTER FOUR =

Five Problems with the American Health Care System

No country's health care system is perfect. Every health care system will have problems, but the way the American system in particular has evolved and is currently structured creates many crippling problems.

The Cost of Being Uninsured

Before the ACA, at least 15% of Americans were, like Wayne and Baltazar, uninsured. This alone seems unconscionable. That one out of 7 Americans lacks health insurance in the richest country in the world, in a country whose GDP is about 22% of the world's total economic output, seems hard to defend. These people are neither lazy nor dependent on the government. Like Wayne and Baltazar, the vast majority are either working or in families in which someone works, but they work for employers that do not provide coverage or are in such low-paying jobs that they cannot afford to pay for health insurance.

As we have seen with Baltazar and his brother, being uninsured does not mean not getting health care. Uninsured Americans do get sick and need health care; they receive about 65% of the care they would receive if they were insured. However, they suffer serious problems because they are uninsured—and we all end up paying for it.

A main reason for health insurance is to provide people financial protection from large, random losses (Chapter 2, page 36). A consequence of being uninsured is running the risk that you may need to spend huge amounts of money on health care that you cannot afford. Most of us could not afford Erin's experience of an unexpected colon cancer surgery; we just would not have the savings to pay over $70,000 for the hospital and surgeon's bills. As the Oregon experiment affirmed, health insurance reduces the likelihood of catastrophic financial outcomes (Chapter 2, page 36).

But most importantly, having insurance improves health. In the 2012 presidential election, Mitt Romney claimed that no one in America died because they lacked health insurance:

> We don't have people that become ill, who die in their apartment because they don't have insurance. . . . No, you go to the hospital, you get treated, you get care, and it's paid for, either by charity, the government, or by the hospital.

It turns out Mitt Romney was wrong. Not having insurance can cost you your life.

People who agree with Mitt Romney might cite the Oregon Medicaid experiment (Chapter 2, page 36). It showed that uninsured people who got Medicaid did *not* see significant improvement in their health compared to those who remained uninsured. Medicaid beneficiaries certainly received more care; for example, among diabetes patients, those on Medicaid were much more likely to have gotten a diagnosis and taken medications to control their blood sugar. But that care did not necessarily translate into better outcomes. After 2 years diabetes patients with Medicaid did not have significantly better blood sugar control than those without insurance.

These results are a bit disturbing. Many people expected—even hoped—health insurance would have a bigger impact on overall health. However, the number of adults with a particular disease and the short amount of follow-up time—just 2 years—are probably too small a sample to result in a big impact. After all, high blood pressure and diabetes are chronic illnesses, and their worst effects often emerge only after many years. Also, the conditions may not normalize immediately. Having people with diabetes in treatment is a good thing and might well improve their health over longer periods of time.

But there is other convincing research that correlates health insurance with better survival. In one important study, Joseph Doyle, a professor at MIT's Sloan School of Management, tracked the health care interventions that car accident victims received. We would expect that health insurance should not affect the emergency care given to a car accident victim. But this is not the case. By carefully examining data from Wisconsin, Doyle showed that an uninsured person received 20% less treatment than the privately insured car accident victim, even after taking into account a whole range of possibly confounding factors, such as neighborhood, type of hospital, and type of car. Of much greater concern, Doyle concluded, "the uninsured are also found to have a substantially higher mortality rate"—in fact, a mortality rate nearly 40% higher than those with private insurance. Being uninsured means your chance of dying in a car accident is 40% higher than that of a privately insured person. Pretty shocking.

Then there is cancer (see Figure 4.1). The American Cancer Society examined cancer patients with and without coverage. They found that for all people with cancer, those who were uninsured had an 8% less chance of being alive 5 years after treatment, compared to Americans who had private insurance. Further, a 2013 study by researchers at Harvard and the University of Massachusetts Medical Schools showed that 5-year cancer survival rates in American counties with high rates of uninsurance are much worse than those counties with low rates of uninsurance, prompting the authors to conclude, "The patients in the higher uninsurance rate counties demonstrated greater mortality (8–15% increased risk on proportional hazards)."

People who side with Mitt Romney might still be skeptical. They might argue that the uninsured have different cancers, more associated with smoking and drinking, such as lung and liver cancer. These cancers are less treatable and more deadly, which would skew the survival rates down. Furthermore, these skeptics might argue that the uninsured are probably diagnosed with more advanced cancers that are less treatable and that they are less likely to adhere to cancer screening tests and to seek treatment promptly when they have worrisome signs and symptoms.

And some of this is true. Patients in high uninsurance counties do show up with larger cancers. (In this way, being uninsured probably influences when an individual decides to go see a physician.) But it is possible to control for these factors—the types of cancers and how advanced they are when the patient presents to the physician. The American Cancer

FIGURE 4.1 Health insurance and cancer survival

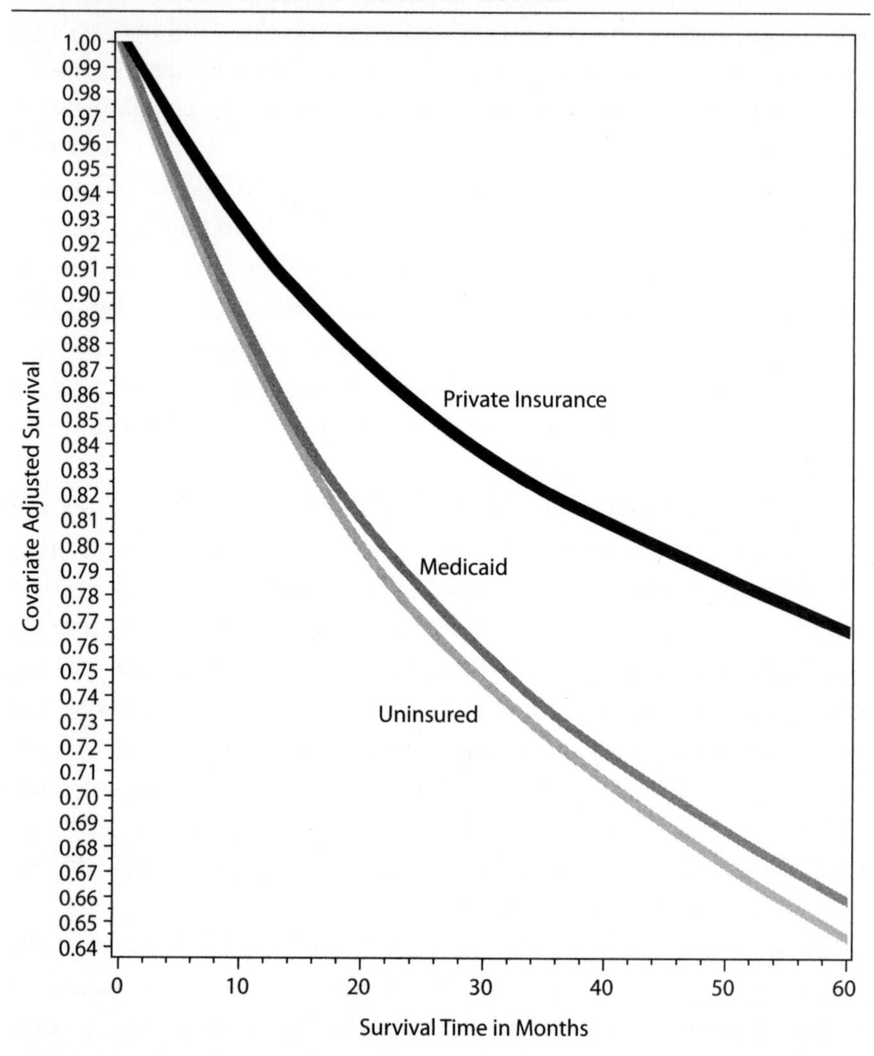

Source: Elizabeth Ward, et al. "Association of insurance with cancer care utilization and outcomes," *CA: A Cancer Journal for Clinicians* 58.1 (2008): 9–31.

Society research shows that even for the same types of cancers at the same size and stage, Americans who are uninsured have a significantly higher chance of dying at 5 years. For instance, among women with stage II breast cancer—that is, breast cancer that has extended to the lymph nodes but not to any other part of the body—those who are uninsured on average survive roughly 10% less than do insured women 5 years after treatment. The pattern persists for Americans with colon cancer.

If an oncologist developed a drug that gave patients an 8% to 10% increased chance of 5-year survival, it would be hailed as a major breakthrough. Consider that the drug Herceptin is viewed as a major breakthrough for certain types of breast cancer, as it provides women a 4% to 5% survival advantage.

No one is sure why the uninsured and Medicaid cancer patients do so much worse than privately insured patients. Part of the reason may be the difficulty and delay uninsured and Medicaid patients experience when they try to see oncologists, get referred for cancer surgery, or get the latest, most costly chemotherapy and radiation therapy.

Regardless of the explanation, the research is pretty clear: at least when it comes to emergency care and cancer, being uninsured does mean you are significantly more likely to die earlier.

But it turns out Mitt Romney is right in one way: uninsured people often do go to the hospital or a physician's office and get treated, and the cost of that treatment is passed onto others. It turns out the "others" are insured Americans. This is *cross-subsidization* (see Chapter 2, page 75), and it means most Americans are paying a hidden tax. Buried in the insurance premium for Americans with health insurance is the cost of providing care for Americans who lack health insurance.

This is how it works. Uninsured patients go to the hospital and get care they cannot pay for. (Unlike Baltazar, they do not pay for it with an installment payment plan.) The hospital still has to pay for the hospital bed, the X-rays, laboratory tests, medications, nursing time, and all the other care the patient receives. Those costs do not just disappear because the patient is uninsured or because Medicaid pays a very low amount of money that does not cover the true costs of care. Instead, the hospital distributes the costs among the bills of all those patients who have health insurance and whose care is paid for. And those higher hospital bills raise the insurance premiums we all see. The hospital is also likely to receive some money for the care it provides to the uninsured from the federal government through the *Disproportionate Share Hospital (DSH)* program (see Chapter 2, page 62). In other words, insured Americans pay for the care the uninsured receive either through higher health insurance premiums or higher taxes that fund DSH payments.

How much is this cross-subsidization? The nonprofit advocacy organization Families USA conducted a study that showed that in 2008 the uninsured received approximately $116 billion in health care. Of that, the uninsured themselves paid for about $43 billion, charity and government paid an additional $30 billion, but the remaining $43 billion comes from the insured. Breaking it down, nearly $1,000 of a family's health insurance premium and $340 of an individual's premium goes to pay for the uninsured's care.

Having nearly 50 million uninsured Americans is bad. It is an unjustifiable moral stain on the country. It increases what insured Americans pay in health insurance premiums and taxes. It puts a financial burden on the uninsured, who are among the poorest but largely working members of American society. And most damningly, it actually kills people.

The Economic Cost of High Health Care Costs

In 2012 the United States spent over $2.8 trillion on health care. This makes the US health care system the 5th largest economy in the world—larger than the entire GDP of France.

The amount the United States spends on health care is out of this world (see Figure 4.2). On a per person basis, even controlling for the country's wealth, the United States spends much more than other developed countries; indeed, the United States spends 40% per person more than the next highest country, Norway. The consulting firm McKinsey and Company, the media and information firm Thompson-Reuters, and the Institute of Medicine all conducted independent studies, and all came to the same conclusion: the United States spends about $700 billion more than it should be spending on health care.

It is not just the level of health care spending that is worrisome; it is also the rate of growth. Since the 1970s spending on health care has consistently grown faster than the overall economy. On average, over the past 40 years heath care costs have grown more than 2% faster than the economy. Economists express this by saying health care spending grows at GDP+2% per year. The consequence is that in 1970 6 cents of every dollar went to health care, and today it is nearly 18 cents. Indeed, as the decades progress the amount of growth in the economy that gets devoted to health care keeps rising (see Figure 4.3), so that over a quarter of the growth in the last decade went to health care. That is scary.

FIGURE 4.2 United States vs. international health spending, 2012

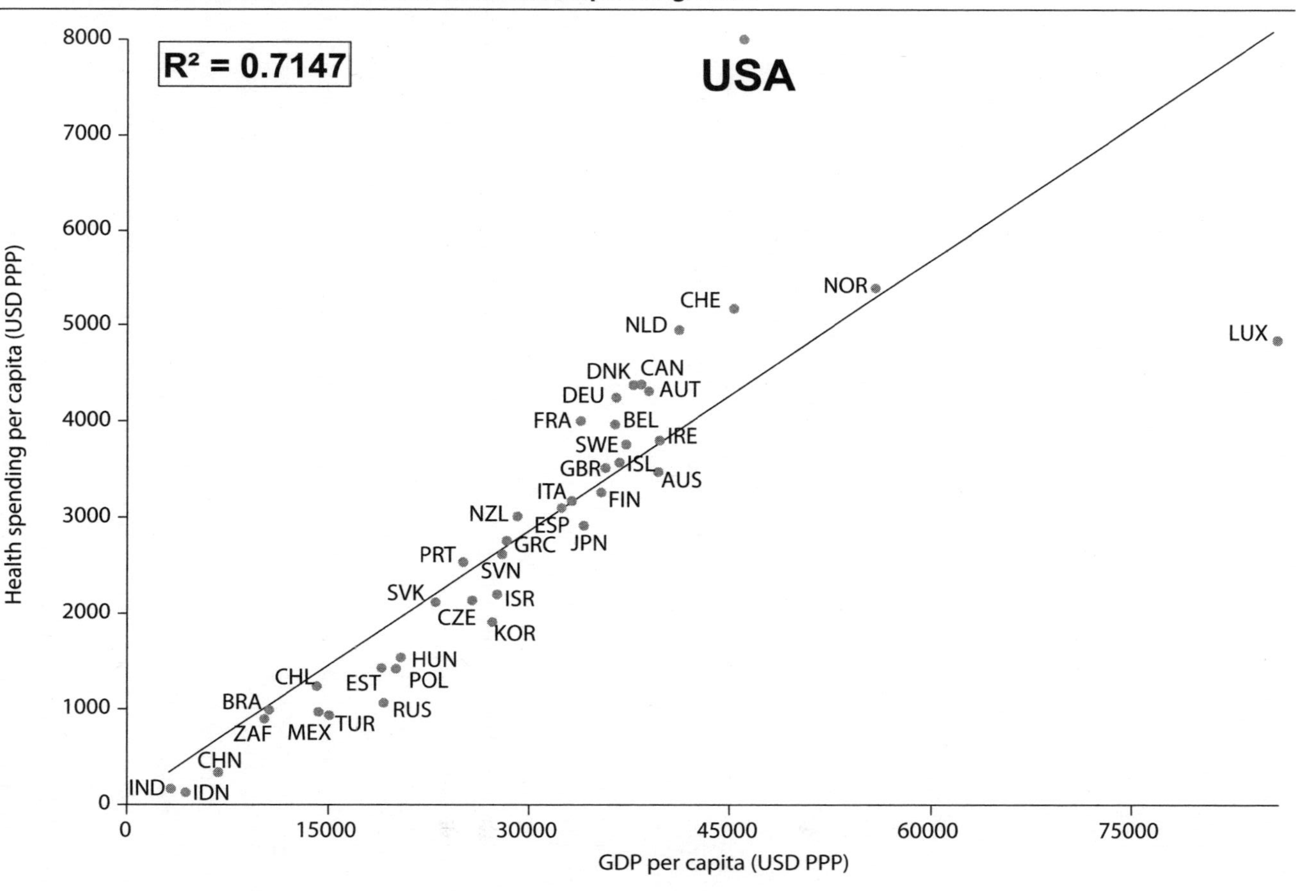

Source: OECD Health Data 2011. WHO Global Health Expenditure Database.

FIGURE 4.3 Annual increase in national health expenditures and their share of gross domestic product, 1961–2011

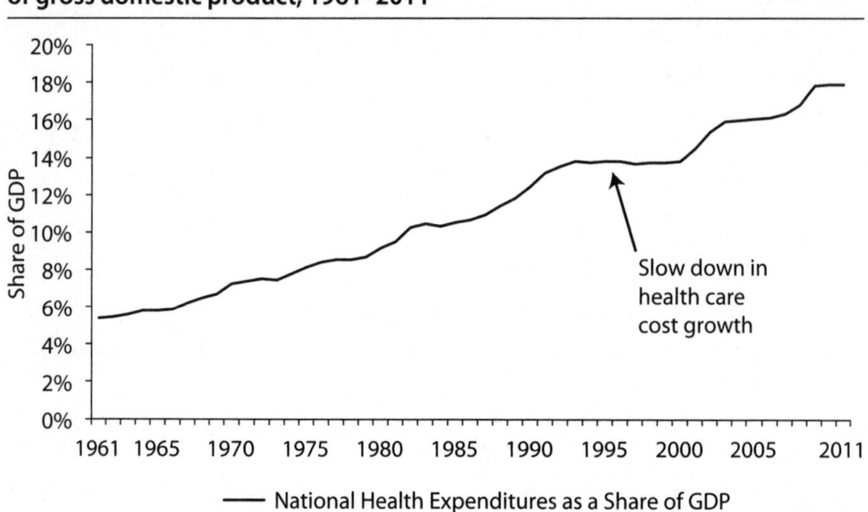

Source: Kaiser Slides, The Henry J. Kaiser Foundation, March 13, 2013. *Data Sources:* Centers for Medicare and Medicaid Services, Office of the Actuary, National Health Statistics Group.

In the mid-1990s, however, health care inflation actually dropped close to matching the growth of the economy (see Figure 4.4). This was right after the failure of the Clinton health care reform initiative and was the time of managed care, in which insurance companies put pressure on hospitals and physicians to lower the prices of health care services and to reduce excess hospital beds and other unrestrained expenses.

This period of cost control lasted just a few years. Americans rebelled against the managed restrictions care. The consequence was a period of relatively high health care inflation beginning around 2000 that has only begun to moderate in the last few years.

This stratospherically high level of health care spending and growth rate have 4 serious, potentially calamitous consequences: (1) more uninsured Americans, (2) cuts to education and other state programs, (3) stagnant wages, and (4) growing federal deficit and debt.

First, there is a direct relationship between high and growing health care costs and the number of uninsured Americans. Since 2000 real health care costs have more than doubled and the number of uninsured

FIGURE 4.4 Average annual growth rates for NHE and GDP, per capita, for selected time periods

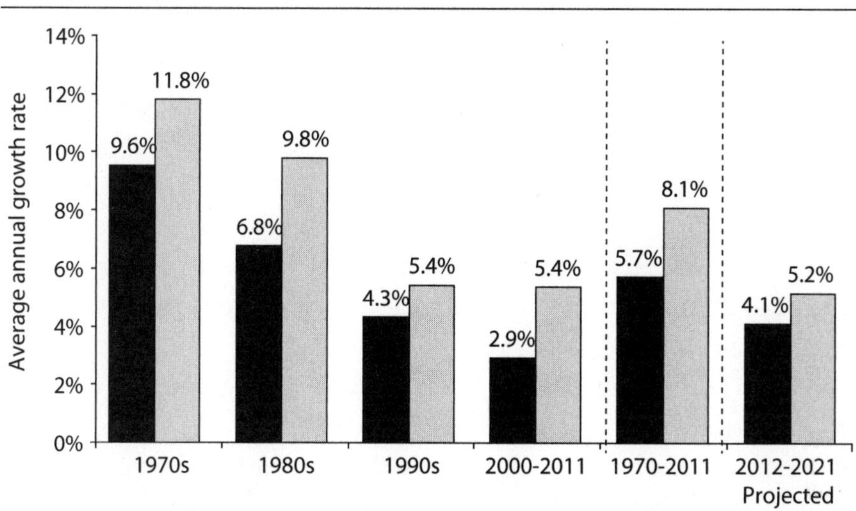

Source: Kaiser Slides, The Henry J. Kaiser Family Foundation, March 13, 2013. *Data Sources:* Centers for Medicare and Medicaid Services, Office of the Actuary, National Health Statistics Group, Bureau of Economic Analysis.

has risen from 36.6 million to 48.0 million, a 31.1% increase. This is not mere coincidence. As prices for insurance increase, some companies, like Baltazar's gardening company, decide they can no longer afford to offer health insurance to their employees and some families decide that even if their employer offers insurance, they cannot afford to buy it. Other individuals who are self-insured also decide they cannot afford the higher premiums. Indeed, several Harvard economists studying this relationship concluded that "each $1,000/year of increased premiums leads to declines in coverage of 2.6 percentage points," even controlling for all other factors such as the robustness of the economy and other policy changes. High and growing health care costs mean millions more men, women, and children go without health insurance.

Many people might think that with enactment of the Affordable Care Act this relationship between higher costs and an increase in the number of people without insurance will no longer be a concern. Unfortunately, although the Affordable Care Act has a mandate that individuals buy health insurance (Chapter 8), it also has an escape clause that recognizes this is only fair if that insurance policy is affordable. Thus, the law states that people are not required to have health insurance if the only plan they can find costs them more than 8% of their household income. Consequently, if health care costs continue to grow at high rates, more and more people may well be uninsured because their employer does not offer coverage and they cannot find an insurance policy that costs them no more than 8% of their household income.

A second problem of high health care costs relates to education and, in particular, increasing tuition costs of public colleges and universities. It probably seems strange to link health care and college tuition, but there is a direct link through state budget squeezes.

States' health care costs typically include 3 components: (1) health insurance for their legislators and state workers, (2) the state's portion of Medicaid expenses not covered by the federal government, and (3) payments for other state health programs such as vaccines, public health measures, hospitals, and payments to hospitals and clinics to compensate for caring for the uninsured. As health care costs go up faster than the overall economy, these costs grow faster than the rise in states' tax receipts. This is known as a budget gap.

Because states are not allowed to run deficits, the governors and state legislators face 3 options: (1) raise taxes to pay for the health care services, (2) cut these health programs, or (3) cut other state services to pay for health care.

Raising taxes in most states is politically impossible. Many states have cut health benefits by restricting Medicaid eligibility, reducing Medicaid payments, shifting Medicaid to managed care, or reducing other programs. But this goes only so far. For instance, shifting Medicaid to managed care or cutting public health programs constitutes a one-time savings. In addition, states do not have unlimited flexibility in cutting their Medicaid program; the federal government has minimums for Medicaid eligibility and benefits, and after a few years there is not much more to cut. Then, only one option is left: cut other state programs.

In 2012, according to the National Governor's Association, collectively the 50 states raised Medicaid spending about $16 billion (see Figure 4.5). This was in part because unemployment and other cuts by private employers meant that more Americans needed Medicaid. To compensate,

FIGURE 4.5 Changes in state general fund spending by category between 2011 and 2012

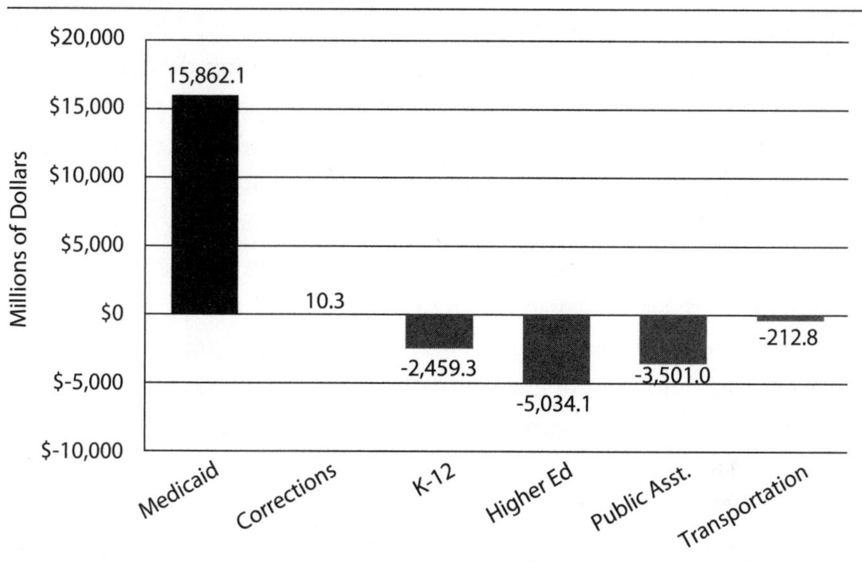

Source: National Association of State Budget Officers. Fiscal Survey of States, Fall 2011.

primary, secondary and college education were reduced—a lot. In 2013 Medicaid went up less, and primary and secondary education funds actually increased, but funds for college education continued to be cut by over $1 billion. The director of Arizona Office of Strategic and Budget Planning characterized the situation: "Medicaid and other health-care expenses are predicted to grow to as much as 40% of the state budget by 2015. That will force the state to cut higher education funding because there are few other options. . . . It certainly seems to be on a collision course." One reason that tuition at state colleges and universities has been going up relentlessly for the last decade is that rising health care costs force states to cut their support for public education.

Paying for Medicaid and state workers' health insurance while cutting public university support does not seem a particularly wise investment for the future, but that is one consequence of health care costs that rise faster than overall economic growth.

A third problem related to high and rising health care costs is the shrinking middle class. Since 1980 average nonfarm wages in the private sector have stagnated; indeed, after controlling for inflation, the average cash wages have actually gone down. There are many reasons for this, but one is that growing health care costs have consumed much of the increase in workers' productivity.

From an employer's perspective there is one number they care about: total worker compensation. This typically encompasses 2 components: cash wages and fringe benefits. Fringe benefits include many things: paid vacation time and sick leave; retirement benefits, whether a pension plan or 401(k) program; life and disability insurance; and other benefits. But the biggest portion of the benefits is usually health insurance. If fringe benefits go up faster because health insurance costs are rising faster, then cash wages cannot rise much. The President's Council of Economic Advisers summarized the data on wages this way: "[Between 2000 and 2009 health care costs doubled while] workers' inflation-adjusted average total compensation per hour increased by 1.3% per year (from $26.23 per hour to $29.39 per hour in 2009 dollars). [However,] workers' average hourly wage and salary compensation increased by just 0.7% per year." Although the increase in total compensation is small—only 1.3% per year—nonetheless, only half went to take-home wages, whereas the other half went to fringe benefits like health insurance. Do we really think that nearly half of every extra dollar we earn should go to health care?

The last major economic impact of high and growing health care costs relates to the financial health of the country itself. In the last years of the Clinton administration the federal government ran budget surpluses that decreased the national debt; indeed, eliminating the debt was within sight. But after President Bush took over, the federal government has run ever-larger deficits. Some of this relates to the Great Recession, but much relates to tax cuts, the wars in Afghanistan and Iraq, and unfunded programs, the largest of which is the Medicare Part D program, instituted in 2006.

Over these years federal health care spending has grown relentlessly (see Figure 4.6). Before the Affordable Care Act, projections into the future were nothing short of dire. Projections in 2010 by the nonpartisan Congressional Budget Office and others showed that the real threat to the federal budget and debt was the growth in Medicare (see Figure 4.7). If health care inflation continued at its historical growth rate of

FIGURE 4.6 Federal health care spending, 2000–2012

YEAR	TOTAL FEDERAL HEALTH CARE SPENDING (IN BILLIONS)	FEDERAL HEALTH CARE SPENDING AS PERCENT OF FEDERAL BUDGET	MEDICARE (IN BILLIONS)	MEDICAID (IN BILLIONS)
2000	$388.9	21.7%	$219.0	$117.9
2001	$428.9	23.0%	$241.1	$129.4
2002	$472.5	23.5%	$256.8	$147.5
2003	$522.5	24.2%	$277.9	$160.7
2004	$568.5	24.8%	$301.5	$176.2
2005	$614.0	24.8%	$336.9	$181.7
2006	$650.5	24.5%	$378.6	$180.6
2007	$716.8	26.3%	$432.6	$190.6
2008	$751.8	25.2%	$452.0	$201.4
2009	$853.0	24.2%	$494.5	$250.9
2010	$916.2	26.5%	$516.8	$272.8
2011	$984.1	25.8%	$563.9	$276.2
2012	$971.8	26.1%	$569.0	$269.1

Source: Altarum Institute.

GDP+2%, then health care would consume about half of the federal budget by 2035. The bipartisan National Commission on Fiscal Responsibility and Reform, the so-called Simpson-Bowles Commission, stated,

> Federal health care spending represents our single largest fiscal challenge over the long-run. As the baby boomers retire and overall health care costs continue to grow faster than the economy, federal health spending threatens to balloon. Under its extended-baseline scenario, CBO projects that federal health care spending for Medicare, Medicaid, the Children's Health insurance Program (CHIP), and the health insurance exchange subsidies will grow from nearly 6% of GDP in 2010 to about 10% in 2035, and continue to grow thereafter.

Indeed, it goes on to state that if nothing is done, "by 2025 [federal tax] revenue will be able to finance only interest payments, Medicare,

FIGURE 4.7 Long-term budget outlook pre-ACA

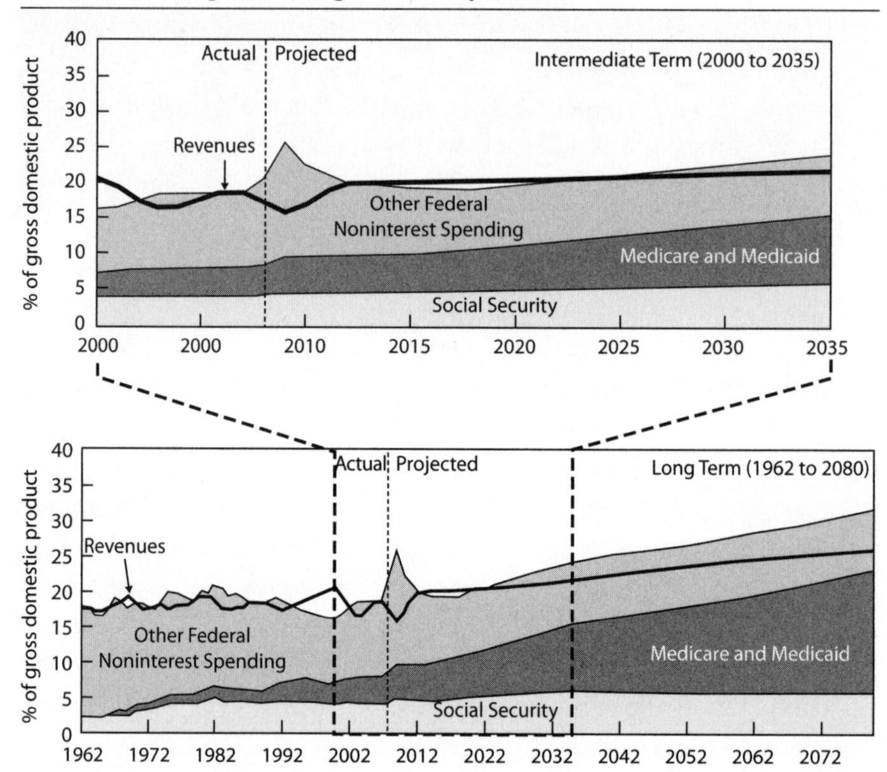

Note: Spending in this figure excludes interest payments on the debt; hence, the gap between federal revenues and noninterest spending shown here does not equal the projected surplus or deficit.
Source: Congressional Budget Office.

Medicaid, and Social Security" and nothing else—not national defense, education, transportation, national parks, or even congressional pay. Controlling health care costs is essential for ensuring the long-term financial health of the United States.

Here is the good news: something was done. There is a growing—but not universal—agreement that over the last few years health care cost growth has moderated and not just because of the Great Recession; indeed, as we will see, a contributing reason for this is health care reform. As one nonpartisan think tank, The Center on Budget and Policy Priorities, put it: "Health reform (the 2010 Affordable Care Act, or ACA) and other developments have significantly slowed the projected growth of Medicare spending." This, in turn, has dramatically improved the long-term outlook for the nation's debt.

But, as the budget experts point out, all of this could change if health care inflation goes back up. That would dramatically increase government health care spending and substantially raise the debt. Keeping health care costs under control is key to maintaining an optimistic long-range budget and debt story. Unless we constantly focus on reducing health care costs, they could imperil the country's fiscal well-being.

Finally, it is worth noting that controlling health care costs is actually good economics. Many people might argue that health care is one of the few expanding areas of the economy and that cutting back might threaten jobs and growth. In reality, however, high and rising health care costs, especially when we spend on low-benefit and marginal care, are a drag on the economy. Not spending that extra dollar on health care does not mean the dollar disappears. The money spent on health care cannot be spent in other ways, such as education, new clothes, new computers, appliances, cars, vacations, and otherwise. But not spending the money on health care would stimulate consumption and growth in other ways. The President's Council of Economic Advisers conducted research showing that reducing health care cost increases by just 1% every year translates into an increase in the GDP of 4% by 2030. That would mean $600 billion more for the overall economy and an extra $7,000 for the average American family. That is a huge economic benefit from controlling health care costs. Thus, controlling health care costs does not slow the economy but instead accelerates it.

The Cost of Poor Quality of Care

For all the extra money the United States is spending on health care, we should be getting much better quality of care than the rest of the world. And proving that the average quality of care in the United States consistently exceeds that in other nations is really impossible.

Doubtless there are pockets of excellence in health care that are the envy of the world. The United States has been the undisputed leader in terms of developing new biomedical tests and treatments. And many people flock to the United States' great academic centers for the latest treatments in cancer, heart disease, prosthetic limbs, and other serious conditions.

But the fact is that what most people need is not the latest and greatest. High blood pressure afflicts 67 million adult Americans and directly contributes to approximately 350,000 deaths annually. We know how to diagnose and treat high blood pressure; it is not high technology we need but rather routine activities, including measuring blood pressure with a cuff, prescribing inexpensive medications that have been used for over 30 years, and routinely monitoring the blood pressure. We should not think this care unimportant. Over the last 50 years average life expectancy of Americans has increased over 7 years. The vast majority of that, nearly 5 years, is because of declines in deaths from heart disease and stroke. And along with declines in smoking, control of high blood pressure is one, if not the biggest factor in reducing stroke and heart disease, more than any other medical intervention. Its impact has been much bigger than all the latest interventions for cancer as well as the bypass and stent operations for heart disease combined. Indeed, all those high-technology cancer treatments developed in the last 50 years have added fewer than 3 months to the average life expectancy in the United States.

Despite these advances, we aren't doing what we should be doing. Fewer than half of American adults with high blood pressure have it well controlled. A few years ago researchers from the nonprofit global policy think tank RAND studied treatments for high blood pressure and 8 other relatively straightforward medical conditions. On high blood pressure they found that among Medicare patients leaving the hospital, blood pressure was left uncontrolled in 58% of patients. They also assessed whether patients hospitalized for community-acquired pneumonia were given a vaccine when they were discharged from the hospital and found that only 36% of patients were vaccinated. Overall, the chances that Medicare patients discharged from hospitals received proven beneficial care were basically the flip of a coin—55%. And when the RAND researchers repeated the study assessing the quality of care delivered to American children, they found that the result was even worse: "On average, according to data in the medical records, children receive 46.5%

of the indicated care." Children received 53.4% of proven care for acute problems like an ear infection or upper respiratory tract infection and even lower levels for prevention, especially if they were adolescents. This does not serve as an endorsement for high-quality care in America.

Another area of poor quality of care in the American health care system relates to hospital-acquired infections and other mistakes. According to the latest study by the Center for Disease Control and Prevention (CDC), 1.7 million Americans, roughly 1 of every 20 people hospitalized, suffers a hospital-acquired infection, causing nearly 100,000 deaths per year. High-quality health care?

But the really disturbing fact is that we know how to prevent many of these infections, and very little of it involves high technology: washing hands, putting in intravenous lines under sterile conditions, removing urinary catheters after a few days, and keeping patients who are on respirators propped up. Indeed, in a few years, with concentrated efforts, hospitals that focused on the problem were able to reduce bloodstream infections by 33% and other (MRSA) infections by 18%.

Further, pediatric vaccines are not only life saving, they are actually cost saving. They are one of the few medical interventions that actually reduces spending. Over recent years the United States has dramatically improved, but in all but hepatitis B the French do better (see Figure 4.8).

FIGURE 4.8 Pediatric immunization rates

VACCINE	UNITED STATES	FRANCE
Diphtheria, Pertussis Tetanus	94%	99%
Polio	93%	99%
Haemophilus Influenza Type B (HiB)	80%	97%
Hepatitis B	90%	42%

The list can go on and on. Even for a condition that the United States prides itself on for being at the technological forefront—namely, cancer—the results on the quality of care are not overwhelming. Research in the Seattle area assessed how often a very high-technology and high-cost test, positron emission CT scans, were used for women with early-stage breast cancer. Cancer professional societies recommended *against* using this test because it does not improve the care or survival for these women; it is unnecessary care. The research found that there was wide variation in use of the test. Some physicians hardly used the test—once for every 10 patients—whereas others used it for almost every single patient even though it would not improve their outcomes.

For many people the frequency of the use of diagnostic tests when not medically necessary is not the most important indicator of the quality of cancer care; rather, use of life-saving chemotherapy and survival are. Research on these metrics paints a mixed picture. A research team from Harvard and RAND, funded by the American Society of Clinical Oncology (the professional society of cancer physicians), reviewed patients' charts and showed that, overall, breast cancer patients received 86% of the right quality of care, and colon cancer patients received 78%. Focusing in on chemotherapy treatments showed that breast cancer patients got the right ones 82% of the time and colon cancer patients just 64% of the time. This is not an A-level grade. For life-and-death treatments, this is not impressive.

Second, even the advocates acknowledge that the better US performance in cancer survival is concentrated in a few cancers such as leukemia and prostate cancer, for which the United States is known to have significant overdiagnosis and overtreatment—which is hardly a good thing, as treatments all have undesirable side effects, such as impotence and incontinence. Meanwhile, European countries have made greater survival gains in other cancers such as colon and uterine cancer.

Finally, the variation in quality within the United States is significant; that is, in some places the quality of care is much better than it is in other places. For instance, considering colon cancer survival among women in the United States, places like Hawaii have a nearly 10% better survival rate compared to places like New York (see Figure 4.9).

In heart disease the story is much the same. In a 2013 report to Congress the Department of Health and Human Services summarized key measures for prevention and treatment of heart disease. They were not high-technology interventions but rather simple diagnostic tests combined with well-tested medications. The results suggest failing grades (see Figure 4.10).

Even when it comes to the use of high technology in heart disease, the quality is not what we should be proud of. Recently research from

FIGURE 4.9 Five-year survival of colorectal cancer by state (women)

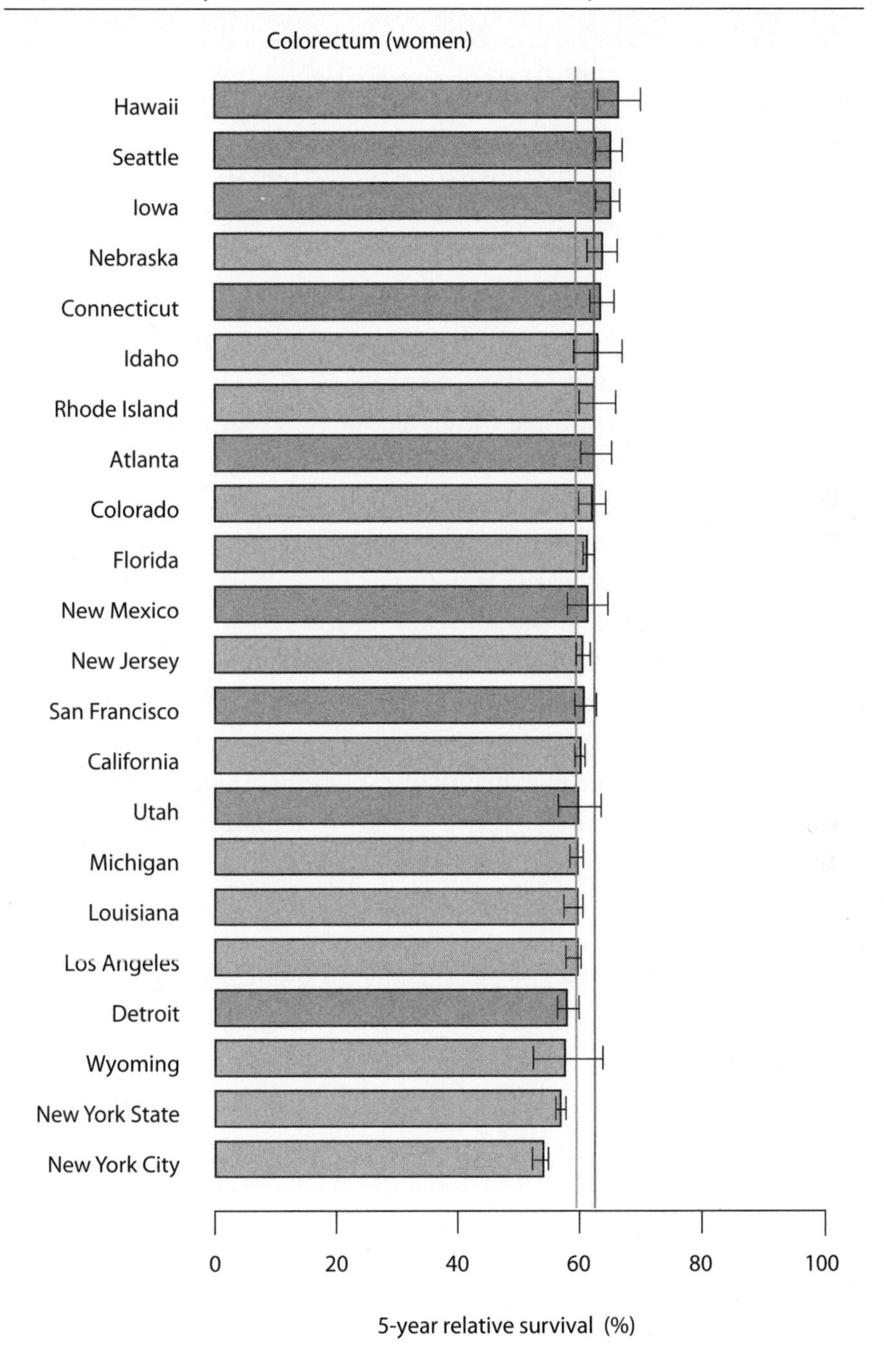

FIGURE 4.10 Quality of prevention and treatment practices for heart disease

MEASURE/ FOCUS	KEY MEASURE NAME/DESCRIPTION	CURRENT RATE
Aspirin use	People at increased risk of cardiovascular disease who are taking aspirin	47%
Cholesterol management	People with high cholesterol who have adequately managed hyperlipidemia	33%
Smoking cessation	People trying to quit smoking who get help	23%

the American College of Cardiology that tabulated data on the use of stents in almost all cases in the United States show that for the nearly 150,000 percutaneous coronary interventions—treatments like stents—placed for nonacute reasons, such as persistent chest pain, only half were medically appropriate. A total of 11.6% of interventions were clearly inappropriate and unnecessary—for instance, patients did not have chest pain or were not on any medications to treat the chest pain. In the other cases the appropriateness was unclear. Thus, at least 15,000 Americans a year—and maybe as many as 75,000—are getting stents and undergoing other procedures that entail serious risks, and yet the procedure neither improves survival nor quality of life.

And the list goes on. The quality of care in the American health care system can be very good at major academic centers for complex, unusual, and rare cases. But these are not the bulk of health care needs. For the vast majority of health care, whether low-technology high blood pressure treatments, vaccines, and hospital infections or high-technology care for cancer and heart disease, the quality is uneven and hardly anything we should be proud of—certainly not when we are paying $700 billion more than other countries.

The Problem of Lack of Transparency in Costs and Quality

A fourth problem relates to the quality of health care and its cost: they are both largely unknown. In Donald Rumsfeld's words, they are unknown unknowns. This is the problem of transparency or, to be specific, the lack of transparency, highlighted by Steve Brill's 2013 *Time* article "Bitter Pill: Why Medical Bills Are Killing Us."

Even people within the health care system do not know the total price of a service. A recent study called around to hospitals to ask about the total price for a hip replacement, including the operating room, hospital, the actual artificial hip joint, and the surgeon's fee for a patient who did not have insurance—this would be the charge master price. Only 45% of orthopedic hospitals and 9.8% of other hospitals could provide that information.

If hospitals cannot give the total price for a procedure, it is no wonder most physicians prescribing a test or treatment have no idea of the price of that test or treatment. Expecting physicians to be cost conscious is difficult if they do not know the prices of what they are ordering for patients.

Upon reflection, this ignorance may not be so surprising. As we saw in Chapter 2, there are multiple prices for any health care service: the charge master price, the Medicare price, the various prices paid by different private insurance companies, the Medicaid price.

What the research shows is that the charge master and commercial insurance company prices for the same test or treatment will also vary substantially even at neighboring medical facilities where, presumably, basic input costs such as rent and wages do not vary substantially. Colonoscopies in New York City can vary fourfold—between $2,025 and $8,700—depending on the hospital.

This variation in price is very hard to justify. Typically, neither patients nor physicians have access to the price, so they cannot shop around for lower prices. Imagine you were shopping for a new shirt but there was no price tag and you could not know until weeks after you bought it whether the shirt cost $25 or $200. This would make shopping a crazy experience.

Even more importantly, just knowing the prices is nearly worthless. How would anyone know whether a low price represents good value when they have no way of knowing whether a doctor or a hospital provides high-quality care or has a penchant for cutting corners? Even if you know that a shirt costs $25 or $200, if you can only see the price tag but not the shirt you are buying, you cannot know whether you will be getting a bargain on a Brooks Brother's shirt or a rip-off one from K-mart. A price tag alone is of limited use.

It turns out there is very little reliable and easily accessible data that compares hospitals and none that really compares physicians on their quality of care. Maybe the best known is the *U.S. News and World Report* Hospital Ranking. But delve into how American hospitals are ranked and you will conclude that the *U.S. News* rankings are so flawed that they are nearly worthless—and may be counterproductive.

Consider that for 12 of the specialties assessed in the rankings, "reputation" makes up about a third of the hospital score. (For the other 4 specialties, the rankings are determined *solely* by reputation.) How does the *U.S. News* assess a hospital's reputation? For each specialty it sends out surveys to 200 randomly selected specialists and then averages the responses over the last 3 years. Here is the shocker: excluding interns and residents, there are over 720,000 office- and hospital-based physicians in the United States. How many physicians provided data on the reputation of the various hospitals? In cancer there are about 10,000 oncologists nationwide. The *U.S. News and World Report* reputation assessment relied on the views of just over 200 cancer physicians in the whole country. Does that sound like a highly trustworthy quality measure?

Another third of the rankings is supposed to be based on a more objective, data-driven metric, survival, measured by "A hospital's success at keeping patients alive was judged by comparing the number of Medicare inpatients with certain conditions who died within 30 days of admission in 2009, 2010 and 2011 with the number expected to die given the severity of illness." Undeniably, 30-day survival should be part of any quality assessment of a hospital. But can one single data-driven measure capture all of the complex activities that go into a hospital's quality? Ridiculous. These data only apply to older patients. Furthermore, 30-day survival has no real significance for many other hospital activities. For instance, in cancer care what matters is 5-year survival. And in other specialties, such as endocrinology or gastroenterology, for which the focus is on chronic care rather than emergency or urgent interventions, 30-day mortality is not a very meaningful quality measure. And then there are a slew of quality measures that the *U.S. News* rankings don't even take into account: hospital-acquired infections, medication errors, pressure ulcers, preventable re-admissions, and so on.

The federal government does a bit better, but it is still far from perfect. The Centers for Medicare and Medicaid Services (CMS) operates Hospital Compare, a website that provides some comparison data on the quality of care for different hospitals. The data focuses on 3 key medical problems—acute heart attacks, heart failure, and pneumonia—as well as surgical care standards and patient satisfaction. Unfortunately, even in these categories there are few actual measures: 2 for pneumonia and 3 for heart failure. There is only one area assessing the quality of pediatric care—pediatric asthma. Recently additional information has been added on hospital infections, surgical complications, and readmissions.

But go to the Hospital Compare website (www.medicare.gov/hospitalcompare/search.html), and you might be frustrated. First, there are many things patients care about that are either not transparent or not reported at all, such as cancer care, heart rhythm problems, any stomach or colon problems, or any neurologic or psychiatric problems.

Even for conditions Hospital Compare does report on there are big holes limiting the ability to compare. In July 2013 I searched 3 university-affiliated hospitals in the Washington, DC, area and tried to compare their quality of care for heart attacks. For many quality indicators, such as heart attack patients getting drugs to break up clots within 30 minutes, interventions like stents within 30 minutes, or aspirin or statin at discharge, these large academic hospitals often had data "not available" or "too few cases." That was shocking, as heart attacks are pretty common and there should be a lot of cases and data. There were more data for hospitals in the Boston area, but the amount of missing data from the major Chicago-area hospitals was like the missing data for Washington, DC, hospitals.

Second, the national averages are suspiciously high (see Figure 4.11). Almost all averages are in the A range. It is Lake Wobegon or having almost every car evaluated by *Consumer Reports* scoring over 90. If every hospital is in the 95th percentile, then it makes no difference which hospital you are treated at. Somehow that seems a bit unbelievable.

There are a variety of explanations for such outstanding hospital performance. The positive interpretation is that hospitals are being measured and, therefore, are focusing on improving their care and are proving they can, when focused, achieve great success. That would suggest

FIGURE 4.11 National averages on quality measures from CMS Hospital Compare

AREA	QUALITY INDICATOR	NATIONAL AVERAGE
Timely and effective heart attack care	Outpatients with chest pain or possible heart attack who got drugs to break up blood clots within 30 minutes of arrival	58%
	Average number of minutes before outpatients with chest pain or possible heart attack who needed specialized care were transferred to another hospital	58 minutes
	Outpatients with chest pain or possible heart attack who got aspirin within 24 hours of arrival	97%
	Average number of minutes before outpatients with chest pain or possible heart attack got an ECG	7 minutes
	Heart attack patients given aspirin at discharge	99%
	Heart attack patients given fibrinolytic medication within 30 minutes of arrival	61%
	Heart attack patients given PCI within 90 minutes of arrival	95%
	Heart attack patients given a prescription for a statin at discharge	98%
Effective heart failure care	Heart failure patients given discharge instructions	93%
	Heart failure patients given an evaluation of left ventricular systolic (LVS) function	99%
	Heart failure patients given ACE inhibitor or ARB for left ventricular systolic dysfunction (LVSD)	97%
Effective pneumonia care	Pneumonia patients whose initial emergency room blood culture was performed prior to the administration of the first hospital dose of antibiotics	97%
	Pneumonia patients given the most appropriate initial antibiotic(s)	95%

the importance of significantly expanding the quality measures and public reporting to many other diseases. The alternative explanation is that there is some gaming of the reporting. Hospitals may be sending in data selectively or, as suggested by my search of the Washington-area hospitals, not reporting adverse data. This explanation would suggest the need to expand data collection to include all cases on the measures being tested. Frankly, both seem necessary.

FIGURE 4.11 ***(continued)***

AREA	QUALITY INDICATOR	NATIONAL AVERAGE
Effective surgical care	Outpatients having surgery who got an antibiotic at the right time (within one hour before surgery)	97%
	Outpatients having surgery who got the right kind of antibiotic	97%
	Surgery patients whose urinary catheters were removed on the first or second day after surgery	96%
	Patients having surgery who were actively warmed in the operating room or whose body temperature was near normal by the end of surgery	100%
	Surgery patients who were taking heart drugs called beta blockers before coming to the hospital, who were kept on the beta blockers during the period just before and after their surgery	97%
	Surgery patients whose doctors ordered treatments to prevent blood clots after certain types of surgeries	98%
Effective preventive care	Patients assessed and given pneumonia vaccination	88%
	Patients assessed and given influenza vaccination	86%
Effective pediatric asthma care	Children who received reliever medication while hospitalized for asthma	100%
	Children who received systemic corticosteroid medication (oral and IV medication that reduces inflammation and controls symptoms) while hospitalized for asthma	100%
	Children and their caregivers who received a home management plan of care document while hospitalized for asthma	86%

Source: CMS Hospital Compare, www.medicare.gov/hospitalcompare/.

The difficulties in trying to obtain quality data are even worse when assessing physicians or groups of physicians. The CMS Physician Compare website is almost totally worthless. It lists physicians by specialty and whether they take Medicare payment, but it offers no transparency on physician quality. Although there are organizations trying to address the data problem, some efforts are worthwhile but others are probably not that helpful.

The problem is that we just do not have transparency when it comes to cost and quality of medical care. This makes it almost impossible for both physicians and patients to access high-value health care. Not only do physicians not know the price of tests and treatments so as to be cost conscious for their patients without reducing their quality of care, but they also rely on reputation or word of mouth when it comes to referring their patients to hospitals and other physicians. And even as physicians lack the price and quality data, patients are even worse off.

Uwe Reinhardt, one of the most respected health policy experts in the United States, once made the analogy that asking patients to shop on price and quality today is like blindfolding them, releasing them in Macy's, and telling them they had to buy the cheapest white dress shirt. Can you really blame them when they show up at the check-out counter with the most expensive purple underwear?

The Problem of Medical Malpractice

One of the biggest concerns for physicians is medical malpractice. It agitates them so much that it is often hard for them to focus on anything else, and it is not hard to be sympathetic to their concerns. A 2011 study in the *New England Journal of Medicine* showed that for physicians in "low risk" specialties, such as family medicine, dermatology, and pediatrics, the chances of being sued for malpractice over a lifetime of practice were about 70%. And for "high risk" specialties, such as neurosurgery and cardiac surgery, the chances were a certainty—nearly 100%. It is true that few of those suits actually go to trial and even fewer result in conviction and payment; indeed, over the course of a lifetime only 5% of all low-specialty physicians and 30% of high-specialty physicians actually paid a malpractice claim. Nonetheless, simply being sued, even for a case that gets dismissed, is time consuming, psychologically traumatic, and distracts physicians from being able to provide their best-quality care.

Medical malpractice is also expensive for physicians. Although there are many factors that influence the malpractice premiums—and the chances of being sued are just a small part of those—the costs can be astronomical. An obstetrician in Florida is often forced to pay more than $100,000 annually in malpractice premiums.

If, pretty much regardless of what you do, you know you are going to be sued in the course of your career and the annual malpractice premiums are in the tens if not hundreds of thousands, it is pretty hard not to be affected by, much less be obsessed with, medical malpractice and fixing it.

This should be reason enough to reform the malpractice system. But there is also a reason from the patient perspective. Experts contend that the medical malpractice system has 3 purposes: (1) to provide prompt and timely compensation to people who are harmed by mistakes; (2) to hold hospitals, physicians, and other providers accountable for their mistakes; and (3) to provide an incentive for providers to take action to reduce the mistakes and improve the quality of care they provide.

It turns out that the current system does a poor job of achieving any of these 3 goals. A massive study involving over 30,000 medical records in the state of New York examined how well the system functioned. In particular, by reviewing hospital records and asking experts to evaluate the cases, Harvard researchers determined how often adverse events happened to patients, how often the adverse event occurred because the physician and/or hospital was negligent, how often physicians and hospitals were sued when mistakes happened, and how often they were sued when no mistake happened (frivolous law suits) (see Figure 4.12).

FIGURE 4.12 Frequency of medical mistakes and malpractice suits, New York State study

MEASURE	NUMBER (%)
Total number of cases reviewed	30,195 (100%)
Total number of adverse events	1,133 (3.75%)
Total number of adverse events due to provider negligence	280 (0.93%) (or 24.7% of all adverse events)
Total number of malpractice suits	47 (0.16%)
Total number of adverse events due to negligence that resulted in a malpractice suit	8 (2.86% of adverse events due negligence)
Total number of malpractice suits that were *not* caused by negligence	39

Source: A. R. Localio et al. "Relation between malpractice claims and adverse events due to negligence: results of the Harvard Medical Practice Study III." *New England Journal of Medicine* 325.4 (1991): 245–251.

About 4% of cases had an adverse event. In most of these the adverse event was unrelated to the physician's or hospital's performance. About a quarter of those adverse events—or 1% of all cases—were due to negligence by a physician, hospital, or other provider.

But here is the crazy part. Of the negligence cases only 3% resulted in a malpractice suit. That means 97% of the time when a physician or hospital commits a mistake that harms a patient, there is no lawsuit. Conversely, of all the malpractice cases filed, over 80% of malpractice suits are not related to an adverse event that was caused by a physician, hospital, or other provider mistake. Other studies show that even after a case goes to court, there is little relationship between the extent of injury and the amount awarded to patients.

The malpractice system is also not efficient. According to a health research brief published by RAND, the average time to settle a malpractice lawsuit is 20.3 months. Further, only about 40 cents of every dollar in malpractice premiums paid by physicians goes to injured patients; the rest is absorbed in administrative and litigation costs and insurance company profits. Finally, there is scant evidence that malpractice suits lead to improved care in the health care system. As one expert put it, "The tort system tends to be defended primarily on the basis of its deterrent effect, but the available evidence suggests that deterrence of medical error is limited at best."

From any perspective the malpractice system is not working. From the patient perspective, most who have been harmed by preventable medical negligence do not sue and are not compensated. This may be because suits, even when justified, take a long time and are very, very costly. And the malpractice system does not seem to improve the overall quality of health care.

From the physician perspective it is almost inevitable that any given physician will be sued in the course of their career. And yet it appears that about 80% of these suits are "frivolous" in the sense that they are not the result of a preventable mistake by the physician or the hospital.

Finally, there is the cost issue. Many physicians are convinced that the high rate of medical malpractice suits encourage high levels of defensive medicine and excessive costs, such as MRIs of the head after mild trauma that are unnecessary according to professional guidelines but are done just in case of a lawsuit, or multiple ultrasounds for a normal pregnancy. Ascertaining the amount of health care spending directly attributable to defensive medicine is difficult because physicians do not have to offer a single reason why they are ordering a test or treatment.

Even if the cost of defensive medicine to the total health care system is small, the malpractice system is clearly defective. It fails to achieve any of its 3 goals: it does not fairly compensate patients harmed by physician and/or hospital negligence, it does not settle cases quickly or cost effectively, and it holds a guillotine over physicians who are likely to be sued no matter how conscientiously they practice and in which many of the suits are frivolous. Finally, there appears to be little impact on improving health care. A worse system is hard to imagine.

There have been multiple proposals to reform the malpractice system. The University of Michigan has introduced a program to encourage all hospital employees to report adverse events. These are investigated, and any malpractice is immediately reported to the patients and a standard compensation offer is provided. This program has reduced lawsuits, led to more prompt resolution of cases, and lowered costs. In 2006 Barack Obama and Hillary Clinton sponsored legislation to encourage hospitals and others to adopt this kind of approach.

Others, myself included, favor a "safe harbors" approach. Physicians and hospitals would be presumed innocent if they implemented electronic health records with algorithms to help them provide high-quality care and provided care consistent with guidelines as determined by professional societies. Patients could still sue if they demonstrated that the guidelines were not followed or that, for some reason, the guideline treatment was not appropriate. I like this approach because it encourages adherence to established quality of standards.

And there are many other proposals, such as specialized malpractice courts. Regardless, there is always a challenge in adopting malpractice reform. Because malpractice oversight is not the responsibility of the federal government, malpractice laws are enacted at the state level, making national, widespread change difficult. Indeed, President Bush advocated for malpractice reform. For 6 of the 8 years of his presidency the Republicans controlled both houses of Congress, and yet President Bush failed to enact any medical malpractice reform.

House Speak John Boehner and the Republican Senate leader Mitch McConnell, among many others, claim that the United States has "the finest health care system in the world." By any metric this statement is almost certainly false. There are places and specific diseases for which the care available at particular US hospitals or by particular US physicians is outstanding, but that is very different from having the finest *system* in the world.

The American health care system is incredibly complex and far and away the most costly in the world: 40% more expensive per person than that of the next most costly system, Norway. And yet, prior to the ACA, there were nearly 50 million uninsured Americans, most of whom are working or are in families in which there is a worker. The actual quality of the system is uneven at best. This is true whether measured in terms of low-technology but life-saving care, such as the control of high blood pressure or the use of vaccines, or of high-technology care for cancer or heart disease. The US health care system is not consistently delivering A much less A+ care. There is little transparency on prices or quality. Physicians are obsessed with medical malpractice and seem to have good reason for being so.

Access, cost, quality, transparency, and malpractice are each in themselves a good justification for health care reform. Together, however, the case is overwhelming. The system needs improving. And people have been trying to reform it for a very long time. But as we will see in the next chapter, those efforts have repeatedly failed. Why?

Part II

HEALTH CARE REFORM

= CHAPTER FIVE =

The Surprising History of Health Care Reform in the United States

The United States has been trying to reform health care for 100 years. It finally got its chance on March 23, 2010, with the enactment of the Affordable Care Act. The history of previous failed efforts to enact legislation is full of unexpected twists: when physicians supported universal coverage but unions opposed it, when Republicans championed comprehensive reform and Democrats stymied change, and when health care reform gave birth to paid public relations campaigns to oppose legislation. A major reason to focus on this history is that the last battle shapes the future war. Previous failed reform efforts have shaped subsequent efforts. When it comes to health care reform, the past is truly prologue.

The First American Health Coverage Bill

There was compulsory health coverage in Revolutionary America. In 1790 the very first US Congress enacted a law requiring owners of ships of more than 150 tons to buy medical insurance for their seamen. The law required "all such advice, medicine, or attendance of physicians, as any of the crew shall stand in need of in case of sickness" and to do it "without any deduction from the wages of such sick seaman or mariners." According to Harvard Law professor Einer Elhauge, this is the first case of compulsory health coverage in the United States. Elhauge argues that in 1798 Congress went further by closing a loophole, the need for hospitalization, and enacted a law requiring seamen to buy hospital insurance for themselves.

Then not much happened regarding compulsory health coverage for another 120 years.

Teddy Roosevelt and the First Attempt to Achieve Universal Coverage

The year 1883 is, in the history of health care reform, a pivotal date. In that year Germany became the first country to enact a health care reform proposal that guaranteed workers health coverage, the Health Insurance Bill of 1883. This revolutionary piece of social policy was championed by a conservative, some would say reactionary politician and member of the Prussian aristocracy, Otto von Bismarck. Bismarck was worried about the potential growth of socialism and the Social Democratic party in Germany. To blunt the appeal of socialism, Bismarck instituted a comprehensive set of welfare programs covering old-age pensions, unemployment, and accident insurance. He also developed health care coverage. (Interestingly, the German Socialists voted against Bismarck's welfare proposals, fearing these would undermine workers' support for their party. Politics is never separate from health care reform in any country.)

Initially, Bismarck wanted the state to be responsible for coverage to win workers' loyalty to the state. Suspicion of Bismarck and expanding state power transformed the policy into compulsory insurance through independent, nonstate insurers called *sickness funds*. Through payroll deductions, both employers and employees contributed to the sickness funds, and the government provided supplemental funding. Recognizing the problem of adverse selection with voluntary insurance, coverage was made compulsory but initially only for industrial workers. Many segments of German society, such as farmers, pensioners, and civil servants, were not included in the health coverage. Now, all Germans have to have coverage through the sickness funds, although the rich can pay a penalty and buy private insurance instead of relying on the sickness funds.

Bismarck's model, based on employment, financed by payroll deductions, and with compulsory coverage through independent insurers, is clearly not socialized medicine or socialist. The state neither provides nor controls the sickness funds, and it neither owns the hospitals nor employs the physicians and other health care workers. Many other European countries, such as Austria in 1888, Hungary in 1891, and Norway in 1909, adopted Bismarck's model. In 1911 Britain enacted its National Insurance Act that provided medical care and replacement of some lost wages if a worker became ill. However, this did not extend to the worker's family.

During the progressive era in the United States health insurance became a national issue. Model health coverage proposals were developed by groups such as the American Association of Labor Legislation (AALL), whose members included some of the nation's leading economists as well as Teddy Roosevelt's personal physician. In the 1912 presidential campaign national health insurance was part of Roosevelt's campaign program. After Roosevelt's defeat progressives pushed for state laws that would provide for all hospital and medical expenses, the cost of maternity labor and delivery as well as replacement income, funeral expenses, and maternity leave. The cost was to be split between employers, workers, and states.

The AALL solicited physician backing, and initially leaders of the American Medical Association were supportive. Indeed, in 1916 the AMA actually authorized a committee to work with the AALL. According to Princeton sociologist Paul Starr, "[T]he AMA and the AALL formed a united front on behalf of health insurance."

But there was also opposition. Fraternal orders, which often provided funeral benefits, opposed state laws. Somewhat surprisingly, so did organized labor. Samuel Gompers, president of the American Federation of Labor, was generally opposed to state welfare policies. He thought unions could do better for workers through their direct negotiations with business. Indeed, Gompers was opposed to state laws related to minimum wage, unemployment insurance, and pensions, fearing workers would look to the state and not the unions for benefits.

Probably the final strike against this phase of health reform came as a result of the United States' entry into World War I. Everything associated with Germany became tainted. Universal health insurance was a "German" idea and, thus, died with the beginning of the war.

In the 1920s, as medical care was becoming more effective and there were fewer physicians (Chapter 1, page 19), costs increasingly became a problem. In 1926 several prominent physicians, economists, and public health officials, including a former president of the AMA, formed the Committee on the Costs of Medical Care (CCMC), a private and privately funded group to study the health care system and develop policy proposals. In 1932 the CCMC issued its recommendations, which rejected compulsory health insurance because of the excessive costs and need for government subsidies. Instead, a majority of the CCMC endorsed voluntary insurance that would promote group practice organizations and prepayment. A minority dissented, opposing group practice in favor of the primacy of individual medical practitioners. The minority endorsed government funding for care of the indigent, thus "relieving the medical profession of this burden." The AMA rejected the majority's proposal and instead embraced the minority's opposition to group practice. There was no agreement on reform.

Franklin Roosevelt

The Great Depression offered the next major opportunity for enactment of universal health coverage. In 1934 President Franklin Roosevelt appointed the Committee on Economic Security (CES), chaired by his secretary of labor, Frances Perkins, the first woman to serve in the US cabinet. The committee's charge was to examine and make recommendations to Roosevelt on the type of social welfare legislation that he should introduce. The committee created a Medical Advisory Committee to study "practical measures for bringing about the better distribution of medical care in the lower income groups." One of the Medical Advisory Committee members was the famed father of neurosurgery, Harvey Cushing, whose daughter had married Franklin Roosevelt's son. Cushing, a Republican who was a fierce defender of the medical profession's prerogatives, ended up endorsing a compromise position, recognizing the inevitability of health insurance but urging local experimentation.

In its report to Roosevelt the Committee on Economic Security strongly supported old-age pensions and unemployment insurance. Although the committee reached a consensus on the importance of health insurance, there was disagreement about its political feasibility. A major source of this disagreement was determining the potential strength of the medical profession's opposition to some form of national health insurance. The conflict over the CCMC's recommendations suggested caution, while the American College of Surgeons' endorsement of compulsory health insurance in 1934 seemed encouraging. But the AMA and other physician leaders came out strongly against compulsory health insurance. For instance, in early 1935 the AMA held a special meeting that affirmed its opposition to compulsory health insurance. Perkins and other Committee members were worried that if comprehensive social welfare legislation included health insurance, opposition by physicians would torpedo the entire bill, including the provisions for Social Security. Ultimately, the Social Security Act was passed in August 1935. Its summary states that it is:

> an act to provide for the general welfare by establishing a system of Federal old-age benefits, and by enabling the several States to make more adequate provision for aged persons, blind persons, dependent and crippled children, maternal and child welfare, public health, and the administration of their unemployment compensation laws; to establish a Social Security Board; to raise revenue; and for other purposes.

Conspicuously, there is no mention of health insurance; for political reasons, it was never included. Opposition from organized medicine blocked any New Deal health insurance legislation. Then, the Republicans' significant gains in the 1938 mid-term election stymied any further effort at health care reform.

In 1943 Senators Robert Wagner (D-New York) and James Murray (D-Montana) and Representative John Dingell (D-Michigan) introduced a bill for comprehensive, compulsory health insurance through the Social Security system. The bill proposed to establish a medical care and hospitalization fund that covered all physician care and 30 days of hospitalization. Medications and dental care were excluded. Patients would be free to choose their physician from any participating doctor, and the fund would pay the bill. The fund was financed by a 1.5% payroll tax on the first $3,000 of income on both employers and employees. Unions and farm organizations supported the Wagner-Murray-Dingell Bill, but the AMA and organized medicine opposed it. The bill never came to a vote in Congress in 1943.

Throughout his presidency Roosevelt waffled on his support of compulsory health insurance. Ever the politician weighing what policies he would support by whether he could enact them, FDR often privately voiced support for compulsory health insurance but seemed to have viewed it as politically dangerous. Even as he sometimes seemed on the brink of pushing for legislation, as in 1938, Roosevelt never consistently endorsed and threw his political support behind health insurance. However, in his 1944 presidential election campaign he began calling for an "Economic Bill of Rights" that included the right to adequate medical care. And in January 1945 his budget called for an expansion of Social Security to include medical care.

Paul Starr, a Princeton sociologist of the American health system, succinctly summarizes the first 2 attempts at health care reform: "Just as the AALL's campaign ran into the declining fortunes of Progressivism and then World War I, so the campaign of the thirties ran into the declining fortunes of the New Deal and then World War II."

Republican Support for Health Care Reform

In California a Republican governor, Earl Warren, called for comprehensive, compulsory health insurance in his 1945 State of the State Address. Having consulted with the California Medical Association (CMA), Warren thought he had their support. Instead, however, the CMA hired Whitaker and Baxter, the first ever political consulting firm, to run a campaign opposing Warren's plan. The CMA, with Whitaker and Baxter, mobilized physicians to write to newspapers and give public speeches against compulsory health insurance with the slogan "Political medicine is bad medicine." They ran slews of ads against Warren's plan and proposed an alternative: voluntary health insurance.

In 1945 the bill for compulsory health insurance, which the California public strongly supported, lost by one vote in the California legislature.

Reintroduced the next year, Whitaker and Baxter defeated it again. This defeat by a well-financed, powerful special interest group was a major cause of Earl Warren's shift to being a strong civil rights liberal.

In 1946 Richard Nixon ran his first campaign, defeating a 5-term Democratic congressman. His campaign included what became characteristic for him: red-baiting charges that his opponent, Representative Jerry Voorhis, was linked to Communist organizations. Nixon had grown up poor, and 2 of his brothers had died of tuberculosis. Because of this, one of Representative Nixon's early initiatives was focused on health care. With Representative Jacob Javits (R-New York), he cosponsored the National Health Care Act of 1950. The main purpose of the bill was "to enable voluntary pre-payment health services plans to make their services generally available in the communities which they serve at charges based on the income of subscribers." The Javits-Nixon proposal used federal money to partially support state programs that provided income-linked subsidies for up to $5,000 of income for Americans to purchase prepaid health coverage from not-for-profit health plans—it was voluntary, not compulsory.

The Democrats spurned this approach.

Harry Truman and the Charge of "Socialized Medicine"

On both civil rights and health care Franklin Roosevelt hardly pushed or risked any political capital and, thus, may have missed some key opportunities. Conversely, on both issues, Truman took bold and politically risky positions for which history has lionized him. Indeed, Truman was probably the president who was the strongest advocate for comprehensive, compulsory health insurance.

In April 1945 Roosevelt died of a stroke, and Truman became president. The Wagner-Murray-Dingell Bill was then reintroduced in May 1945 with some modifications. On November 19, 1945, 3 months after the end of World War II, President Truman sent a special message to Congress urging they enact national health legislation that included compulsory health insurance under the Social Security system to cover medical, hospital, nursing, laboratory, and dental care (see Figure 5.1). Truman

FIGURE 5.1. Landmark dates in the history of health care reform

DATE	ACTION
November 19, 1945	First time a president (Truman) sends a bill for universal health care insurance, National Health Insurance, to Congress.
March 1960	First time the House Ways and Means Committee votes on a government health insurance bill. Defeated.
September 26, 1960	First time Senate votes on a government health insurance bill. Both Forand's Medicare and Javits's "insurance subsidy" bills are defeated. The Kerr-Mills Eldercare bill with federal-state financing of services for indigent elderly is passed and ultimately enacted as law.
September 2, 1964	First time a chamber of Congress, the Senate, passes a government health insurance plan, King-Anderson Medicare Bill 49–44.
April 8, 1965	First time the House passes a government health insurance plan, Mills Medicare and Medicaid bill, Social Security Amendments of 1965, 313–115.
July 30, 1965	First piece of national health insurance legislation is signed into law in Independence, Missouri.

also asked for support of medical research, grants to states to support maternal and child health programs, and funds for the construction of hospitals and other health facilities. Truman sent Congress a redrafted Wagner-Murray-Dingell Bill. The proposal was called National Health Insurance and was integral to Truman's Fair Deal program. This was the first time in American history that an administration had introduced national health insurance legislation.

Even though it was controlled by Democrats, the House Ways and Means Committee refused to hold hearings on Truman's bill, while the Senate's hearing became bogged down in debates about whether the bill was "socialistic." Simultaneously, Britain enacted the National Health Service Act to form "a comprehensive health service designed to secure improvement in the physical and mental health of the people of England and Wales and the prevention, diagnosis, and treatment of illness." Britain's National Health Service was implemented in 1948.

In 1946 Congress passed the Hill-Burton Act to fund hospital construction (Chapter 1, pages 20–21). But the 1946 elections halted Truman's reform proposal. For the first time since 1932 the Republicans gained control of Congress, having run in opposition to Roosevelt's New Deal and Truman's Fair Deal with the slogan "Had Enough?"

Subsequent events shifted national attention away from health insurance. Unions became embroiled in a fight against Republican efforts to curtail their power through the Taft-Hartley Act. (The unions lost.) The Cold War began in earnest and the Truman administration was actively promoting the Marshall Plan to rebuild Europe as a bulwark again Communism. Consequently, President Truman's 1948 State of the Union Address omitted any reference to his National Health Insurance proposal.

Throughout 1948 the chances for health care legislation were not taken seriously. Truman was widely perceived to be a lame-duck president, the Cold War was raging, and the 1948 Democratic platform failed to include Truman's National Health Insurance program. Nevertheless, during the campaign Truman frequently called for passage of his health insurance proposal and attacked the "do nothing" Republican Congress for its failure to address health care. Truman's emphasis on health care was probably less aimed at Republicans and more at keeping liberals from defecting to Henry Wallace, the third-party candidate of the left.

Because few people believed Truman would win, his victory—and his restoration of Congress to Democratic control—was huge, and some interpreted it as a strong endorsement of his health insurance program. Panicked, the AMA responded by assessing each member an extra $25 so they could hire the Whitaker and Baxter political consulting firm to oppose Truman's plan. The firm summarized its campaign objectives this way:

> 1. The *immediate objective* is the defeat of the compulsory health insurance program pending in Congress. 2. The *long-term* objective is to put a permanent stop to the agitation for socialized medicine in this country by (a) awakening the people to the danger of a politically controlled, government-regulated health system; (b) convincing the people, through a Nation wide campaign of education, of the superior advantages of private medicine, as practiced in America, over the State-dominated medical systems of other countries; (c) stimulating the growth of voluntary health insurance systems to take the economic

shock out of illness and increase the availability of medical care to the American people.

In the end Whitaker and Baxter spent nearly $5 million in AMA money to defeat Truman's plan. They collected key endorsements from the American Bar Association, American Dental Association, and American Legion and were able to "flip" the Catholic Church from supporting national health insurance to opposing it. They effectively deployed the charge of "socialized medicine" against Truman's plan. This charge also resonated with the nation's growing anticommunism and its great fear when, in 1949, the Soviet Union unexpectedly exploded its first atomic weapon and, in 1950, when Communist North Korea invaded South Korea.

The 1950 US elections saw the defeat of several key senators who supported the reform. In addition, an increasing number of middle-class Americans were getting health insurance through their employers (Chapter 1, page 31). Thus, by the middle of 1951, interest in compulsory national health insurance legislation was petering out and the AMA was declaring victory.

Kennedy Versus Nixon in 1960: Who Supported Comprehensive Health Care Reform?

Beginning in the mid-1950s, 2 trends pushed health reform back on the national stage: the growing costs of health care, especially hospital care, and the increasingly apparent fact that an employer-based health insurance arrangement would inherently exclude certain groups. One particularly sympathetic group was the elderly who were no longer working and could not be covered through employers.

In 1957 Aime Forand (D-Rhode Island), who sat on the House Ways and Means Committee, sponsored a bill called Medicare. The proposal would include coverage for hospital costs in Social Security and pay for it through a payroll tax. In 1958 Congress began holding hearings on health coverage for the elderly. The American Hospital Association endorsed the bill because hospitals were increasingly bearing the burden of providing uncompensated care to the elderly. As part of its strategy to oppose the legislation, the AMA urged physicians to voluntarily reduce their bills to the elderly. Many other organizations also opposed the legislation, including the US Chamber of Commerce, the National Association of Manufacturers, the pharmaceutical companies, and the newly formed Health Insurance Association of America.

Over the next few years congressional hearings on the issue of health care for the aged helped galvanize public support. However, the congressional committees with jurisdiction over health care were controlled by conservatives, who stymied efforts to enact legislation. Finally, in March 1960, Forand forced a vote in the House Ways and Means Committee. Although his bill was defeated, the vote was a symbolic victory; it was the first vote on health insurance ever by this powerful committee. Importantly, the defeat did not diffuse pressure for some kind of coverage for the elderly (see Figure 5.1).

In response to persistent public pressure, Republicans began developing an alternative approach. Eisenhower's secretary of health, education, and welfare, Arthur Flemming, offered a proposal outside of the Social Security framework. His plan provided for sliding-scale subsidies for low-income elderly to voluntarily purchase private health insurance. Senator Jacob Javits introduced Flemming's so-called subsidy plan into Congress, and Vice President Nixon swung behind the proposal and persuaded President Eisenhower, who had long avoided health reform issues, to endorse it.

Also responding to the continuing pressure, Representative Wilbur Mills (D-Arkansas), chairman of the Ways and Means Committee, sought to find a compromise. In collaboration with Senator Kerr (D-Oklahoma), his modest program provided federal grants to states, which could then provide health coverage to the aged poor. This was known as Eldercare.

Throughout the spring and summer of 1960 there was a deadlock between the Democrats' Medicare proposal, the Republican plan for the voluntary purchase of private insurance, and the Kerr-Mills Eldercare plan. Then, in an unusual postconvention August session, all 3 bills were debated and voted on in the Senate. The Republican subsidy plan was defeated on a party-line vote: 67 to 28. Medicare, supported by the

Democratic presidential and vice presidential candidates, Kennedy and Johnson, was defeated by a coalition of Republicans and conservative Democrats, 51 to 44. Finally the Kerr-Mills Eldercare bill passed 91 to 2. Although Eldercare fell far short of universal coverage for the elderly, this marked the first time a compulsory health insurance bill of any kind, Medicare, was brought to a congressional vote.

Interestingly, this vote did not remove health care as an election-year issue. The September 26 Kennedy-Nixon debate focused on domestic issues. Both candidates agreed on the need to address health care coverage, especially for the aged, but they clashed on the specifics of their respective proposals.

In 1961 Forand left Congress, but Cecil King (D-California) modified the Medicare Bill to cover inpatient hospital services, skilled nursing home services, home health services, and outpatient hospital diagnostic services for Social Security beneficiaries over 65. Payment would be the "reasonable" cost of services.

Also in 1961, then-actor Ronald Reagan released a 10-minute record attacking the Medicare Bill, arguing that "one of the traditional methods of imposing *statism* or socialism on a people has been by way of *medicine*. It's very easy to disguise a medical program as a humanitarian project, most people are a little reluctant to oppose anything that suggests medical care for people who possibly can't afford it." He ended by asking his listeners to write to Congress with the message, "We do not want socialized medicine." The American Medical Association secretly financed Reagan's recording and its distribution.

Unsolved, health care remained an issue on the national agenda. In part this was because after 18 months only about half of the states had opted into Eldercare. And, as a 1963 report by the Senate's Special Committee on Aging wrote damningly, "After 3 years of operation, the Kerr-Mills Medical Assistance for the Aged (MAA) program [Eldercare] has proved to be at best an ineffective and piecemeal approach to the health problems of the Nation's 18 million older citizens."

Responding to public pressure, moderate Republicans led by New York Governor Nelson Rockefeller and, again, Senator Javits were moving to accept the Social Security framework either to cover hospital admissions or to buy private insurance. President Kennedy continued to press for Medicare, most notably in a nationally televised address from Madison Square Garden on May 20, 1962. The AMA continued to strenuously fight against it. Ultimately, there was still insufficient support on the Ways and Means Committee to pass the Medicare bill.

Then, President Kennedy's assassination in November 1963 generated huge national interest in completing his legislative agenda, particularly health care. Indeed, in his first speech to Congress President Johnson urged the passage of Medicare. Quickly thereafter, in February 1964, he sent a special health care message to Congress, claiming Americans want, need, and can afford "the best of health not just for those of comfortable means, but for all our citizens old and young, rich and poor." Johnson proposed hospital insurance based on Social Security payments for seniors, a 5-year expansion of Hill-Burton to build more hospitals, as well as long-term care facilities, a new program to provide grants for establishing medical group practices, and support for more nursing schools.

Nothing happened. The House Ways and Means Committee would not budge. So, using his unparalleled knowledge and skill of the legislative process, President Johnson engineered a mechanism to force a vote. The House had just passed an increase in the Social Security benefits. Bypassing the Senate Finance Committee, which was opposed to Medicare, Johnson had the Medicare proposal included as an amendment to this benefit bill on the Senate floor. The amendment passed on September 2, 1964, and marked the first time in history a chamber of Congress passed a government-based compulsory health insurance bill. Senator Barry Goldwater, the Republican presidential candidate, voted against it. However, because the House had not voted on the Medicare bill, it had to go to a conference committee, which ended up being deadlocked, so the bill never became law. Another defeat.

Medicare and Medicaid

It was not until Lyndon Johnson's and the Democrats' stunning electoral victory in the 1964 election that Congress began to move—indeed, run—on health care. Johnson won a smashing victory with 61.1% of the vote—the highest percentage of popular votes since the 1820 election—and 486 electoral votes. In addition, the Democrats picked up 2 Senate seats, for a total of 68, and 37 House seats, giving them a two-thirds House majority, the largest since Roosevelt's 1936 landslide. This victory changed everything.

On January 4, 1965, with the new Congress, Representative King's modified version of Medicare was the first bill introduced in both the House and Senate—H.R.1 and S.1. On January 7, 1965, in his first address to Congress, entitled "Advancing the Nation's Health," President Johnson vowed to extend Social Security to include health coverage of the elderly and to enact a program to cover health services for low-income children.

Spurred by the election, Representative Mills took personal control of drafting the health care legislation. Representative John Byrnes, the ranking Republican on the Ways and Means Committee, offered a plan to create a federally administered health insurance program that was voluntary—the elderly could opt to join or not. The government would provide income-linked subsidies to enable the elderly to pay the premiums. Funding would come from general revenues rather than a Social Security–like payroll tax.

In just 2 months Mills amalgamated all the proposals into the Social Security Amendments of 1965, otherwise known as Medicare and Medicaid.

1) Medicare Part A that covers hospitalization was a version of the original Forand and King proposal. Employer and employee payroll taxes contributed to a trust fund that paid for hospital-based care. The benefit was 90 days of hospital care, 100 days of nursing home care, and 100 home nursing visits in each illness episode. It also covered hospital outpatient services.
2) Medicare Part B that covers physician office visits and other outpatient care was a gesture to the Republicans. It used Byrnes's government-subsidized voluntary insurance framework to pay for physicians' fees, additional home nursing services, diagnostic and laboratory work, certain kinds of therapy, and ambulance, if necessary.

3) Medicaid was the original Kerr-Mills Eldercare program expanded to the nonelderly indigent. This was a means-tested, shared federal-state program with comprehensive coverage of health services.

Of course, not everything changed. After the 1964 election the AMA held a meeting and reaffirmed its opposition to any compulsory government-sponsored health insurance program like Medicare. Its alternative was a modified version of the old plan in which the federal and state governments would provide subsidies for the poor elderly to purchase private insurance.

On March 23, 1965, less than 3 months after the new Congress convened, the Ways and Means committee voted 17–8 for the Mills Bill. After 1 single day of debate Medicare and Medicaid passed the House of Representatives, 313–115. After 3 days of debate the Senate passed the legislation, 68–21. A conference reconciled differences between the House and Senate versions, and on July 30, 1965, just over 6 months after President Johnson's inauguration, he flew to Independence, Missouri, and signed Medicare and Medicaid into law with President Truman sitting at his side.

Angry and suspicious, physicians and hospitals debated boycotting Medicare. To mollify their opposition, the government adopted 2 policies in implementation that were very favorable to them. First, instead of paying directly, the government paid through private insurance companies. Blue Cross became the "fiscal intermediary" for Part A, processing claims and providing reimbursement to hospitals, while Blue Shield plans were "carriers" to pay for physician services. This was a classic case of path dependence: it utilized the existing insurance-provider relationships and ensured Medicare was amalgamated to the existing health-financing infrastructure. Second, and more importantly, the government agreed to pay hospitals based on their costs and included depreciation for capital investments in buildings and equipment. This had the effect of incentivizing hospital expansion, because new, expensive facilities received higher payments.

Both these policies were expensive. But they were viewed as necessary to buy off hospitals, physicians, and insurance companies and ensure their cooperation with—if not support of—Medicare during its initial launch. Unfortunately, done for political reasons and momentary expediency, they ended up encouraging perverse incentives, such as the emphasis on hospital expansion, hospital-based care, and fragmentation of the delivery of care.

Eleven months after enactment, on July 1, 1966, people over 65 years of age began receiving Medicare benefits.

Nixon, Kennedy, and Mills

Surprisingly, enactment of Medicare and Medicaid, though major achievements, hardly even slowed the calls for additional, large-scale health care reform. The 1969 National Governors Conference endorsed the need for national health insurance. In 1970 the Senate Finance Committee, chaired by Russell Long (D-Louisiana), hardly a liberal, endorsed a national catastrophic health insurance plan. Simultaneously, Senator Abraham Ribicoff (D-Connecticut), with the support of a Republican, Governor Rockefeller of New York, introduced a Medicare-for-all plan. Making health care his signature issue, Senator Edward Kennedy proposed the Health Security Act. The basic idea was for a single federal health insurance system to replace all private insurance. It would have a budget, consumers would have no deductibles or co-pays, and it would be paid for with a payroll tax.

Simultaneously, the business community was worrying about health care costs. Economy-wide inflation was high, running at about 6%. Both general health care spending and federal health care spending were rapidly rising (see Figure 5.2). To control inflation, in August 1971 Nixon instituted wage and price controls.

Among health policy experts there was increasing interest in ending the use of fee-for-service payment to hospitals and physicians. Paul Ellwood, a Minnesota neurologist, argued loudly against fee-for-service medicine on the grounds that it incentivized doing more interventions while it also disincentivized keeping patients healthy. He advocated for prepaid group practice. But this elicited the ire of the American Medical Association, so he relabeled his idea health maintenance organizations—HMOs.

FIGURE 5.2 Federal and national health expenditure 1962–1971

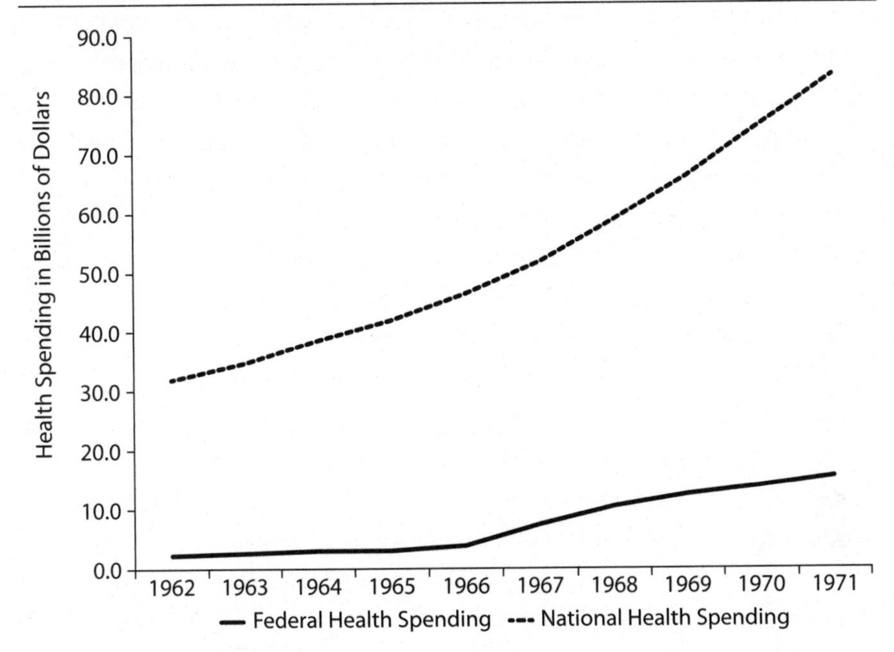

Source: The Altarum Institute.

Worried about health care inflation and the growing advocacy from both Democrats and Republicans for national health insurance, Nixon authorized his staff to develop an alternative. On February 18, 1971, Nixon sent a special message to Congress in which he outlined his national health strategy. It contained 4 key elements:

1) An employer mandate to provide health insurance to employees.
2) A Family Health Insurance Plan to replace Medicaid for the poor, providing them with subsidized health insurance. (Medicaid would be kept for the aged poor, blind and disabled.)
3) Requiring each state to establish insurance pools for people who did not qualify for employer coverage, the family health insurance plan, or traditional Medicare or Medicaid.
4) Encouragement but no requirement to offer health maintenance organizations.

Nixon stated the key elements this way:

> The National Health Insurance Standards Act would require employers to provide adequate health insurance for their employees, who would share in underwriting its costs. This approach follows precedents of long-standing under which personal security—and thus national economic progress—has been enhanced by requiring employers to provide minimum wages and disability and retirement benefits and to observe occupational health and safety standards.
>
> Required coverages would include not less than $50,000 protection against catastrophic costs for each family member; hospital services; physician services both in and out of a hospital; maternity care; well-baby care (including immunizations); laboratory expenses and certain other costs.
>
> The proposed package would include certain deductibles and coinsurance features, which would help keep costs down by encouraging the use of more efficient health care procedures. It would permit many workers, as an alternative to paying separate fees for services, to purchase instead memberships in a Health Maintenance Organization.

This marked a shift in the national debate in 2 ways. First, a consensus that now included Republican Party leaders seemed to emerge that health insurance should be made mandatory and universal, not just voluntary. Second, the Republicans embraced a liberal idea, moving off fee-for-service to prepaid health care. For liberals this was justified by their appeal to cooperatives; for conservatives this was justified as a cost-control measure. Importantly, there was a growing policy consensus.

By July 1971 22 separate health insurance bills were before Congress. Not a single one was ever voted out of committee.

If comprehensive reform could not be enacted, then at least more modest expansions could be. The Social Security Amendments of 1972 expanded Medicare coverage to the severely disabled and Americans with end-stage renal disease needing dialysis. Also, the Medicare Part A payroll tax was increased over a 14-year period from 1.1% to 1.45%. In 1973 the Health Maintenance Organization Act required employers with 25 or more employees to offer federally certified HMO coverage if they offered their employees traditional health insurance. The act also provided grants and loans to develop and expand HMOs.

It looked like 1974 might finally be the year for comprehensive health care reform. In October 1973 Senator Ribicoff and Senator Russell Long cosponsored a catastrophic health insurance bill. In February 1974 Nixon revised his plan and introduced his Comprehensive Health Insurance Plan (CHIP). Every American would be covered in one of 3 ways: through their employer, by Medicare, or through a new health insurance plan that would cover all poor and provide income-linked subsidies for purchasing private insurance. Medicaid would be ended. In addition, Medicare benefits would be expanded to include drugs and an out-of-pocket maximum. Employers would have to cover at least 65% of the health insurance premium. The Chamber of Commerce and other business groups supported Nixon's CHIP plan.

In April 1974 Senator Kennedy and Representative Mills, chair of the House Ways and Means Committee, cosponsored a bill that provided for national health insurance, with private insurers now acting as fiscal intermediaries, basically paying hospitals and physicians. This new bill's benefits were almost identical to those in the Nixon Bill, and it included co-payments and out-of-pocket maximums.

Suddenly, a Republican president, 2 leading Democratic senators, and the most powerful House member on health care seemed aligned. There was a plausible consensus deal. Then it all fell apart for the usual Washington reasons: a scandal. Actually, 2 scandals.

Through the spring and summer of 1974 Nixon became increasingly embroiled in the Watergate scandal. Then, at 2 a.m. on October 7, Fanne Foxe, an Argentine "exotic dancer," fell out of Representative Mills's car into the Tidal Basin. He appeared the next day with a big gash on his face. A sex scandal swept Washington, and Mills was forced to resign in disgrace as chair of the Ways and Means Committee. The strong politician who might have steered a bill through the House was out.

Envisioning a huge election victory in November 1974, unions and other liberal organizations opposed compromising with Nixon. They insisted on Kennedy's original Health Security proposal for a national health insurance scheme with no insurance companies and no deductibles or co-pays.

Ultimately, nothing happened. Everyone insisted on their preferred plan. Everyone thought they had more leverage than others and refused to compromise. After 1974 Senator Kennedy retreated to his more radical Health Security Act. Conservative Democrats stuck to their catastrophic health insurance ideas. Republican support for comprehensive health care reform dissipated. Another moment for comprehensive health care reform evaporated.

After this there was little movement all the way until the early 1990s.

Harris Wofford's Right to a Doctor Epiphany

During the 1980s there was not much attention to health care on the political stage. In the early to mid-1980s CMS changed how it paid hospitals to a lump-sum diagnosis-related groups (DRGs) payment for an episode of care instead of based on hospital bills (Chapter 2, page 70). But there was not a push to reform the whole system. From late 1982 to early 1990, the Reagan years, the economy experienced robust growth. Then, just after the fall of the Berlin Wall, the economy tilted into a recession.

On April 4, 1991, Senator John Heinz, a moderate Republican from Pennsylvania and heir to the Heinz Ketchup fortune, died in a small plane crash. After sounding out a few more promising candidates, the Democratic governor of Pennsylvania settled on his fourth choice, appointing a little-known ex-Kennedy aide and ex-college president, Harris Wofford, to the vacant position.

Under Pennsylvania law a special election was scheduled for the following November to fill out the remainder of Senator Heinz's term. The Republicans were running the former Pennsylvania governor and the first President Bush's sitting attorney general, Dick Thornburgh. He looked like a shoe-in. Conversely, Wofford was a nobody. His campaign was going nowhere and he was down 47% in the polls.

It was clear the election would be, first and foremost, about jobs and the economy. When Wofford's campaign polled the public on what issues mattered to them, jobs rose to the top; health care did not seem to be on anyone's radar. But as Pennsylvania's former secretary of labor and industry, Wofford understood that what was really motivating voters' concern about jobs was actually a concern about health care coverage. Wofford pointed out to his political staff that a key problem for employers was the growing cost of health care and that a key problem for people who lost their jobs or were fearful of losing their jobs was loss of health insurance. As the public labeled the problem jobs, Wofford translated that to be a concern about health care.

For campaign manager Paul Begala, Wofford's logic certainly made sense. But unless he could find a compelling way to sell the issue, barnstorming Pennsylvania to tell voters about a health care plan wouldn't make a dent in the candidate's poll deficit. Then a serendipitous exchange at a campaign fundraiser changed the course of the campaign—and perhaps the next decade of health policy.

After delivering his standard stump speech Wofford was approached by an ophthalmologist looking to bend his ear. What the doctor said was an epiphany for Wofford. "Your intellectual forbearers—lawyers—were the ones who drafted the Constitution," the ophthalmologist argued, "and because law was important to them, they put in a host of *legal* protections, like the right to have an attorney if you break the law. If *my* intellectual forbearers wrote the Constitution, it would have said sick people have the right to a doctor."

Because the candidate was relatively unknown, the campaign pollster tested a few alternative ways to introduce Wofford to the public, gauging the impact of various personas on voters' likelihood to cast a ballot for him. One alternative highlighted his professional experiences as an aide to President Kennedy and Martin Luther King Jr. That one didn't work. Another alternative stressed his lifelong dedication to education and his years as a university president. That one didn't work. Finally, they tested a persona that emphasized his commitment to bringing jobs to the state of Pennsylvania and guaranteeing universal health care coverage. When they used this introduction Wofford's popularity soared past Thornburgh. All they needed to do was deploy the health care message and the 47-point polling deficit would be erased.

In early August the campaign held an important strategy session. The polling data said that by emphasizing health care, Wofford had a shot at winning. The campaign threw a "Hail Mary," gambling everything on the health care message. Soon Wofford's stump speech and commercials were declaring the campaign's new slogan: "The Constitution says that if you are charged with a crime, you have a right to a lawyer. But it's even more fundamental that if you're sick, you should have the right to a doctor."

Wofford ended up defying the early polls and winning with 55% of the vote, a veritable landslide in Pennsylvania. But his victory also changed the 1992 presidential election. First, it made President Bush, who had overseen the fall of the Soviet Union and the Berlin Wall, seem vulnerable, especially on domestic issues. Second, it put health care at the center of the campaign.

Clinton's Health Care Reform Effort

Initially candidate Bill Clinton did not have a health insurance plan. Indeed, at a meeting in November 1991 where he was trying to woo my brother Rahm to be his national campaign finance director, a meeting Rahm invited me to for no obvious reason, Clinton found out what I did and said he would be open to any good ideas I may have about how to reform the health care system. The candidate's first head of health care was a total unknown, Atul Gwande, who was taking time off from being a medical student to work on the campaign.

In the early 1990s health care policy experts were debating Alain Enthoven's managed competition model of health care. Enthoven defined it as a "purchasing strategy to obtain maximum value for consumers and employers, using rules for competition derived from microeconomic principles." The basic idea is that people should choose among a variety of health insurance options in a structured competitive marketplace for insurers. The government or employer contributions are linked to the premium for the lowest- or second lowest–cost plan. If people want a more expensive option, one with a wider network of physicians or more drugs on the formulary, they pay the premium difference. That is, if the insurance option they prefer has a wide choice of physicians and hospitals as well as low deductibles, its premium is likely to exceed their employer's or the government's contribution, and then the consumer must pay the price difference. The idea is to empower people to make prudent health insurance choices that are likely to drive down prices through competition. Enthoven viewed this as working within the employer-based system, so that most of the competitive marketplaces would be run by employers. This approach resonated with Clinton's overall belief that market-based solutions were preferable, and soon he was speaking the language of managed competition.

As one of his first actions as president Bill Clinton established the Task Force on National Health Care Reform under the direction of his wife with the assistance of his old friend, Ira Magaziner. The task force was entrusted to develop a comprehensive health care reform proposal. Over 500 people became involved in the task force's 34 different committees that famously met in secret in the Old Executive Office Building, the one just west of the White House on Pennsylvania Avenue. Tight restrictions on communication with the media and Congress kept the country uninformed about the policy being developed.

Efforts to enact a budget and a tax increase delayed introduction of Clinton's health reform legislation. On September 22, 1993, after 9 months of work, President Clinton outlined his plan to a joint session of Congress. However, the need to pass the North American Free Trade Agreement further delayed health care reform legislation. Finally, in November 1993, the 1,342-page Health Security Act bill was submitted to Congress. The First Lady testified to Congress in a performance that impressed even her critics in her understanding of the details of health economics and the health care system. The legislation's core requirements included:

1) Health alliances would be established as state and substate regional purchasing agents run by states in compliance with federal standards. Alliances would consolidate the purchasing power of small businesses and individuals as well as Medicaid recipients and foster competition among health insurance companies that offered both health maintenance organizations and traditional fee-for-service health plans. Alliances were also supposed to collect and distribute premiums, certify health plans and offer them to consumers, ensure that average premiums grow no faster than federally set limits, and disseminate performance data.
2) Employers would be required to provide health insurance to all of their employees. Very large employers (over 5,000 employees) could opt out of the alliances and negotiate directly with insurers for the plans they would offer. Smaller employers would go

through the health alliances. Employers would pay at least 80% of the insurance premium.

3) Employees could select from among competing health maintenance organizations. Workers would be responsible for up to 20% of the insurance premium.
4) Government would subsidize costs so that large employers would not have to pay more than 7.9% of payroll and small employers would not pay more than 3.5% of payroll in health insurance premiums. Similarly, government would subsidize individuals with incomes below 150% of the federal poverty line who lacked employer-sponsored insurance.
5) Medicare would continue, and seniors would receive a drug benefit.
6) Medicaid would pay for the poor to get insurance through the health alliances.
7) There would be a 7-member, presidentially appointed national health board that would monitor the health alliances' functioning, delineate and modify the standard benefit package with evolving biomedical technology and health needs, and set regional medical spending ceilings.
8) The bill was supposed to cost $331 billion, financed by a 75 cent-per-package cigarette tax along with the proposed savings of $124 billion in Medicare and $65 billion in Medicaid through lower health care inflation.

After Clinton's September speech public opinion strongly supported health care reform and universal coverage. Interestingly the medical profession supported the employer mandate. The business community initially was supportive of reform efforts, especially because of their interest in controlling health care costs. Even the US Chamber of Commerce was momentarily willing to support reform and an employer mandate. Union support, however, was lukewarm; they preferred a single-payer plan over the Health Security Act's more market-friendly approach, but they did not want to oppose a Democratic president openly.

For obvious reasons the health insurance industry was strongly opposed to this reform. Beginning in September 1993 they ran a set of 14 devastating commercials featuring Harry and Louise, a middle-class couple who despaired of the bureaucratic nature of the Clinton health reform plan. The voiceover says, "Government may force us to choose from among plans designed by government bureaucrats." Then Louise declares that "choices we don't like is no choice at all." The couple bemoans that their "old [health insurance] plan was a good one." These ads were heir to the Whitaker and Baxter campaign against Truman's national health insurance proposal in both their antigovernment tone and effectiveness. This time, however, the insurers, not physicians, ran the ads.

Clinton's Health Security Act hit a big roadblock when the Congressional Budget Office (CBO) assessed the costs of legislation. The CBO ruled that there would be almost no cost savings from competition among insurance companies in the alliances. More importantly, the CBO ruled that the insurance premiums that went through the alliances, like Social Security, were part of the federal budget even though they paid for private health coverage. This determination added about $130 billion to the cost of the plan and also seemed to legitimate Republican opposition charges that the health legislation would expand government by 20% and be the biggest tax increase in American history.

The legislation also had a rough time in Congress mainly because of Democrats. First, Representative Dan Rostenkowski, a classic Chicago machine politician, the chair of the House Ways and Means Committee, and a strong supporter of the Clinton plan, became embroiled in his own scandal. (Somehow, ever since Mills guided the creation of Medicare in 1965, the chair of the House Ways and Means Committee always seems to become involved in a scandal when health care reform is on the agenda.) Rostenkowski was alleged to have taken officially purchased stamps for the congressional franking privilege and traded them back for cash. Other charges included paying "ghost" employees and diverting congressional funds for personal use. (The prosecutor was Eric Holder, who, at the time, was an attorney in the criminal division of the Justice Department.) Ultimately the post office charges were dropped, but this scandal curtailed Rostenkowski's political power during the health care debate. This was especially significant because it limited his ability to keep Representative Pete Stark (D-California), a vociferous single-payer advocate on the Ways and Means Committee, from derailing Clinton's bill. Eventually, Rostenkowski was forced to resign in 1994. Other liberals, such as Representative Henry Waxman (D-California), objected to limits on Medicare and Medicaid spending.

Even more problematic was Senator Daniel Patrick Moynihan (D-New York), who was chair of the Senate Finance Committee that has primary jurisdiction over health care reform in the Senate. He was miffed that the Clintons did not engage him and his committee in writing the legislation. As a result, he never strongly supported the bill, and claimed it was too complex and would not work in the real world.

Complicating matters even further were Democrats who offered their own reform proposals. Representative Jim McDermott (D-Washington) and Senator Paul Wellstone (D-Minnesota) sponsored a single-payer plan. Representative Jim Cooper (D-Tennessee), a moderate to conservative Democrat, sponsored a managed competition bill without a mandate.

Senator John Chafee (R-Rhode Island) was appointed chair of the Republican Senate Task Force of Health, with the responsibility for drafting a Republican response to the evolving Clinton proposal. With support of 23 Republican senators, including Minority Leader Senator Robert Dole, he developed a bill with an individual mandate to buy insurance. Senators Don Nickles (R-Oklahoma) and Orrin Hatch (R-Utah) introduced a bill based on the conservative Heritage Foundation's Consumer Choice Health Plan. This would end the tax exclusion and instead give each American family a tax credit "to purchase a basic health insurance package, including catastrophic coverage, to offset the costs of out-of-pocket expenses or to deposit funds into a tax-free 'medical savings account'—a 'medical IRA'—from which families could pay routine medical expenses." Costs would be held down, they argued, because individual choice would force insurers to compete, thus reducing premiums.

In early 1994 business began to get cold feet and reverted to its usual preference for private-sector solutions. The US Chamber of Commerce reversed its position on the employer mandate and universal coverage. Innately suspicious of government, many business leaders became persuaded they could control their costs better with insurers' managed care approach rather than Clinton's plan.

The Republican leader, Senator Dole, quickly abandoned his support for Chafee's health care reform proposal based on an individual mandate. Soon, as pointed out in Chapter 2, Dole began circulating Senator Arlen Specter's complex diagram in order to oppose the Clinton Plan. In the summer of 1994, when prospects for the president's plan were declining, Senator Chafee joined with Senator John Breaux, a conservative Democrat from Louisiana, and other moderate senators to try to develop a mainstream compromise health plan that would break the logjam. The plan rejected any mandate, trying to eliminate the problem of the uninsured by subsidizing their purchase of coverage. The plan included smaller purchasing alliances to give individuals and small businesses (those with fewer than 100 employees) access to affordable insurance plans. It subsidized individuals at up to 240% of the poverty level for the purchase of their health insurance and basically extended the tax exclusion to individuals, making their payments for premiums 100% tax exempt. It created a national health commission with responsibility for reporting to Congress on progress toward universal coverage. If by 2002 more than 5% of the American public remained uninsured, the commission would recommend how to solve the problem. Congress would have to vote on the commission's recommendation or else it would automatically be implemented. Interestingly, the Chafee-Breaux proposal developed its own "Cadillac" tax, placing a 40% tax on health insurance benefits that exceeded a federally defined standard benefits package. A combination of a cigarette tax, the tax on high-cost health plans, and cuts to Medicare financed this bipartisan approach.

The Chafee-Breaux plan was close enough to the Clinton Health Security Act that a compromise should have been possible; indeed, Chafee was probably open to such a compromise. But conservatives found it too liberal, and liberals found it too conservative without a guarantee of universal coverage. It lacked sufficient support among Democratic constituents to provide cover for a compromise. Unfortunately, the White House never compromised with Chafee; nor did the administration negotiate with Representative Cooper.

After about 18 months of work it was clear the Health Security Act was not going to be enacted. Compromise was quickly evaporating as Democrats up for election in 1994, such as Senators John Kerry, Dianne Feinstein, and Joe Lieberman, were running away from the mandate and Republicans, sensing a victory, became more intransigent.

Ultimately, despite starting out with a large majority of Americans supporting universal coverage and health care reform, the moment passed. Neither the House nor Senate voted a single piece of health legislation out of committee.

Although health care reform appeared inevitable after Clinton's victory in November 1992, defeat was overdetermined. First, the long delay in developing the proposal and postponing its submissions to Congress until after the budget and NAFTA were enacted gave time for the opposition to mobilize and present its case. Second, the secrecy of the health care task force, rather than engendering additional public support, raised suspicions as it also alienated opinion leaders who were not part of the task force. They began attacking the proposal mostly out of personal pique.

Third, health care reform was too closely identified with the Clintons, especially because Hillary Clinton was head of the task force. By conflating opposition to the Clintons with opposition to health care reform, Republicans found it easier to oppose reform. Fourth, the bill was developed at the White House, and this offended key congressional leaders who felt excluded, especially Senator Moynihan. Rather than support the bill, they attacked it because it was not their own. Simultaneously, a countervailing political force who might have been able to muscle the bill through, Representative Rostenkowski, was impaired by scandal.

Fifth, support for the Clinton proposal even among Democratic constituents—"friends"—was fragmented. There were many different bills on health care reform, dissipating congressional attention. There were just too many moving parts and ways to appear to be for health reform while opposing it. In addition, unions and liberal groups loathed the market-based Health Security Act, still hoping and campaigning behind the scenes for a single-payer national health insurance plan. This severely fractured supporters of reform, thereby allowing the antireform minority to be more effective. The lack of unity among supporters on the liberal side also constrained the president's ability to negotiate a compromise with conservative Democrats and moderate Republicans like Cooper, Breaux, and Chafee.

Sixth, although enemies were inevitable, the legislation threatened the very existence of the insurance companies, so they were willing to fight with everything to defeat the bill. Seventh, the Health Security Act was very complex. Maybe this is inevitable when trying to reform health care, but it provided an easy target for the "Harry and Louise" ads.

Eighth and finally, the Congressional Budget Office's ruling made the bill much more "expensive" from the way legislation is judged and gave rhetorical ammunition to its opponents, especially Newt Gingrich. In the 1994 congressional elections Republicans, led by Newt Gingrich, ran a national campaign based on opposition to the Clinton health care reform proposal. As a result, the Republicans won back control of the House for the first time in 40 years. This ended any effort to reform the whole system for nearly 20 years.

However, President Clinton, along with Senator Kennedy, was able to pass an incremental reform, the Children's Health Insurance Plan, in 1997. This plan covered children whose families earned too much money to qualify for Medicaid but were uninsured. The program is modeled on Medicaid: it is jointly funded by the federal government and states, administered by states, and the children receive Medicaid-like benefits. Today CHIP covers approximately 8 million children, but it is not universal coverage.

Lyndon Johnson, maybe the greatest legislative strategist in American history, once laid out 6 principles for enacting legislation:

1) Speed
2) Keep the economists quiet
3) Master the congressional process
4) Give Congress the credit
5) Go public and build momentum
6) Passion

Far be it for me to contradict Johnson. Although some of these principles, such as speed and going public, apply to the history of health care reform legislation, there are others specific to health care reform that are not on Johnson's list, perhaps because they are too obvious to mention. But here are the 6 principles specific to legislating for health care.

First, accept that any effort faces long odds. Even when reform appears likely because of a major election victory, such as Truman's and Clinton's, or an unusual alignment of advocates, such as that between Nixon, Kennedy, and Mills, no action is a much more likely outcome than enacting health reform legislation. Since 1912 the United States has resisted any universal coverage or national health insurance program.

Representative Cooper likes to pose the challenge: a congressman runs into the House chamber and a vote is being held. He knows nothing about what is being voted on but has to cast a ballot. How does he vote? Cooper says he must vote No. There are no end of reasons to vote No: "The bill was poorly drafted." "The plan would not have addressed the problem at hand." "A key constituency would have been adversely affected." A Yes vote is always more risky. It is much safer to bet against health care reform occurring than for it.

Second, lack of unity on the part of advocates for health care reform on a specific plan pretty much guarantees failure. Lack of agreement dissipates those in support, thereby allowing a smaller but focused group of opponents to be more effective. The left's insistence on single payer and unwillingness to rally around a more market-based Democratic plan has contributed to the defeat of more moderate but important universal-coverage proposals both in 1974 and 1993.

Third, never underestimate both the power and fragility of Washington egos. Almost by definition elected officials must have strong egos to raise money, campaign, and withstand public and media assaults and even electoral defeats. And like all people, they want to be treated with respect even if not love. Failing to give proper respect to politicians can make them oppose legislation out of resentment rather than policy differences. When Moynihan was not consulted on the Clintons' Health Security Act, it was easy for him to feel insulted and, as chair of the Senate Finance Committee, to obstruct its passage. Similarly, when consulting and paying due homage, it is possible to get people to do things they would otherwise oppose. Robert Caro tells a wonderful story about how, in 1964, Lyndon Johnson gave Senator Harry Byrd of Virginia—chair of the Finance Committee and a strong anti-integrationist—who hated big federal budgets and deficits, his wish for a federal budget under $100 billion. This ended Byrd's opposition to Kennedy's tax cut and also cleared Senate workflow in order to enact the Civil Rights Act of 1964, both of which Byrd deeply opposed.

Fourth, speed is of the essence. The House Ways and Means Committee passed Medicare and Medicaid in 2 months, and the full House voted on it in just over 3 months. The entire process, from convening the new Congress to President Johnson's signature, lasted less than 7 months. Conversely, proceeding slowly means that coalitions for reform can fracture and opposition can coalesce. In Lyndon Johnson's White House tapes in which he strategizes with John McCormack, the Speaker of the House, after the Ways and Means Committee passed the Medicare and Medicaid legislation, he admonishes the Speaker on the issue of a House vote in the earthy manner only Johnson was capable of. Johnson refers to the legendary Sam Rayburn (D-Texas), the longest-serving speaker of the House who was one of Johnson's mentors and surrogate fathers:

> For God sakes, don't let dead cats stand on your porch, Mr. Rayburn used to say, "They stunk and they stunk and they stunk." When you get one [of your bills] out of that committee, you call that son of a bitch up before they [the opposition] can get their letters written.

Fifth, like people and all organizations, Congress does not like new things. Successful legislation must be built on previous templates. Rarely is something truly "new" enacted. In part this is because of the need for speed. The quicker you need to get legislation through, the less time there is to develop and refine it, much less actually write it. No one can write a new 1,400-page bill; they have to borrow heavily from what already exists. Similarly, representatives and senators instinctively oppose the new and are comfortable with what they have already enacted. Having Social Security start at 65 years of age and financed through a payroll tax was ultimately borrowed from Bismarck. Once that was in place, Forand adopted it for his Medicare proposal. And Wilbur Mills used that Social Security platform for Medicare Part A, and then he adopted the Republican proposal for Medicare Part B and the Kerr-Mills structure of joint federal and state financing and state administration for Medicaid. It also explains why trying to develop new ideas, such as Clinton's health alliances, runs into such strong opposition.

Sixth and finally: the opposition. The opposition to any health care reform in the United States is always couched in antigovernment slogans, whether they are about "socialized medicine" or the bureaucracy telling Americans what to do. This line of attack is tried and true—it taps into the traditional American suspicion of government. Any chance of passage must try to counter this line of attack. Furthermore, certain groups—physicians, insurers, and business—are pretty reliable opponents for any health care reform. Physicians, long opposed to anyone who comes between them and the patient, were opposed to health insurance for physician expenses even if it were private. Once insurance became a reality and they became used to it, however, physicians could tolerate voluntary insurance but opposed any plan to make insurance mandatory. Since organized medicine, the AMA in particular, was defeated by Johnson on Medicare and Medicaid and they learned to like the Medicare payments, their opposition to health care reform has been more muted.

Any reform has to overcome these 6 hurdles and whatever other ones the moment in history brings. So how was Obama able to enact the Affordable Care Act? Which of these lessons did he heed?

= CHAPTER SIX =

Enacting the Affordable Care Act

After 100 years of trying, the United States finally enacted comprehensive health care reform that included universal health care coverage as well as many other ways to improve the health care system. Although health care reform legislation had failed in 1912, 1935, 1946–1949, 1965, 1974, and 1993, it finally succeeded on March 23, 2010. This was a historic event.

How did it happen?

With the events so recent, there are many excellent and detailed accounts of the peregrinations toward ultimate signature on March 23, 2010. Here I shall focus on 3 themes. First, how the 6 lessons of history elucidated in Chapter 5 were addressed—or not—in the campaign to enact the Affordable Care Act. Second, the essential but not widely understood role of the Congressional Budget Office in the legislative process. Third, by examining how 3 particular elements of health care reform came to be—or not be—in the final bill, we can learn something about how policy, politics, and interest groups interact during the legislative process in general and health care reform in particular.

Overcoming the 6 Impediments to Enact the Affordable Care Act

Like every election since 1992, health care was an important but not the dominant issue in the 2008 election. And after Obama's victory the freefalling economy was the #1 issue and getting a stimulus bill—the American Recovery and Reinvestment Act (ARRA)—was the top priority. ARRA included some health care reform—financial incentives for physicians and hospitals to install and use electronic health records. After stimulus was enacted on February 17, 2009, health care was next in line. The leading Democratic contenders had all developed detailed health reform proposals. The main difference involved whether to require individuals to purchase health insurance—the "individual mandate." Initially, Senator John Edwards and Senator Hillary Clinton supported the individual mandate and Senator Barack Obama opposed it, which was the more centrist approach. Senator John McCain's campaign adopted the Heritage Foundation's proposal from 1993 that called for the government to eliminate the tax exclusion for health insurance payments while giving families and individuals tax credits—worth $5,000 for a family—to purchase their own policies. The McCain/Heritage plan also allowed people to buy insurance plans across state lines, and this, they argued, would lower costs by increasing competition.

In a rerun of 1993, after the November election the prospects for enacting health care reform appeared promising. Health reform was an important campaign issue, and there was a stark difference between the Obama and McCain proposals. Even more promising, the 2008 returns gave the Democrats control of both chambers of Congress, including a filibuster-proof 60 votes in the Senate—if you include the 2 Independents that caucused with the Democrats.

Some Obama administration officials, particularly my brother Rahm and Vice President Joe Biden, were focused on the desperate economic situation and plummeting employment, so they favored an incremental approach rather than comprehensive health care reform. But the president saw health care in economic terms. He was convinced that the rise in health care costs was a major threat to the United States' long-term economic viability—to the middle class and to the federal government's fiscal stability.

Maybe most importantly, Obama had a sense of his own transformative opportunity. He defied the very long odds to become the first African American president, so he would defy the odds again in enacting comprehensive health care reform. Indeed, in July 2009, when opposition to his health care reform plan was solidifying, he told a number of health care aides that he felt "lucky" and was convinced comprehensive reform would pass.

For many Democrats, perhaps including the president, there was also a hope of enacting comprehensive reform for the dying Ted Kennedy. Universal coverage had been Kennedy's signature—but always elusive—issue over the course of nearly 50 years in the Senate. He had managed to secure incremental reforms, such as the CHIP program for uninsured children, but he never reached his ultimate goal: universal coverage. By 2008 Kennedy was dying of brain cancer. This would be his last attempt.

There is no doubt that the president was the one who insisted on making reform comprehensive not incremental. Every time anybody wavered, every time it looked like comprehensive reform was faltering and the incremental approach might be more feasible, the president was the one who insisted on not going down the Medicare and Medicaid route but instead pushing for comprehensive reform. Obama accepted the long odds and the gamble, and multiple times he stepped in to save the reform effort through galvanizing speeches and other acts.

Here is how the administration approached the 6 barriers to all the previous attempts at health care reform.

Lack of unity among the supporters for health care reform. There were several fissures within the pro-health reform camp. One was over the public option. Liberals always preferred a single-payer approach, whether it is called a national health insurance plan or Medicare for all. As in 1993, liberals viscerally opposed a market-based plan, and their way of holding onto at least some remnant of a national health insurance program was the public option. This created a public insurer that would compete in the exchanges against private insurance companies. Not surprisingly, the public option was an anathema to many more market-oriented people in the Obama administration, commonly referred to as the "Economic Team," who were under the leadership of National Economic Council director Larry Summers and Office of Management and Budget director Peter Orszag. Keeping the public option open was critical to retaining liberal support.

Speaker of the House Nancy Pelosi (D-California) performed another critical set of moves to forge unity among supporters. Her challenge was that, traditionally, the Ways and Means, Energy and Commerce, and Education and Labor Committees have jurisdiction over parts of health care. They could fight, pass disparate bills, and divide the supporters of reform. So she had to thwart this possibility. At each session of Congress John Dingell (D-Michigan), the longtime chair of the Energy and Commerce Committee, had reintroduced his father's national health insurance plan. Worried that Dingell might not fully endorse the president's approach, Pelosi engineered his replacement as chair by Henry Waxman (D-California). This signaled both her resolve to get health reform enacted as well as her power, thus diminishing the proclivity of representatives to advocate for their favorite approach. Even more importantly, she insisted that the 3 committees work together and produce one health care reform bill. Having 3 strong chairs submerge their egos and come up with what would be called the Tri-Committee Health Reform bills was a major challenge, but it was necessary to avoid fracturing reform supporters.

Another essential element to keep unity was undertaken by Senator Max Baucus, chairman of the Senate Finance Committee, which had jurisdiction over health care reform. Whether the committee would vote on any health care bill was unclear. (By contrast, the Senate's Health Education, Labor and Pensions Committee, the one chaired by Senator Kennedy, was certain to support health care reform.) As chair of the Finance Committee, Baucus was critical.

Just days after President Obama won the election, Baucus issued a nearly 100-page white paper, appropriately entitled, "Call to Action: Health Reform 2009." It purported to be Baucus's outline for health care reform, in which he stated,

> It is not intended to be a legislative proposal. Nor is it an exhaustive exploration of every health care issue that should or needs to be addressed, or that will be considered. Rather, it details my vision for health care reform.

But it was not a detailed vision or proposal; instead, it read like a melting pot. It mopped up as many ideas as it could from every possible constituency so as to keep them on board. It was for comprehensive reform. It included insurance exchanges but also a public option. It implied mandates. It eliminated insurance companies' preexisting condition restrictions in the exchange. It had subsidies for families living under 400% of the federal poverty line to buy insurance. It had patient-centered medical homes and value-based purchasing. Everyone could find one of their ideas in Baucus's white paper. And because it was not yet a legislative proposal and presumably could still be shaped, at least at the early stages of the process, everyone in health care complimented the senator and embraced it.

Finally, it appeared as though most of the Democrats and their supporters had learned the pragmatic lesson that not getting reform would be the biggest defeat. Health care reform advocates came to widely accept the message that standing on principle and torpedoing a reform bill because it did not include something you loved was wrong. The liberal blog Daily Kos announced, "Whatever the final piece [of legislation], it will need to be passed. Something that cannot pass is useless." This was a huge psychological and practical victory, and it prevented supporters from undermining reform because they believed they could get more in the future.

Managing the egos. Maybe the most critical lesson drawn from the Clinton effort was the importance of congressional deference. The Obama administration let Congress lead or, at least, appear to lead the debate. The marching orders were to give the committees in both the House and Senate power to draft legislation. This was especially important on the Senate side, where, in theory, just one senator could derail the plan. It helped to ensure the support from critical people at the start and, therefore, throughout the process.

As with all legislation this led to including proposals in the bill that were favorites of particular legislators that prudent policy making might not have supported. Take the SHOP exchanges—exchanges exclusively for small businesses to buy insurance with subsidies: they really are not necessary. Small businesses could let their employees buy insurance in the individual exchanges. Furthermore, every previous effort to create effective small business exchanges had failed; indeed, Massachusetts, which has had a very successful individual exchange, has never really been able to establish a vibrant small business exchange. Nevertheless, because key congressional leaders had sponsored SHOP exchange legislation as an incremental step, these exchanges were included in the Affordable Care Act. (Ultimately, they remain so unworkable that implementing the SHOP exchanges under the Affordable Care Act has had to be delayed, and they will likely never be an important element in expanding coverage.)

Senator Ron Wyden (D-Oregon) was probably the senator who had studied health care the most. In 2007 he had proposed the Healthy Americans Act. It was a reform proposal that drew important Republican support; it was cosponsored with one of the more conservative senators, Senator Bob Bennett (R-Utah). (He would eventually be defeated in a Republican party primary by an even more conservative Tea Party leader, Michael Lee, because of his support for President Bush's bank bailout bill.) Wyden wanted acknowledgement for his extensive work on health care and had many provisions he wanted included in the ACA. For instance, he wanted a safety valve for individuals who would have to pay too much for employer-based coverage to enter the exchanges and get subsidies. He got his safety valve, but certain people in the White House who strongly supported employer-based insurance were never happy about this. After its inclusion in the ACA, this provision was subsequently eliminated in another piece of legislation.

The deals cut to overcome the reluctance of two moderate senators, Joe Lieberman (I-Connecticut) and Ben Nelson (D-Nebraska), probably most clearly demonstrated the concern for congressional egos. Although liberals heavily favored the public option, Lieberman was strongly opposed to it and insisted on deleting it from the bill. Because his vote was essential, the Senate bill contained no public option.

Ben Nelson wanted the guarantee that states could prohibit insurers from covering abortions in their own exchanges. But he also wanted a sweetheart deal for Nebraska on its Medicaid expansion. Instead of the federal government paying 100% for 3 years then having that funding level slowly decline to 90% for the remainder of the decade, he wanted Nebraska to get 100% federal funding indefinitely. It added about $100 million to the cost of the bill, just about 0.01% of the total cost. Because Nelson's was the 60th vote, he got what became known as the "Cornhusker Kickback" in the Senate bill. Eventually, however, embarrassed by the negative publicity surrounding the deal, he agreed to have it stripped from the law. (Ironically, Justice Scalia brought it up in the Supreme Court's hearings on the Affordable Care Act in the spring of 2012, apparently not realizing it was not in the final legislation. No one in the courtroom had the courage to correct the justice.)

Speed is of the essence. This may be the most important of all imperatives for legislation. Anytime a legislator demands that a bill be slowed down for more hearings or debate, you know they are trying to kill it. So when Republicans demanded that the ACA be slowed down, the euphemism was clear. Early in 2010, after nearly a year of work, Senator Lamar Alexander (R-Tennessee) argued, "We think to do that we have to start by taking the current bill and putting it on the shelf and starting from a clean sheet of paper." Starting afresh after 12 months of work would have ensured no legislation would be voted on.

The White House and Democratic leadership in Congress accepted the imperative for speed, but it was constantly challenged. In all, it took 14 months for health reform to pass. Much less time had been required to pass Medicare and Medicaid in the pre-Internet 1960s. This slowness almost killed the ACA multiple times.

How did supporters try to adhere to this speed imperative? Initially, President Obama fixed summer 2009 as his deadline for passage of health care reform. Within the White House whenever there were policy disagreements, the oft-repeated mantra was "Let's just get it passed. We will work it out in conference." (Conference is the reconciliation process by which different versions of a bill passed by the Senate and House are melded into one bill that both chambers then enact.) Phil Schiliro, head of legislative affairs in the White House, repeatedly insisted that policy differences should not be permitted to delay the bill. A bill that is not perfect was better than delay that increases the odds of no bill at all. Schiliro's approach always frustrated the policy wonks—me included—but it was probably right for enacting any legislation. It certainly kept the process moving as quickly as possible.

Similarly, in the House the tri-committee approach was done in part for speed. And Speaker Pelosi was effective in enforcing discipline. By July 2009 the 3 House committees had all voted out the same bill that the House then passed, 220–215, on November 7.

Still, there were delays. The first was no one's fault. Former Senator Tom Daschle was supposed to head the White House reform effort, but a personal tax problem forced his resignation. The search for a replacement in the White House delayed the administration's ability to coordinate its own activities on health care reform.

Initially, Senator Baucus pledged to act quickly, stating, "I'd like to have us ready for the floor by June or July, before the August recess. I'd say June." For months Baucus was meeting with various Republican members of the Finance Committee, trying to forge a bipartisan approach. Beginning in mid-June Baucus and 2 other moderate Democratic senators began meeting with 3 Republicans, including the ranking Republican on the Finance Committee—composing the so-called Gang of Six—to see whether a bipartisan compromise was possible. There were scores of meetings, consuming months of precious time.

It is unclear whether the inability of the Republicans on the Gang of Six to agree to reform was intended all along as a way to delay the bill and thereby kill it or was based on genuine policy differences. Nevertheless, the delay worked. By the August recess the Finance Committee had not passed a bill. Members of Congress went home enduring town hall meetings where voters challenged them on every aspect of the issue and sometimes veered into conspiracy theories. The most vocal and vitriolic attacks, which came from those aligned with the Tea Party, scared many members of Congress and almost doomed health care reform.

After 8 months of work only the combination of 3 actions saved health care reform. Tired of delay, Obama officials pulled the plug on Baucus's discussions with Republicans. They would push forward with a Democratic bill. Then, on August 25, 2009, Senator Kennedy died. This had the effect of rallying Democrats to get something done in his memory. On September 9, 2009, after Congress returned from the unnerving summer recess, the president addressed a joint session of Congress, what became the infamous "you lie" speech, when Representative Joe Wilson (R-South Carolina) shouted out, "You lie!" when the president stated the legislation would not mandate coverage for undocumented immigrants. Ever the clutch hitter, Obama nonetheless declared his continued commitment to enacting comprehensive health care reform. The speech reinvigorated reform's supporters and steadied those wavering from the August attacks.

The Senate delay also had an effect on the House. Even after the 3 committees passed the ACA in July, the full House did not want to take a controversial vote on health care reform without assurance that the Senate would enact something too. House Democrats had recently taken a highly controversial vote on energy legislation only to have the Senate do nothing. They resented that they were "left out to dry" by the Senate and were not going to allow this to happen on health care. Thus, the full House waited for months to take a vote until the Senate Finance Committee had passed health care reform legislation and they were sure the full Senate would vote on the measure. Delay bred delay.

Even after both the House and Senate passed the bill there was delay centered on resolving outstanding issues, such as whether there should be one national exchange or 50 state exchanges. This delay almost proved fatal. On January 19, 2010, in the special election to replace Kennedy in the Senate, Scott Brown, a Republican, won a seat the Democrats had held for decades. This victory eliminated the 60-vote filibuster-proof Democratic majority. It also caused some moderate Democrats, such as Senator Jim Webb (D-Virginia), to call for suspension of any action on health care.

Use old templates rather than new ideas. One of the president's key principles guiding his health reform effort, repeatedly pledged to the American public during the campaign, was, "If you like your health care plan, you can keep it." Many people now feel as if this pledge was not fulfilled. But it was meant to communicate that the legislation itself would not require the discontinuation of specific health plans, or, as had occurred in previous proposals, total elimination of private insurance plans (Chapter 5). This pledge of stability limited the types of reforms that could be enacted. Basically it forced the bill to retain as much as possible the existing complex financing mechanisms, including employer-based health insurance, Medicare, Medicaid, the VA, and the rest.

The opposition nonetheless deployed the well-worn charges of socialized medicine. Opponents to health care reform typically include physicians, insurers, and pharmaceutical manufacturers, all of whom typically invoke socialized medicine and the meddling of government bureaucrats in the physician-patient relationship. In this regard the battle for the Affordable Care Act was no different. Even as the socialized medicine charge was used frequently, it was also refined, based on focus groups and polling, to "the government takeover of healthcare." Frank Luntz, the Republican message magician, circulated his memo on "The Language of Healthcare 2009," with its subtitle, "The 10 Rules for Stopping the 'Washington Takeover' of Healthcare."

During the 2008 general election the libertarian Cato Institute had declared, "Obama's health care plan would socialize medicine even further. Reasonable people can disagree over whether Obama's health plan would be good or bad. But to suggest that it is not a step toward socialized medicine is absurd."

Various Republican politicians argued that the health reform legislation was a bigger threat to the United States than terrorists. And even after the ACA was passed, Republicans continued in this vein. As late as summer 2013 the chairman of the Republican National Committee claimed that the ACA imported "European, socialist-style health care" to the United States. Some attacks just never die.

Opponents of reform also invoked a new charge: death panels. This phrase and its power reflected an intense battle for the support of the elderly, a key electoral constituency. They had government-supported health insurance, Medicare. And they did not see much in health care reform for themselves. They were not very supportive. The Democrats tried to rally them by improving Medicare's drug benefit, Part D, by eliminating the so-called donut hole (Chapter 2, pages 59) and eliminating co-pays for preventive services.

In August 2009, making a play to turn seniors against the ACA, Sarah Palin claimed that the legislation had a provision for death panels for Medicare beneficiaries. The attack distorted an idea reform advocates discussed, that physicians might be paid for an office visit to discuss end-of-life care preferences with their patients. Ironically, this idea had previously garnered significant Republican support. Newt Gingrich, for instance, had supported it. Senator Johnny Isakson (R-Georgia) had introduced legislation on the matter. When she was governor of Alaska, Palin herself had supported a month-long push to have residents complete living wills. But the battle over the ACA was about politics, not policy, so she raised the idea that there would be death panels:

> Government health care will not reduce the cost; it will simply refuse to pay the cost. And who will suffer the most when they ration care? The sick,

> the elderly, and the disabled, of course. The America I know and love is not one in which my parents or my baby with Down Syndrome will have to stand in front of Obama's "death panel" so his bureaucrats can decide, based on a subjective judgment of their "level of productivity in society" whether they are worthy of health care. Such a system is downright evil.

Leading conservative commentators, such as Rush Limbaugh and Glenn Beck, repeatedly echoed Palin's charge. After the idea of paying for physician-patient discussions on end-of-life care was dropped, Republicans transferred the death panel charge, claiming instead that there was a committee, the Independent Payment Advisory Board, that would decide what care seniors would get. In December 2009 Representative Michele Bachmann reiterated the death panel charge: "And it's the part dealing with the Medicare Advisory Board—what many people have labeled the death panels—because these unelected bureaucracies will decide what we can and can't get in future health insurance policy. That's why they're called death panels."

The notion of death panels was quickly expanded to attack me personally, labeling me as Dr. Death. I was, it was claimed, an advocate for euthanasia of the elderly and disabled. Bachmann made the charge against me from the floor of the House: "The president's adviser, Dr. Emanuel, believes communitarianism should guide decisions on who gets care. He says medical care should be reserved for the nondisabled. So watch out if you're disabled."

Every responsible party who has examined the issue of death panels and the Dr. Death charge has concluded that they are totally false. As PolitiFacts.com concluded,

> But to make the sensational claim that Emanuel says health care should not be extended to the disabled is a gross distortion of his position, lifted out of context from an academic paper in which he poses philosophical ideas but doesn't necessarily endorse them. Emanuel's hefty medical record also counts for something, as well his unequivocal public position against euthanasia and doctor-assisted suicide. We rule Bachmann's statement False.

Yet Palin's and Bachmann's charges were potent. Within a few weeks polls showed that nearly 90% of the public had heard of death panels. As late as 3 years after enactment of the Affordable Care Act a Kaiser Family Foundation survey showed that 39% of the public still believed death panels were part of the ACA. And despite the claim being definitively rejected as false, the Republicans were still invoking the idea in August 2013. Reince Priebus, chairman of the Republican National Committee, revived the claim that "what people don't want are government panels deciding whether something's medically necessary."

The Obama administration clearly understood the importance of neutralizing key elements of the traditional opposition. On March 5 the president held an East Room meeting with 150 people that included representatives of the AMA, US Chamber of Commerce, insurance companies, and drug manufacturers to discuss health care and reform. Early in 2009 Nancy-Ann DeParle, who was the White House health reform leader, began meeting with insurance, drug and device companies, and others traditionally in the opposition. The goal was threefold: neutralize their opposition; secure, if possible, their support for reform; and gain pledges on how much they could be taxed to help fund reform. Ironically, the most cooperative of the traditional opposition groups turned out to be the drug companies. In part, this was because the head of the Washington lobbying group, PhRMA, the Pharmaceutical Research and Manufacturers of America, was Billy Tauzin, a former Louisiana congressman who understood deal making. But it was also a cold cost-benefit calculation. The drug companies estimated that because of the ACA, as more insured people would buy more drugs, drug company revenues would expand to about $120 billion over the next decade. Thus, they were willing to be taxed $85 billion to fund health care reform, leaving the companies with a net profit of $35 billion. To help push the ACA forward, they would give seniors drug discounts and spend money running ads in favor of the health care reform legislation. By mid-June there was a deal, and it stuck even as House members objected to "special deals" and others wanted to extract more from the drug companies. Of all the actors in the health reform debate, the pharmaceutical industry never wavered. Their deal set a template for hospitals. Negotiations were more protracted with insurers, however.

Other key groups signed on to support the reform efforts. Especially important were the nurses who, it turns out, the American public trusts the most regarding health care issues. Then there was the American Medical Association. The power of the AMA had slipped since its defeat on Medicare. Its membership was down to less than 30% of practicing physicians. Nevertheless, inside Washington the AMA remained the mouthpiece for physicians. Many physicians, including senior leaders of other organizations, were strongly for reform. And this time, unlike the past reform efforts—whether 1935, the Truman effort, or even the fight over Medicare—the AMA certainly was not assessing members with special dues to run a big campaign against reform and socialized medicine. That change itself was a huge victory.

But the administration did not merely neutralize the AMA; it got their endorsement—repeatedly. At a critical time in early September, despite the angry August attacks in congressional districts, the president of the AMA sent an open letter stating,

> On behalf of America's physicians and their patients, we strongly urge you to reach agreement this year on health system reforms that include the following 7 critical elements:
>
> - Provide health insurance coverage for all Americans
> - Enact insurance market reforms that expand choice of affordable coverage and eliminate denials for preexisting conditions
> - Assure that health care decisions are made by patients and their physicians, not by insurance companies or government officials
> - Provide investments and incentives for quality improvement, prevention and wellness initiatives
> - Repeal the Medicare physician payment formula that will trigger steep cuts and threaten seniors' access to care
> - Implement medical liability reforms to reduce the cost of defensive medicine
> - Streamline and standardize insurance claims' processing requirements to eliminate unnecessary costs and administrative burdens

The letter, with its opening endorsement of universal coverage and eliminating preexisting condition exclusions—and only later comments about keeping government out of decision making and liability reform—was an important change from a traditional opponent. Then in December 2009 the AMA sent an even stronger letter to Senator and Majority Leader Harry Reid: "The American Medical Association (AMA) remains committed to achieving enactment of comprehensive health system reform legislation that improves access to affordable, high-quality care and reduces unnecessary costs. We do not believe that maintaining the status quo is an acceptable option for physicians or the patients we serve."

Ironically, for its support of the ACA, the AMA did not receive very much. The public option was not included in the bill, and there were provisions for administrative simplification. But the AMA's biggest concern, the Sustainable Growth Rate formula (SGR) (Chapter 3, page 83), was not fixed in the Affordable Care Act. And, as we shall see later in this chapter, medical malpractice was only peripherally addressed in the ACA.

It seemed the administration and Democrats were successful at neutralizing and even garnering support from the traditional opposition to health care reform. But in 2010 the Catholic Church raised one of the most important obstacles. Catholics had long favored universal coverage of the poor. However, in the struggle over the ACA the Church became more obsessed about public financing for abortion than it was concerned about universal coverage for the poor and middle class. The president was willing to accept the traditional proviso to health legislation that "no federal dollars would be used to fund abortion." But that did not resolve the issue. The Church expanded its demands. The bishops of the Church wanted the Stupak Amendment, named after the Democratic congressman from Michigan, Bart Stupak, who insisted on a provision prohibiting federal funds not just from paying for abortion but even from subsidizing "premiums for a health plan that includes abortion coverage." Catholic nuns, strong supporters of universal coverage, publicly broke with the bishops on the abortion issue and supported the Affordable Care Act. Eventually, the Stupak Amendment was included in the House bill but not in the Senate one.

The final near-death experience of the Affordable Care Act occurred with Scott Brown's January 2010 victory. At this point both the Senate and House had enacted health care reform bills, but they were different bills. Although there were negotiations about how to reconcile their differences, after Scott Brown's victory the White House was like a funeral; everyone was depressed. Twelve months of hard work and near victory seemed to go up in smoke.

Given the situation, there was only one legal and feasible way forward. The House had to accept the Senate's bill. The House hated this option. The 2 chambers maintain a deep rivalry. And representatives often feel slighted and disrespected by their Senate colleagues, even those from the same party. Accepting a Senate bill without even the face-saving chance to integrate some House modifications was very difficult for the Representatives to swallow. Many commentators were arguing it would not happen. The liberal commentator Mark Shields wrote,

> It is both silly and unrealistic to propose, as some health care supporters have, that House Speaker Nancy Pelosi ask her House colleagues to pass the Senate bill. For House Democrats, to vote for the Senate bill with its widely publicized special deals, including the Louisiana Purchase to secure the vote of Democrat Sen. Mary Landrieu and the Nebraska Auction to win the backing of Democratic Sen. Ben Nelson, would be political suicide.

For 2 months House Speaker Nancy Pelosi had tried to rally her fellow Democrats, but they were in no mood. Then, in February 2010, the for-profit insurance company Wellpoint announced a 39% rate increase for some California customers in the individual market. Everyone was outraged, energizing reform supporters. Repeatedly the president declared that the Wellpoint rate hikes starkly illustrated the necessity for reform. This persuaded the House to embrace the idea that after 14 months of work and the potential for a major legislative achievement, having no reform bill would be worse than enacting the imperfect Senate health care reform bill. On March 21, 2010, the House voted 219–212 to enact the Senate's version of the ACA. Some modifications in the Health Care and Education Reconciliation Act were also passed quickly after the ACA was adopted.

On March 23, 2010, President Obama signed the Affordable Care Act into law.

FIGURE 6.1 President Obama signs into law the ACA. © Doug Mills/*The New York Times*/Redux Pictures

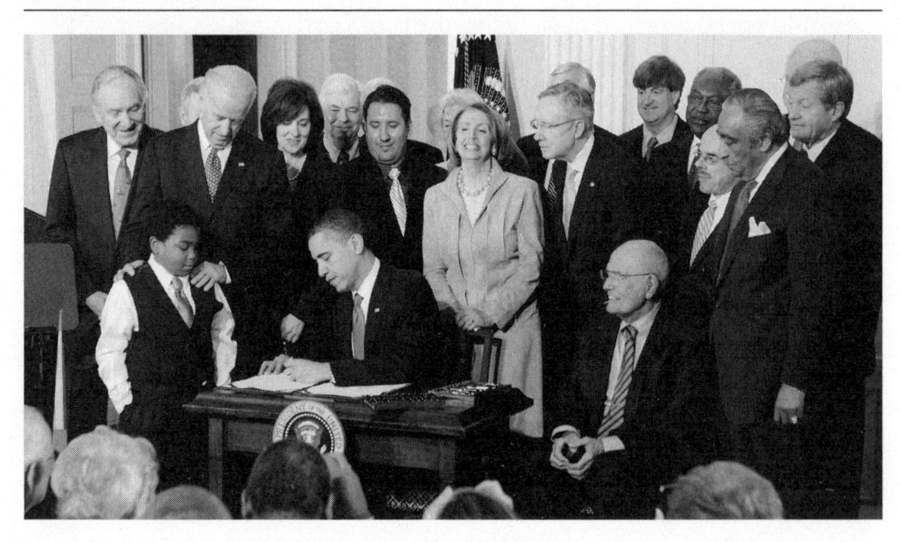

The Pivotal but Little-Known Role of the Congressional Budget Office

Although frequently mentioned, the Congressional Budget Office (CBO) is one of the least understood actors in the legislative process, and it played a vital but underappreciated role in the adoption of the ACA.

The CBO was created in 1974 to provide objective, nonpartisan analyses to inform Congress's economic and budgetary decisions. The Speaker of the House and president pro tempore of the Senate jointly appoint the CBO's director based on recommendations from the respective budget committees.

The CBO's most important activities relate to providing baseline projections for the federal budget over the next 10 years and "scoring" proposed bills. This scoring function means that the "CBO provides formal, written estimates of the cost of virtually every bill 'reported' (approved) by Congressional committees to show how the bill would affect spending or revenues over the next 5 or 10 years." Importantly, a CBO score specifies the cost—or savings—of legislation over the next 10-year window. It is not a per-year estimate but rather a per-10-year estimate. (This timeframe is often lost when Washington insiders talk to people outside the Beltway.)

CBO scoring is tyrannical. Legislation rises or falls by its score. Whenever talking to congressional staff or politicians about potential legislation, their first question and almost sole focus is, "Does it score?" By which they mean, "Will the proposal save money?" If a bill costs money, funds will have to be found either by raising taxes or cutting other programs—usually a deathblow to a proposal. Even proposals that are valuable and worthy but neither save nor cost—"don't score"—are not of much interest. Conversely, changes that "score"—that is, save money—are much more likely to be enacted.

Although the CBO's scores are objective and nonpartisan, they are frequently wrong. Performing this scoring function is extraordinarily difficult. Predicting how people will respond to new government programs is as much art as it is science. It is fraught with challenges and mistakes. Indeed, predicting the costs and savings of many programs, especially those with few precedents, is nearly impossible. For instance, scoring on health care requires predicting how physicians and hospitals will react to changes not only in payment but also in the marketplace. The score depends on estimating how insurers will change their policies and premiums. It also hinges on whether employers insure more people or stop providing insurance, whether individual Americans buy insurance, and if so, what kind, or whether they pay the penalty. The sheer number of variables, and the number of variables with little historical data on which to base predictions, is staggering, making prediction almost a complete guessing game.

Furthermore, there is an inherent institutional bias at the CBO to be cautious—that is, to overestimate costs and underestimate savings. This bias seems natural when you consider that if the CBO is wrong and a program costs too much, it may put the federal budget further into debt and opens the CBO to substantial criticism. Conversely, if a program costs less than the CBO projected, the federal budget is in better shape, and few people complain. An institutional proclivity to minimize criticism means the bias at CBO is to underestimate savings. This bias also can create real harm by placing significant roadblocks for important and worthy legislation that are projected inaccurately as either generating high costs or little to no savings. But this aspect of the process is often overlooked because the legislation that fails to be enacted is often never noticed or remembered.

When it comes to health care, over nearly 3 decades the CBO bias has been validated. For instance, in the 1980s CBO's estimates for the savings of DRGs was 18% too low. In the 1990s the actual savings from the Balanced Budget Act of 1997, the act that contained the Sustainable Growth Rate formula (SGR) (Chapter 3, page 83) as well as changes to payment for home health visits, turned out to be 50% higher in 1998 and 113% higher in 1999 than the CBO estimated. Most memorably, the CBO estimate for the cost of Medicare Part D, the drug benefit, turned out to be 42% too high. And we will never really know about the many proposals that could have improved the health care system but were given scores that ensured they would not be considered, much less enacted. Nevertheless, there has to be an objective, official scorer, and the CBO is it. Only the CBO's estimates on revenues and savings matter when debating legislation like the Affordable Care Act.

The health care reform legislation contained at least 3 critical elements that affected the score and can be adjusted to change the score. One is expenditures, which, in turn, depend upon subsidy levels, the nature and "richness" of the essential benefits, the federal payment level for the expansion of Medicaid, and factors such as what the premiums are likely to be in the exchanges. The score also depends on the savings anticipated from modifications in government programs, such as penalizing hospitals for having a high level of readmissions. Finally, the score depends on revenue raised: taxes on industries and penalties for not having insurance. These, in turn, depend on people's behavior, such as how many Americans will not purchase health insurance.

Although the CBO scores are objective and nonpartisan, politicians often use CBO scores as partisan weapons. Republicans can try to get scores that have high costs or low savings so as to embarrass Democrats and vice versa. Adverse scores can literally kill a bill. Conversely, a good score, especially if unexpected, can boost the chances for legislation. Consequently, parties trying to develop major legislation are likely to want to know the result before they ask for an official CBO score. Therefore, both to rapidly assess the impact of policy alternatives and to minimize political risks, before asking the CBO for its official determination, the Democrats needed to create a model and accurately predict the CBO score. In this regard, it helped the administration that Peter Orszag, who had directed the CBO and understood its inner workings, was now director of the Office of Management and Budget (OMB).

During the development of the ACA the administration undertook 2 major efforts to create a shadow CBO "score" function. First, the Department of Health and Human Services contracted with Jonathan Gruber, an economist at MIT, to predict the CBO score. Gruber was picked largely because he had developed an economic model of the health care system that the CBO borrowed and refined to create its own model. The second shadow scoring function was a model developed for the White House by Jeffrey Liebman, a professor of public policy at Harvard University who served as the chief economist in the OMB, and Gordon Mermin, an economist on his staff. Liebman and Mermin's model turned out to be ridiculously simple. The two were able to put it together in less than 2 weeks, and it turned out to predict the CBO score within a fraction of 1%.

During the process of developing the ACA the president and Rahm Emanuel established a very firm maximum-cost limit. They wanted the cost of coverage—payments for Medicaid expansion, subsidies for the exchange, and enhancements to various programs—to total no more than $1 trillion over 10 years. In addition, the president specified that approximately half of the money needed to pay for the bill should come from savings in government health programs and half should come from new revenues. Finally, the legislation was not to add to the deficit in the 10-year budget window; it would have to be revenue-neutral or be in surplus.

The CBO's score of the Senate bill that was passed on December 24, 2009, was minus $118 billion. In other words, in the 10 years from 2010 to 2019 the ACA was projected to *save*—and, thus, *reduce* the national debt by—$118 billion. The CBO estimated that costs for expanding coverage would be $836 billion over the 2010–2019 window, but savings from changes in programs, such as reducing payments to Medicare Advantage plans, and new revenue, such as taxing the drug companies and tanning salons, would amount to $954 billion. Contrary to Republican claims, such as those by Paul Ryan, the CBO's initial estimate was that the ACA would reduce the federal debt over its first decade of enactment.

The Fate of Three Issues

Three elements of reform—the "Cadillac tax" limiting the tax exclusion, payment reform, and medical malpractice—illustrate the complex interplay between policy, politics, and interest groups in the context of enacting major legislation such as the ACA. I recount these 3 cases because from January 2009 to January 2011 I served as the senior adviser on health care to the director of the OMB in the White House, working on the reform effort and was engaged on these issues.

The Tax exclusion and the Cadillac tax. The IRS institutionalized the tax exclusion for health insurance premiums in 1954 (Chapter 1, page 31). Employers' contributions to health insurance premiums are not included when computing an employee's income tax and both the employee's and employer's payroll taxes. Functionally, it makes an additional $1 of health insurance more valuable, because it is not taxed, than an additional $1 of wages, which is taxed.

Economists, whether liberal or conservative, denounce the tax exclusion. It is grossly inequitable, giving significantly greater benefits to the rich than to those less well off. It is also thought to be a major driver of higher health care costs, and it keeps cash wages down. Further, as the single-largest tax break, it lowers government revenues by about $250 billion per year (Chapter 2, page 46).

During the 2008 presidential election John McCain proposed eliminating the tax exclusion and replacing it with a $5,000 per family tax credit for purchasing health insurance. In response, Obama's campaign ran over $100 million worth of ads attacking McCain on this very issue. Some of the ads said, "McCain would make you pay income tax on your health insurance benefits. Taxing health benefits for the first time ever. And that tax credit? McCain's own website said it goes straight to the insurance companies, not to you, leaving you on your own to pay McCain's health insurance tax. Taxing health care instead of fixing it. We can't afford John McCain."

There was significant disagreement within the White House about the tax exclusion. Members of the health reform team from the NEC and OMB were largely in favor of reducing it. The political team was against touching it in any way. Indeed, David Axelrod created a video montage of the various commercials the campaign had run on the tax exclusion and showed it to the health reform team at the end of a meeting. The stated purpose was to remind the health reform team, especially those from NEC and OMB, that changing the tax exclusion was a major issue in the campaign and that Obama had clearly opposed this change.

The president himself repeatedly reiterated a major principle of his administration: fidelity. One of the president's core beliefs was that the American public should be able to trust what he said. Consistency was a virtue. Indeed, Obama frequently made clear to his staff that the things he said on the campaign and as president were not to be contravened unless there was a very, very good rationale. Frequently, when confronting a decision, he would ask, "What position did we take on that?" to be sure that his current decision would be consistent with his past declarations. The video showed the candidate's position clearly.

The economic team thought it had good reasons for a change in position, but the political team rejected them. There was a standoff. Given the president's principle of fidelity, the political team had the upper hand.

One day in mid-July 2009 key members of the health care team, Nancy-Ann DeParle, Peter Orszag, Gene Sperling, Jason Furman, Bob Kocher, Jeanne Lambrew, a few others, and myself, were meeting in Phil Schiliro's second-floor White House office. Toward the end of the meeting Schiliro left the office and returned with the president. Obama sat at the head of a small table surrounded by 8 members of the team, with a few others sitting on Schiliro's couch and side chairs. It was supposed to be a combination of a Friday afternoon "thank you for your hard work" appreciation and pep talk about the importance of completing the health care reform effort.

For some reason, probably because the policy wonks were inexperienced at and uncomfortable with small talk, the discussion moved from pleasantries to substance. I took the opportunity to argue for altering the tax exclusion. It was clear the president understood that changing it would be a terrific source of revenue. But it was equally clear that raising money to fund reform alone was not going to move him to modify his campaign pledge.

I made the case that the tax exclusion was the single-most effective instrument the president possessed to control and reduce private-sector health costs. As the discussion evolved it appeared this was an argument the president seemed not to have heard before.

Early the next week OMB and NEC arranged an Oval Office meeting with 3 economists to further solidify the president's thinking about the link between the tax exclusion and cost control. After this meeting the economic team delineated a variety of policy options for reducing but not eliminating the exclusion. One approach was a cap on the amount of the exclusion that higher-income families, those earning over $250,000 per year, could take. Another approach was to limit the exclusion to only apply to health premiums below a certain threshold. A third approach was more circuitous, limiting expensive health plans by taxing them when they rose over some threshold.

The political team remained adamantly opposed to any change, as did several of the president's core group of supporters, especially unions. For decades unions had secured substantial health benefits for their workers, and many of their insurance plans had no or low deductibles and few restrictions. Consequently, these were some of the highest-cost plans in the country. Unions vigorously defended these plans and viewed any alteration of the tax exclusion as a direct assault on their core benefits won through collective bargaining.

Ultimately, good policy rationales in favor of cost control—not revenue generation—overcame the president's past statements. He decided to go forward with a proposed tax on the portion of the health insurance premium over some threshold rather than a direct limit on the tax exclusion. The specific provision requires that in 2018 sponsors of insurance, not the beneficiary—that is, employers not employees—would pay a 40% tax on the portion of the premium that surpassed a threshold; this was $27,500 for a family plan and $10,200 for an individual plan. There are various changes desired by unions and others opposed to the exceptions (see Chapter 8, pages 223).

This change is having its intended effect even years before its implementation in 2018. Insurers and employers are working to reduce the cost of the insurance products to avoid the "Cadillac tax."

Physician payment reform. A second example illustrates how the federal bureaucracy can influence the substance of legislation.

Members of the White House economic team firmly believed that physician payment change was critical for controlling health care costs and improving quality of care. The fee-for-service payment system still dominated, accounting for about 85% of payments to physicians. It strongly incentivizes physicians to order more tests and recommend other interventions. As the colloquial saying goes: fee-for-service incentivizes volume over value, quantity over quality. Peter Orszag, the director of the OMB, was adamant that to "bend the cost curve," payment change was absolutely necessary. Although alone it may not transform the delivery system, the economic team was certain that payment reform had to be part of the ACA.

As members of this group, Bob Kocher, a physician and the health policy expert at the NEC, and I believed that the easiest way for physicians to move off of fee-for-service health care and to incentivize quality was through bundled payments. Bundled payments are best understood by analogy to menu pricing. If fee-for-service is ordering à la carte, bundled payment is *prix fixe*. It puts all of the costs for a defined unit of care together for one price. For instance, a bundle payment for a hip replacement would cover the preliminary X-rays, the operating room time, the orthopedic surgeon's fee, the anesthesiologist fee, the actual artificial hip, laboratory tests, and rehabilitation and physical therapy as well as other services needed after the operation. In this situation negotiating a low price on the hip implant or using lower-cost but equally effective out-of-hospital rehabilitation services would translate into more money retained for the physicians and hospital. Similarly, the team would want to do everything to reduce the chance of expensive postsurgical wound infections and other adverse events. Thus, bundled payments incentivize physicians and hospitals to be efficient and eliminate unnecessary care but also not stint on care that might cause costly complications. The bundled payment idea goes beyond DRGs paid to hospitals (Chapter 3, page 70) because the DRG payment does not include physician fees, posthospital services, and other items that are included in bundles.

Medicare had some limited but valuable experience with bundled payments. In the 1990s Medicare had run an experiment using bundled payments for coronary bypass procedures (CABGs). The program both reduced costs and improved quality, but Medicare had never widely implemented it. Nevertheless, we thought this experience made bundles a very promising approach.

Furthermore, because the bundle covers discrete events rather than an open-ended whole year of care and because it involved only a few providers, it should be easier for physicians and hospitals to implement. Further, after gaining experience with a few bundles, Medicare, physicians, and hospitals could create bundles for more medical interventions to include chronic conditions, the largest part of health care costs. The guidelines created by professional societies, rather than anything the government imposed, could serve as a basis for creating the bundles.

Dr. Kocher and I presented this idea to the rest of the white House health team and received strong support from Peter Orszag. Larry Summers, a cancer survivor, was a bit more hesitant because he worried about the tendency to stint on care. However, he permitted us to proceed, especially if we had good, quality metrics to minimize the chances for low-cost, low-quality care.

Conversely, Medicare was much more skeptical, arguing that it was too difficult to create bundles, especially for chronic conditions. To counter this, Dr. Kocher and I organized a meeting at the White House with experts who had experience in creating bundles.

After several months of discussion we had a final conference call to determine the administration's position. The Medicare officials raised 3 main objections. First, bundles would have to be developed and tested before they could be used widely. They could not commit to a set of bundles, especially for chronic conditions; there was just too much uncertainty. Second, they did not have the computer infrastructure to pay physicians and hospitals on the basis of bundles. CMS's operations were structured for efficient fee-for-service payment; they had never developed any computer software for bundled payments. Indeed, CMS was paying by paper and pencil rather than electronically for the bundled payment demonstration projects it was experimenting with. Finally, CMS argued that physicians and hospitals were not organized to handle bundles. There were not enough providers who could actually take a lump-sum payment, create efficient delivery models that would save money, and distribute the money without killing each other.

These objections did not seem insurmountable. Professional guidelines could serve as the backbone for developing bundled payments, and specifying a defined timeline for introducing bundles afforded opportunities to work with the physicians and hospitals to refine them. The computer software problem was a classic "chicken and egg" challenge: Medicare would not develop the software unless it was certain bundles would be implemented, but without the software, bundles could not be widely implemented. If, however, there were a defined timeline for introducing bundles, the software would be developed. Finally, without bundled payments there was no financial reason for physicians and hospitals to negotiate and develop ways to provide high-quality, efficient care within a bundled-payment structure. Yet if they had to, both groups were plenty smart and would figure it out if there were a financial incentive to work together.

The arguments went back and forth. But Medicare was adamantly opposed to any binding timeline for implementing bundled payments, much less any other payment models to replace fee-for-service. Ultimately the ACA legislation authorized 10 demonstration projects, with the important proviso that any successful model could be introduced to all of Medicare without the need to go back to Congress for additional legislation.

Medical malpractice. The fate of medical malpractice reform shows the political limits of interest groups and how politics can frequently trump policy. There were good reasons to think that health care reform would contain some kind of malpractice reform. The AMA supported health care reform and desperately wanted malpractice reform, so getting it would seem to be a reasonable price to pay for their support. It was a great bargaining chip to help move physicians in the direction of accepting and adopting payment reform. In addition Larry Summers and Peter Orszag both strongly supported malpractice reform. They believed that, done properly, it could reinforce incentives to improve quality of care.

Most importantly President Obama strongly favored malpractice reform. In 2006, when a senator, Obama and Hillary Clinton coauthored an article in the *New England Journal of Medicine* advocating malpractice reform. They delineated the Medical Error Disclosure and Compensation (MEDiC) Bill:

> The MEDiC program would provide federal grant support and technical assistance for doctors, hospitals, and health systems that disclose medical errors and problems with patient safety. . . . If a patient was injured or harmed as a result of medical error or a failure to adhere to the standard of care, the participant would disclose the matter to the patient and offer to enter into negotiations for fair compensation.

Early in the process of developing the ACA there were many discussions inside the White House about malpractice reform. Nancy-Ann DeParle, head of the White House health reform office, authorized a small group that included 2 lawyers, Susan Sher and Danielle Gray, as well as Dr. Kocher and myself to explore it. One important legal fact hampered this process: medical malpractice is largely a state, not a federal responsibility. The federal government cannot directly legislate to reform malpractice laws. Any legislation would have to incentivize states, such as with grants or subsidies or some other mechanism, to change their malpractice laws.

The group delineated the pros and cons for a wide variety of policy options, ranging from caps on damages and specialized health courts to early disclosure, apologies, and standardized compensation. What became clear was how little empirical research there was to guide policy toward one option over another. For instance, material on caps for damage awards, with restrictions on statutes of limitations, suggested some modest moderation of malpractice premiums, and there were limited data on whether this saved money by reducing defensive medicine practices. There were also limited data on health courts that specialized in malpractice cases, and what there was seemed to show no savings in overall costs. Prereview of cases by an expert panel that supposedly permitted only worthy cases to proceed seemed to have no impact on cost, quality, or improving the malpractice system. What the group realized is that we needed a lot more data to make an informed policy choice, and there would be no data without additional research.

Several reform team members, including myself, favored so-called safe harbors, in which physicians who implement electronic health records with decision supports and follow approved guidelines have a presumption of not having committed negligence. Safe harbors would, the group believed, improve the system of care, make guideline care more routine, and protect physicians who did not order MRIs for headaches or back pain.

One afternoon late in the summer during this policy development process I wandered into my brother's office just to check in with him. Rahm asked me about some analyses I was doing for him. Then, looking down at the two papers on his otherwise clutter-free desk, he asked in his usual staccato, "What else is going on, Zeke?"

"I'm also working on the medical malpractice proposal I told you about," I began to explain.

He immediately cut me off: "Shut the f*** up! We are not doing malpractice. Period. Every time the AMA comes in here they don't talk about malpractice. It is SGR #1, 2, and 3 with those guys. We don't need to do malpractice for the doctors, and I am not alienating the president's base for nothing. Stop it."

And that told me everything about the politics and policy of medical malpractice. Democrats would do malpractice reform under 2 circumstances: if they needed to include reform to keep the physicians, especially the AMA, supporting the ACA legislation, or if they needed to attract Republican support for the larger reform bill. Neither was the case. The AMA was supporting the bill, and regardless of what they were saying in public, when they met with the senior administration leaders they were not emphasizing malpractice reform; instead, the AMA lobbyists were focused on fixing the SGR and physician payment (Chapter 3, page 83). And not a single Republican was interested in negotiating and compromising about anything related to health care reform. So there was no need to develop a malpractice proposal to attract Republican support. Without these political imperatives there was no rationale for Democrats to consider malpractice reform. Between foregoing the public option that alienated liberals, changing the tax exclusion that offended unions, and making deals with drug companies that pissed everyone off, the president did not need to antagonize the plaintiff bar for no gain.

Despite the politics, the president remained committed to malpractice reform. In preparing for the important speech on September 9, 2009, before a joint session of Congress Obama wanted something on malpractice reform. The small team was asked whether there was something that could be done to push the agenda. There were not many options without legislation, but a team member discovered the ability to use patient safety funds for demonstration projects, arguing that changes in malpractice practices should improve the quality of care. Toward the end of the speech the president expressed his thinking on malpractice:

> Now, finally, many in this chamber—particularly on the Republican side of the aisle—have long insisted that reforming our medical malpractice laws can help bring down the cost of health care. (*Applause.*) Now—there you go. There you go. Now, I don't believe malpractice reform is a silver bullet, but I've talked to enough doctors to know that defensive medicine may be contributing to unnecessary costs. (*Applause.*) So I'm proposing that we move forward on a range of ideas about how to put patient safety first and let doctors focus on practicing medicine. (*Applause.*) I know that the Bush administration considered authorizing demonstration projects in individual states to test these ideas. I think it's a good idea, and I'm directing my secretary of health and human services to move forward on this initiative today. (*Applause.*)

This speech occurred after the administration had given up on finding bipartisan compromise after nearly 8 months of fruitless work by Senator Baucus. This was not an offer based on political calculations. Instead, the president was doing whatever he could on malpractice reform despite the politics. Indeed, the administration went further: the original grant program was more likely to get hospitals and health systems to change how they handled malpractice cases but was not targeted at states to change their malpractice laws. Therefore, a provision in the ACA provided 5-year grants for state demonstration projects that implemented changes in medical malpractice laws. Priority was given to reforms that would improve patient safety and enhance the availability of affordable malpractice insurance. The hope was that there would be some interesting experimentation and production of some much-needed empirical data to inform future policy discussions on malpractice reform. These 2 acts were more than any politician, Republican or Democrat, had ever done to advance medical malpractice reform.

Ultimately, despite strong initial support from the White House and from the president himself, there was insufficient rationale for implementing comprehensive malpractice reform. There was no definitive policy rationale linking malpractice reform to substantial cost control or patient safety to appeal to. And the politics were against it. Because the AMA did not make malpractice reform one of its top 3 agenda items in negotiations with senior administration officials and because Republicans were not interested in finding a compromise on health care that included malpractice reform, there was not enough political justification to antagonize Democratic constituents over the issue. So comprehensive medical malpractice reform is absent from the ACA.

Despite 100 years of failure, violating some of the 6 key lessons on enacting health care reform legislation, and multiple near-death experiences, March 23, 2010, was historic. Maybe the vice president put it most succinctly:

"This is a big f***ing deal."

But it wasn't the end of the fight. Immediately after President Obama signed the ACA, lawsuits were filed to block it. Before it could even be implemented, the US Supreme Court would have its say.

= CHAPTER SEVEN =

What the Supreme Court Said

The Constitutionality of the Affordable Care Act

The passage of the Affordable Care Act was filled with drama: the drama of the August 2009 recess, when representatives and senators were attacked by Tea Party opponents of reform; the drama of the Senate's Christmas Eve vote for the ACA, in which Majority Leader Reid mistakenly voted to oppose the Senate's bill; the drama of Vice President Biden whispering the famous expletive to President Obama at the signing of the act.

As though this were not enough, the drama continued with 3 days of Supreme Court arguments in March 2012, and then the ultimate drama of June 28, 2012, when the Court ruled. And the drama was further heightened by CNN's mistake in trying to be the first to report the Court's decision—but calling it wrong. Their call stopped hearts and sowed confusion for 10 minutes or more until the real facts could be circulated.

Ultimately, the Court ruled that the ACA was constitutional as an application of Congress's power to tax. It also created a complication for rolling out the Medicaid expansion, limiting the powers the federal government can use to persuade states to adopt certain policies.

But how did the ACA get to the Court in the first place?

The ACA's Path to the Supreme Court

On March 23, 2010, minutes after President Obama signed the ACA into law, Florida along with more than 20 other states filed a lawsuit challenging the ACA's constitutionality. Later the National Federation of Independent Businesses and a few individuals who did not have health insurance at the time joined the lawsuit. Additionally, there were as many as 30 other constitutional challenges filed.

These challenges from conservatives were a bit surprising in themselves. They focused on the individual mandate. But it was not a liberal invention. Democrats adopted it from a platform the Heritage Foundation, a conservative think tank, put forth around the time of the Clinton reform. As long as Republicans were advocating the mandate, no conservatives ever raised the question of its constitutionality, but this changed when Democrats were on the verge of enacting it as part of the ACA.

By November 2011 there were 4 federal circuit court rulings with different interpretations of the act's constitutionality. In the Florida case 9 district court judges ruled the ACA unconstitutional. On appeal, the 11th Circuit Court concurred, ruling that the individual mandate exceeded Congress's lawful authority but that the Medicaid expansion was constitutional as a "valid exercise of Congress's power under the Spending Clause of the Constitution (Article 1, Section 8, Clause 1)."

In the Virginia case the 4th Circuit Court ruled that the lawsuits must be dismissed under an arcane federal law governing tax collections, but 2 of the judges made clear that they would uphold the constitutionality of the ACA, one on the basis of Congress's power to regulate commerce and one on the basis of Congress's power to tax.

In an Ohio case the 6th Circuit Court also upheld the constitutionality of the ACA's individual mandate. Judge Jeffrey Sutton, a conservative judge who clerked for Justice Antonin Scalia, wrote a principled opinion endorsing the ACA's constitutionality. It may have scuttled any chance he has for a Supreme Court nomination by a Republican administration. It was a profile in courage.

Most importantly, the DC Circuit Court, a court widely viewed as second only to the Supreme Court in its ability to shape the law, also upheld the ACA's constitutionality. Judge Lawrence Silberman, a Reagan appointee who was awarded the Presidential Medal of Freedom by President Bush, wrote that although the ACA limited individual liberty, it did so in a constitutional manner because Congress has the power to regulate commerce:

> [The ACA] certainly is an encroachment on individual liberty, but it is no more so than a command that restaurants or hotels are obliged to serve all customers regardless of race, that gravely ill individuals cannot use a substance their doctors described as the only effective palliative for excruciating pain, or that a farmer cannot grow enough wheat to support his own family. The right to be free from federal regulation is not absolute, and yields to the imperative that Congress be free to forge national solutions to national problems, no matter how local—or seemingly passive—their individual origins.

Like Sutton, Silberman offered a principled defense of judicial restraint. Thus, by November 8, 2011, there were split circuit court decisions on the individual mandate but consensus that the federal government could use its powers to expand Medicaid. When there is disagreement among appellate courts, the Supreme Court generally agrees to take up the case to resolve the conflict and establish a uniform law of the land. So on November 14, 2011, the Supreme Court agreed to hear an appeal of the 11th Circuit Court's decision in the Florida case.

The Constitutional Arguments Over the ACA

Constitutionality of the Individual Mandate

There were 2 issues brought before the Supreme Court. The first was the constitutionality of the individual mandate, or the requirement that individuals have minimum essential coverage or otherwise face a financial penalty. In Section 1501 of the ACA, individuals who do not have health insurance by January 1, 2014, must pay a penalty unless they are otherwise exempt for religious reasons, because they are Native Americans, incarcerated, or fit some other exempt category. The IRS collects the penalty through an individual's tax return, and it amounts to $95 or 1% of an individual's income, whichever is greater (capped at $285) in 2014, $325 or 2% of income (capped at $975) in 2015, and $695 or 2.5% of income (capped at $2,085) in 2016, and subsequently rising with cost of living. In no case can the penalty be greater than the cost of health insurance.

Those claiming the ACA was unconstitutional had a simple argument. Although the constitution gives Congress the power to regulate commerce, opponents claimed that by requiring people to buy health insurance or else pay a penalty, Congress was *forcing* people to enter into commerce. In other words, Congress could regulate activity—the purchase of health insurance—but could not regulate inactivity—the nonpurchase of health insurance. As Paul Clement, the brilliant lawyer arguing before the Supreme Court on behalf of those opposing the ACA, said,

> The individual mandate rests on a claim of federal power that is both unprecedented and unbounded: the power to compel individuals to engage in commerce in order more effectively to regulate commerce. This asserted power does not exist.The power to compel a person to enter into an unwanted commercial relationship is not some modest step necessary and proper to perfect Congress's authority to regulate existing commercial intercourse. It is a revolution in the relationship between the central government and the governed.

Opponents warned darkly that Congress would start with health insurance and then require any purchase it deemed fit. As Judge Sutton of the 6th Circuit Court put it, "If Congress can require Americans to buy medical insurance today, what of tomorrow? Could it compel individuals to buy health care itself in the form of an annual check-up or for that matter a health-club membership? And if Congress can do this in the healthcare field, what of other fields of commerce and other products?"

The conservative rallying cry was clear: If the Court accepts the fact that Congress can require people to purchase health insurance, why couldn't it require that people buy broccoli to be healthy? In her Supreme Court opinion, Justice Ruth Bader Ginsburg called this "the broccoli horrible." Accepting the ACA would threaten to undermine individuals' ability to make their own decisions about how to lead their lives.

Proponents of the constitutionality of the ACA countered with 3 arguments. The first was an invocation of the Commerce Clause. According to Article 1, Section 8, Clause 3 of the Constitution, Congress has the right to regulate commerce: "[The Congress shall have Power] To regulate Commerce with foreign Nations, and among the several States, and with the Indian tribes." The Necessary and Proper Clause of the same section further amplifies this power: "The Congress shall have Power To make all Laws which shall be necessary and proper for carrying into Execution the foregoing Powers [including the Commerce power], and all other Powers vested by this Constitution in the Government of the United States, or in any Department or Officer thereof."

According to proponents of the ACA, Congress enacted the law to address problems in the health care marketplace involving nearly 18% of the GDP. The Commerce Clause clearly grants Congress the authority to regulate such large markets as that of health care, which is unique in its size and significance and, thus, not like the broccoli market at all. With broccoli, the market works regardless of whether any individual buys or does not buy the vegetable. With health insurance, however, the market fails because of adverse selection, in which only the sick buy insurance, driving the premium to unaffordable levels unless there is a mandate balancing the sick and the healthy (Chapter 2, page 41). The mandate is the only way insurance companies can offer all Americans—including those with preexisting conditions—affordable coverage regardless of health status.

The Obama administration countered the argument that the individual mandate was forcing people to engage in commerce by pointing out that everyone will eventually need health care: either they pay for it themselves or they shift the costs to someone else who pays for them. Like it or not, every American—except, maybe, hermits—will engage in the commerce of health insurance and health care. It is inevitable. Congress was simply regulating when people paid for that health coverage and took measures to prevent them from free riding on other Americans and raising everyone else's insurance premiums. This regulation, the administration argued, makes the market more stable, efficient, and affordable. Thus, the supposed activity-inactivity distinction the opponents raised was a false distinction. Regulating when people pay for an inevitable purchase is not regulating inactivity.

In a second argument the Obama administration pointed out that the Necessary and Proper Clause gave Congress the power to do whatever is necessary to ensure its power to regulate commerce. The Constitution therefore sanctions the mandate because Congress thought it necessary to impose it in order to have a well-functioning health insurance marketplace. As the administration noted, nothing in the Constitution limits the means by which Congress can choose to exercise its powers granted by the Constitution. They had a surprising source of support for this argument: Justice Scalia, one of the most conservative justices. In a case involving federal marijuana regulation, he wrote, "Where Congress has the authority to enact a regulation of interstate commerce, it possesses every power needed to make that regulation effective."

The government had a backup argument. The individual mandate penalty was a tax. Based on Article 1, Section 8, Clause 1, Congress has the power to tax: "The Congress shall have Power to lay and collect Taxes, Duties, Imposts and Excises, to pay the Debts and provide for the common Defence and general Welfare of the United States." Thus, the individual mandate is constitutional because it functioned just like any other tax law. Just as Congress can give tax benefits to homeowners or people with children, it can also tax people who have insurance at a lower rate than people who do not. There was, of course, an irony in the administration's argument about the mandate and the power to tax. During the debate over the mandate Republicans insisted that the mandate was a tax, and Democrats insisted it wasn't. As soon as President Obama signed the bill, both sides reversed their positions: the Democrats claimed it was a tax and, therefore, was justified by Congress's constitutional power to tax, and the Republicans insisted it wasn't a tax and, therefore, couldn't be justified by the taxing power. In the end the Supreme Court ignored these contortions, which are specious "legislative history"—that is, the shifting arguments representatives and senators offer on the floor to justify their votes.

Constitutionality of the Medicaid Expansion

There was a second issue related to the constitutionality of the Medicaid expansion. Many commentators were surprised that the Supreme Court took this issue. Constitutionally, the federal government cannot order states to adopt certain policies, but it can "bribe" states by conditioning the receipt of federal funding on compliance with federal rules. For instance, the federal government could not order states to raise their drinking age to 21 years, but it could make the states' receipt of federal highway funds contingent on adopting the higher age requirement.

In one case, *South Dakota v. Dole* (483 U.S. 203, 1987) the Court ruled that such linkages are constitutional. But the Court also noted that sometimes these inducements might cross the line, becoming coercive and, thus, unconstitutional, stating, "The financial inducement offered by Congress [to states could be so excessive they would be] coercive as to pass the point at which 'pressure turns into compulsion.'"

Florida and the other states invoked this coercive theory. They noted that if a state did not expand Medicaid, the ACA required the federal government to withhold all Medicaid money, not just the Medicaid money for the expansion. For many states Medicaid constitutes the largest-single budgetary item. Further, the federal portion of Medicaid constitutes the largest federal transfer of funds to the states. If the federal government withheld all Medicaid funds from any state, it would strap that state's budget, endangering every other program, from education to corrections. Thus, the states argued that withholding all Medicaid funds constitutes not inducement but rather compulsion and coercion, and this made it unconstitutional. Interestingly, according to the 11th Circuit Court's review, never before had any federal court invoked this coercive theory to limit a federal law. So having the Supreme Court entertain an objection to the ACA based on this theory was surprising.

Both the Federal District Court and the 11th Circuit Court rejected this state coercion argument. The 11th Circuit Court made 4 points in its rejection of this claim. First, when Congress enacted Medicaid in 1965, it reserved the right to amend the program's requirements and has done so many times. States were on notice that Congress could and would change this program over time. Adding an expansion was neither new nor unprecedented. States had full warning.

Second, the Medicaid expansion is a minimal burden on the states. The federal government is bearing 100% of the costs for the first 3 years, and the proportion slowly declines until the federal government assumes 90% of the Medicaid costs. The states get a huge financial benefit for minimal financial payment. This hardly seems coercive.

Third, the Medicaid expansion was slated to begin nearly 4 years after enacting the ACA, giving the states plenty of time to make alternative arrangements if they objected. Medicaid itself is a voluntary program. The states are not legally required to keep it at all.

Fourth, the law does not require the federal government to withdraw all Medicaid funds. That is the ultimate penalty, but it is not the only penalty. The secretary of the Department of Health and Human Services (HHS) can withhold lesser amounts.

The Supreme Court's ACA Ruling

Chief Justice John Roberts wrote the majority decision. On the matter of the individual mandate the Court ruled 5 to 4 that Congress's power to regulate commerce did not support it. However, the majority did rule that the individual mandate was a lawful exercise of the taxing power. On the matter of the Medicaid expansion, 7 to 2 ruled that the threat to remove all federal Medicaid funds was coercive.

Chief Justice Roberts's decision was strange in at least one way. He extensively explained why the Commerce Clause did not apply to the mandate. Typically, when the Supreme Court upholds a law, the justices do not weigh in on questions that they were not required to resolve in order to decide the case. There is a great deal of argument about why Justice Roberts devoted so many pages to the Commerce Clause argument. (The most plausible explanation is that he switched his vote to strike down the ACA after drafting the commerce clause opinion.) He justifies this by claiming he had to explain why he invoked the taxing power as the basis for the decision. Justice Ruth Bader Ginsburg admonished his disingenuousness. There always are innumerable arguments that do *not* justify a position, and it is not customary for a justice to rehearse why each of them fails.

As for the Commerce Clause argument, Chief Justice Roberts basically sided with the states and the 4 other conservative justices, Scalia, Clarence Thomas, Samuel Alito, and Anthony Kennedy, in affirming the activity-inactivity distinction. He argued that Congress did not have the power to regulate inactivity. Based on prior decisions, the Court recognized that Congress has the power (1) to regulate activity that substantially affects interstate commerce, even if that activity is not interstate commerce itself, and (2) to regulate smaller activities that affect interstate commerce only when aggregated with similar activities. But he argued,

> Congress has never attempted to rely on that power to compel individuals not engaged in commerce to purchase an unwanted product.The power to *regulate* commerce presupposes the existence of commercial activity to be regulated.The language of the Constitution reflects the natural understanding that the power to regulate assumes there is already something to be regulated.

The reason the Commerce Clause does not justify the individual mandate, he argued, was that

> [the mandate] compels individuals to *become* active in commerce by purchasing a product, on the ground that their failure to do so affects interstate commerce. Construing the Commerce Clause to permit Congress to regulate individuals precisely *because* they are doing nothing would open a new and potentially vast domain to congressional authority.

Chief Justice Roberts addressed the administration's claim that the activity-inactivity distinction is untenable especially when someone will certainly become sick and use the health care system at some future point. But rather than argue the point, Roberts merely stated that his reading "reflect[s] the natural understanding" and that "the distinction between doing something and doing nothing would not have been lost on the Framers, who were 'practical statesmen,' not metaphysical philosophers."

It is worth noting here that this comment was a bit ironic, as the main objection to the activity-inactivity distinction was, as Chief Justice Roberts himself acknowledged, made not by philosophers but by practical economists. The Chief Justice was the one who was invoking subtle distinctions like a metaphysical philosopher, not a skeptical statesman.

Finally, Chief Justice Roberts argued that if the government is allowed to regulate inactivity, it could indeed mandate people to buy broccoli. After all, Americans who eat an unhealthy diet increase overall health care costs and, through the insurance system, transfer those costs to others. If we accept the view that Congress can regulate inactivity, Chief Justice Roberts said, "Congress could address the diet problem by ordering everyone to buy vegetables." The Chief Justice never considered that there is an obvious solution to such unwise policies, and it is not the Supreme Court. Americans can rebel at the ballot box by voting out politicians who require them to buy broccoli.

Having rejected the Commerce Clause argument, Chief Justice Roberts did accept that the individual mandate is a tax and, therefore, justified by Congress's taxing power. Rather than commanding individuals to buy health insurance, the individual mandate can be seen as a tax on people who fail to buy insurance:

> [The individual mandate] makes going without insurance just another thing the Government taxes, like buying gasoline or earning income. And if the mandate is in effect just a tax hike on certain taxpayers who do not have health insurance, it may be within Congress's constitutional power to tax.

This view, he claimed, is bolstered because of the characteristics of the payment: it is made to the Treasury when taxpayers file their income tax returns, does not apply to individuals who do not file income tax because their income is too low, is modified based on income and number of dependents, and generates revenue for the government, albeit a comparatively small amount, projected to be just $4 billion in 2017. But these characteristics were enough for Chief Justice Roberts to argue that for Congress to impose such a tax in the form of the individual mandate was constitutional.

Roberts then responded to the 4 conservative justices' argument that Congress did not label the individual mandate a tax and, therefore, it cannot be considered a tax. Citing many previous rulings, Chief Justice Roberts declared the fact that Congress did not call the penalty payment a tax was immaterial for the constitutional question: "That constitutional question was not controlled by Congress's choice of label." Furthermore, he noted that not having health insurance was not viewed in the ACA as "unlawful" and, thus, worthy of criminal prosecution or other punishment. In this sense, although Congress called the payment a penalty, it did not view it as a violation of federal law. Thus, it is more natural to view the payment as a tax.

Finally, when it came to the expansion of Medicaid, Chief Justice Roberts wrote for 7 justices that it went too far. Under the spending clause, everyone agrees: Congress can require states to adopt certain programs in exchange for federal monies. This was affirmed in the *South Dakota v. Dole* case conditioning federal highway funds on states raising the drinking age.

It was Chief Justice Roberts's opinion that in any such policy-change-for-federal-money deal states must be able to accept it freely: "The legitimacy of Congress's exercise of the spending power 'thus rests on whether the State voluntarily and knowingly accepts the terms of the 'contract.'" In other words, the states must not be coerced into accepting the deal; they must be able to reject the deal if they do not like the policy they are being asked to adopt:

> In the typical case we look to the States to defend their prerogatives by adopting "the simple expedient of not yielding" to federal blandishments when they do not want to embrace the federal policies as their own.

Chief Justice Roberts argued that, based on *South Dakota v. Dole*, Congress can withhold funds for a program—in that case, highway money—if the states do not adopt a policy—raising the drinking age to 21—if the amount is small enough not to be coercive. The problem with the ACA, he argued, is that the amount of money the federal government was threatening to withhold was not only excessive but also the funds from another program. Federal Medicaid funds now account for more than 10% of state budgets. Threatening to withhold that amount, he stated, is not a

> "relatively mild encouragement"—it is a gun to the head. A State that opts out of the Affordable Care Act's expansion in health care coverage thus stands to lose not merely "a relatively small percentage" of its Medicaid funding, but *all* of it. The threatened loss of over 10% of a State's overall budget, in contrast, is economic dragooning that leaves the States with no real option but to acquiesce in the Medicaid expansion.

Thus, the large amount of federal funding at risk for not expanding Medicaid made a state decision involuntary.

The administration countered that the states had been forewarned about changes to Medicaid's eligibility rules as far back as the initial 1965 legislation and that many changes had been instituted over the years. Chief Justice Roberts countered that although it uses the same name—Medicaid—the ACA in fact "accomplishes a shift in kind, not merely degree." The original program was a categorical program (Chapter 2, page 47). It applied to the blind and disabled, children, pregnant women, and poor elderly. The program under the ACA, however, is a means-tested program applying to everyone under 65 with income below 133% of poverty. "[Medicaid] is no longer a program to care for the neediest among us, but rather an element of a comprehensive national plan to provide universal health insurance coverage," Roberts wrote. In this case 7 justices felt that the ACA transformed Medicaid into a new program. Thus, Congress cannot withhold money to fund the old categorical Medicaid program if states do not adopt the Medicaid expansion.

Although the Supreme Court did affirm the constitutionality of the ACA, at least a few constitutional scholars, such as Akhil Amar of Yale Law School, have warned that people should "look at the dark cloud behind the silver lining." He was worried that the ruling restricts the federal government's power in at least 2 ways: (1) limiting what Congress can do under the commerce clause, and (2) limiting how closely it can link federal funds to the adoption of certain policies. For the moment these restrictions do not apply to the health care system, but they might at some point in the future.

After the June 28, 2012 Court ruling, the ACA was clearly the law of the land—passed by Congress, signed by the president, and upheld as constitutional by the Supreme Court. Yet opponents have not stopped trying to prevent its implementation. They have repeatedly attempted to repeal the ACA. They have fought to prevent funding of the ACA. And they have brought additional lawsuits against the ACA. In every attempt they have failed.

The ACA is being implemented, albeit with glitches, challenges, and problems.

But what, in fact, is in the ACA? What precisely is being implemented? And what does the ruling against the Medicaid expansion mean for achieving universal coverage?

= CHAPTER EIGHT =

What Is in the Affordable Care Act?

The Substance of Health Care Reform

The Affordable Care Act is 906 pages long. That is the official version from the Government Printing Office. In addition to the 55 pages in the Health Care and Education Reconciliation Act of 2010 that amended certain portions of the ACA, the entire act runs under 1000 pages, with 422,018 total words. The entire American health care system, the 5th-largest economy in the world, was repaired in fewer than 1,000 pages—not much longer than Stephen King's *11/22/63* novel. Not bad and far less than the claimed 1,200 or even 2,400 pages, neither of which was ever true. (That enormous figure was based on a proposed bill that had numerous other provisions and potential amendments that were never enacted.)

But the real question about the ACA is what do those words say and, more importantly, mean?

The ACA is divided into 10 different titles (or, rather, chapters or parts) (see Figure 8.1). The first 2 relate to access and expanding coverage. The 3rd contains provisions addressing both cost and quality. The 4th is about public health matters. The 5th addresses workforce issues. The 6th relates mostly to pursuing fraud and abuse but also contains some provisions on quality improvement. The 7th pertains to changing laws so as to speed up access to new drugs and setting a legal framework to get expensive, branded biological compounds, such as antibodies, to market as cheaper generics. The 8th implements a new long-term care insurance program that was subsequently repealed. The 9th title addresses the act's financing and raising revenue, and the 10th reauthorizes the Indian Health Care Improvement Act.

FIGURE 8.1 Ten titles of the Affordable Care Act

Title I: Quality, Affordable Health Care for All Americans	• Prohibits insurance companies from denying coverage based on preexisting conditions • Caps out-of-pocket expenditures • Extends dependent coverage for young adults to age 26 • Requires full coverage of preventive care and immunization • Creates individual and small-business insurance exchanges • Establishes tax subsidies for individuals up to 400% of the federal poverty level (FPL) and employers • Establishes individual and employer mandates and penalties • Caps insurance company nonmedical, administrative expenditures—the medical-loss ratio
Title II: The Role of Public Program	• Expands Medicaid to 133% of the federal poverty level • Simplifies enrollment for Medicaid, CHIP, and the exchanges
Title III: Improving the Quality and Efficiency of Health Care	• Launches value-based purchasing program in Medicare • Extends Physician Quality Reporting Initiative (PQRI) • Establishes Center for Medicare and Medicaid Innovation (CMMI) to develop pilot programs aimed at encouraging high-quality, efficient care • Provides incentives for Accountable Care Organizations (ACOs) • Closes the "donut hole" in Medicare Part D • Creates the Independent Payment Advisory Board (IPAB) • Establishes payment adjustments (penalties) for hospital-acquired conditions such as hospital-acquired infections • Establishes the hospital readmission reduction program
Title IV: Prevention of Chronic Disease and Improving Public Health	• Creates the National Prevention, Health Promotion, and Public Health Council, an interagency body charged with developing a national public health strategy • Requires calorie counts on menus at chain restaurants • Provides small-business grants for workplace wellness programs • Improves access and availability of preventive services
Title V: Health Care Workforce	• Establishes a National Health Workforce Commission to review needs and advise Congress and the administration • Modifies the Federal Student Loan Program to provide scholarships and repayment to primary care doctors and nurses • Invests in grant programs that support training of primary care doctors • Provides payment bonuses to primary care doctors

Title VI: Transparency and Program Integrity	• Requires drug and device manufacturers to report gifts to physicians and other providers • Establishes stricter transparency and ethics standards for nursing homes • Creates the Patient-Centered Outcomes Research Institute (PCORI) • Establishes procedures to screen providers and suppliers who participate in Medicare, Medicaid, and CHIP to reduce fraud • Encourages states to develop and test alternatives to the existing civil litigation system for medical malpractice
Title VII: Improving Access to Innovative Medical Technologies	• Streamlines the FDA licensing process for products that are biosimilar to a product that has been on the market for at least 12 years • Provides drug discounts for children's hospitals and underserved communities
Title VIII: Community Living Assistance Services and Supports	• Establishes a voluntary, self-funded insurance program for community living assistance services and support (CLASS)
Title IX: Revenue Provisions	• Imposes the "Cadillac tax" on high-cost, employer-sponsored health plans • Imposes a medical device tax on the device manufacturing sector • Imposes an annual flat fee on pharmaceutical manufacturers • Imposes an annual flat fee on health insurers • Imposes an excise tax on indoor tanning services • Imposes an excise tax on elective cosmetic surgery • Eliminates the deduction for employer Part D subsidies • Increases additional 0.9% Medicare tax for high-wage workers
Title X: Reauthorization of the Indian Health Care Improvement Act	• Extends the Indian Health Care Improvement Act, which expired in 2000 • Modernizes and streamlines care delivery for the Indian Health Service, which cares for 1.8 million American Indians and Alaska Natives

One thing that becomes clear just from the mere listing of the 10 titles is that, contrary to claims, the ACA is not just about access and universal coverage. It is not even 90% about access. Only titles 1 and 2—222 pages of the 906 pages of the ACA—deal with expanding Medicaid and creating the exchanges, and even of that, only about 39 pages really focus on these topics. However you count the pages, under a quarter of the bill can be said to be about access; the vast majority of the legislation addresses other matters.

Additionally, legislation is not necessarily logically organized, or at least the logic might escape an intelligent citizen. For instance, provisions related to improving the quality of the health care system are spread out over at least 3 titles.

Because of this, rather than delineate the content of the ACA's 10 titles, this chapter will explore themes, analyzing the major changes the act makes through 8 distinct categories:

1) Access—particularly expanding Medicaid and creating health insurance exchanges
2) Cost control—including accountable care organizations (ACOs) bundled payments, the "Cadillac" tax, the Center for Medicare and Medicaid Innovation, and the Independent Payment Advisory Board
3) Quality improvement—including reduction in hospital-acquired infections and readmissions, electronic health records, and the establishment of the Patient-Center Outcomes Institute
4) Prevention—including the coverage of preventive services without co-payments, menu labeling, and employer wellness programs
5) Workforce—including support for nursing schools and changes in loan forgiveness for physicians entering the National Health Service Corps
6) Revenue—including device, cosmetic surgery, and tanning salon taxes
7) Other important odds and ends—including administrative simplification, medical-loss ratio, and transparency of financial relationships between drug companies and physicians
8) The CLASS Act—that would have created a voluntary long-term insurance program, but it was subsequently repealed

This chapter is meant to serve as the definitive resource for finding out what is in the ACA. Probably the main reason to elaborate the details of the ACA is that this act establishes the institutional framework that will structure the American health care system for at least the next 30 years. Given how difficult comprehensive health care legislation is to enact in the United States, this act will define the country's overall approach to access, cost, and quality for our and perhaps our children's lifetimes. This may seem daunting, but understanding the insurance exchanges, accountable care organizations, bundled payments, and the rest is critical to understanding how we will get health insurance and be cared for the rest of our lives.

ACCESS

A major objective of health care reform was to achieve universal coverage. Because the president promised that people who were satisfied could keep their insurance if they wanted to, the ACA sought to provide coverage to the 15% of uninsured Americans through existing programs.

One popular and successful expansion of access applies to young adults. Beginning 6 months after the ACA was signed into law, section 2714 requires insurance companies to allow young adults to stay on their parents' insurance plan until the age of 26. Most plans terminated children at 18 or, if they were students, until they graduated college. This change permitted more than 3 million young adults to become insured. Many insurance companies actually extended coverage to young adults before they were legally required to do so on September 23, 2010.

Another important provision was aimed at increasing the actual purchase of coverage when insurance was offered. Relying on the insights of behavioral economics, section 1511 of the ACA requires employers with more than 200 full-time employees to enroll workers automatically in health insurance and to continue current workers in health insurance unless they explicitly opt out. In many other contexts, such as retirement accounts, using this type of opt-out mechanism—you are enrolled unless you actively exclude yourself—significantly increases uptake. This provision was supposed to go into effect in 2014, but the Department of Labor has delayed its start.

But the 2 most important reforms related to access involve expanding and transforming Medicaid for the poor and establishing insurance exchanges or web-based marketplaces where people could select private health insurance policies with government subsidies. Importantly, creating the exchanges not only provides access for the uninsured, like Wayne and Baltazar, but it also substantially improves the options for Americans like Erin who previously had purchased insurance in the individual marketplacc. In the exchanges Americans like Erin can frequently find more choices and avoid the preexisting condition exclusions that previously made coverage for cancer survivors either impossible or very expensive. And many will also be eligible for subsidies to make health insurance more affordable.

The coverage expansion began on January 1, 2014 (Title I, sec. 1253, 1311). The nearly 4-year delay in implementing the Medicaid expansion and the exchanges from when the ACA was signed into law was necessary for both financial and practical reasons. Financially, by putting off expanding access to 2014, the total 10-year cost estimate of the ACA came in under the president's $1 trillion threshold. As the glitches and problems in opening the exchanges have demonstrated, it takes time to launch such complex endeavors. Insurance companies need to create products, computer software needs to be developed, call centers need to be established and personnel trained, and a host of other activities need to be organized. To put it mildly, enrollment in the federal exchanges was filled with inexcusable and infuriating website problems and failures. Several state exchanges, such as those in Kentucky, Connecticut, and California, performed much better. Hopefully, over the next months and year, these website failings will be eliminated and the user experience will be optimized.

Importantly, the 12 million undocumented immigrants were excluded from getting health insurance through the ACA. Contrary to Representative Wilson's "you lie" claim during President Obama's September 9, 2009, speech to a joint session of Congress (Chapter 6, page 166), undocumented immigrants are excluded from Medicaid expansion and purchasing coverage in the exchanges, even if they pay the full premium.

Access Part 1. Medicaid Expansion

There are 4 major aspects to the Medicaid expansion. First, the ACA changes Medicaid's eligibility requirements. Originally, Medicaid was created as a means-tested, categorical program (Chapter 2, page 47) to

FIGURE 8.2 Modified adjusted gross income (MAGI)

MAGI is one of those technical bureaucratic categories that only lawyers and accountants could create to ensure lifetime employment. It is determined in a 3-step process. First, gross income includes wages, interest, dividends, and the like. Second, adjusted gross income (AGI) subtracts over 20 deductions such as health savings account (HSA) contributions, alimony, and allowable IRA contributions. Third and finally, modified adjusted gross income (MAGI) then adds back some of those deductions, such as the IRA contributions and student loan interest, and some other income, such as tax-exempt interest.

provide coverage to various categories of poor people—children, pregnant women, mothers of young children, the disabled, the very poor elderly. States were free to alter the eligibility requirements as long as they met a federally set minimum.

On January 1, 2014, the ACA established nationwide eligibility standards. Every American up to age 65 with income below 138% of the federal poverty line (in 2013 $32,550 for a family of 4 and $11,490 for individuals) is entitled to Medicaid unless they get health insurance through their employer or some other source (Title II, Sec. 2002).* This income threshold is based on a family's modified adjusted gross income (MAGI, see Figure 8.2). This transforms Medicaid into a strict means-tested program with uniform national standards.

Second, what benefits are the additional people entitled to? The expanded Medicaid program is supposed to offer a new benefit package that fulfills the requirements of the "essential benefits" that is the basis of health insurance options in the exchanges (Title II, Sec. 2001). This is less than the traditional, very comprehensive Medicaid benefits.

The third relates to the benefits package that was an important change in payment to physicians. One of the big complaints about Medicaid is that it provides comprehensive benefits on paper but not in reality. Given the low payment rates (see Chapter 3, page 73), most physicians refuse to see Medicaid patients or limit the number they do see. To

*Some people have felt confused, seeing many claims stating that people with incomes up to 133% of the federal poverty line are entitled to Medicaid. This is caused by an across-the-board 5% of income disregard. So although the law states 133% of the poverty level (Sec. 1331), effectively the threshold is 138%. Welcome to legislation that keeps lawyers fully employed.

counter this the ACA mandated that primary care physicians, specified as family medicine, internal medicine, and pediatrics, be paid at Medicare rates for 2013 and 2014 (Health Care and Education Reconciliation Act of 2010, Title I, Sec. 1202). The federal government was picking up the full price for this payment increase. Ironically, the problem of access for Medicaid patients is less severe for primary care physicians. The serious access problems are for specialists, particularly pediatric specialists, who are already in very short supply. For specialists, the ACA contains no mandated increase in Medicaid payment.

The fourth and final aspect concerns how this expansion is financed. The federal government could not require states to adopt the Medicaid expansion. The states must proactively enact legislation to expand their Medicaid program. And yet they are resistant because Medicaid is becoming such a burden on state budgets (Chapter 4, page 105). Thus, the ACA needed to sweeten the deal sufficiently to persuade the states to adopt it. Thus, the federal government pays for almost all of the cost of this Medicaid expansion (see Figure 8.3).

This level of federal funding makes the Medicaid expansion a great financial deal for states; indeed, states actually will save money (see Figure 8.4). Previously states paid for the health care costs of the uninsured in at least 2 ways. First, there is the cost shift (Chapter 3, page 99). The insurance premiums the states paid for their employees and legislators include added payments to hospitals and physicians for services they render to the uninsured that are not otherwise paid for. Furthermore, states and localities often fund programs to provide health care services to the uninsured, whether through county hospitals, free clinics, or other facilities. With Medicaid expansion most of the uninsured would have coverage, and these hidden costs and programs would be reduced. Instead of absorbing the unpaid bills associated with caring for the uninsured, the hospital bills would be paid by Medicaid. Research by the President's Council of Economic Advisers revealed that even states that spend very little to help the uninsured, such as Nebraska and Wyoming, still save money by accepting the Medicaid expansion (see Figure 8.4).

The ACA requires states to have *Maintenance of Effort (MOE)* (Title I, Sec. 1101). Before the ACA, the federal government paid an average 57% of the Medicaid costs, with poorer states getting a higher percentage of

FIGURE 8.3 Federal financing of the Medicaid expansion

YEAR	PERCENT OF MEDICAID EXPANSION COST PAID FOR BY THE FEDERAL GOVERNMENT
2014–2016	100%
2017	95%
2018	94%
2019	93%
2020 and beyond	90%

their costs covered. There would obviously be a substantial financial incentive for states to pare back their Medicaid beneficiaries between 2010 and 2014 and then add poor people back once the federal government covered 90% of their costs. To counter such gimmicks, the ACA requires MOE: that states keep in place the eligibility requirements for adults they had on March 23, 2010, the date the ACA was signed into law.

One last point relates to how CHIP is treated in the ACA. The law requires states to maintain their eligibility standards for CHIP (and children on Medicaid) until 2019 (Title II, Sec. 2101). There is no change in benefits. In addition, beginning in 2015 the federal government is increasing the proportion it pays, up to 100% of all CHIP costs (Title II, Sec. 2101). This is a substantial benefit for state budgets and protects children's coverage.

The CBO estimates the ACA will add 9 million new Medicaid beneficiaries in the first year and 12 million by 2020.

Access Part 2. Creation of Health Insurance Exchanges

The second—and more interesting, far-reaching, and transformative—mode of expanding access in the ACA was the creation of state-based insurance exchanges. Basically, these are marketplaces in which insurance companies offer different plans with different hospitals, physicians, drug formularies, and co-pay and deductible levels. The plans are standardized to 4 price points—bronze, silver, gold, and platinum. People then shop, comparing these plans, and they select the one they prefer. People earning up to 400% of the federal poverty line (in 2013 $94,200 for

FIGURE 8.4 Projected state savings by adopting Medicaid expansion

STATE	SPENDING ON EXISTING HEALTH PROGRAMS FOR UNINSURED ($ MILLIONS)	HIDDEN TAX ON STATE EMPLOYEE HEALTH INSURANCE PREMIUMS	ESTIMATED STATE COST FOR UNCOMPENSATED CARE	STATE COST OF MEDICAID EXPANSION AT 90% FEDERAL PAYMENT, POST-ACA	NET STATE SAVINGS WITH 90% OF FEDERAL PAYMENT, POST-ACA
Arkansas	$6.2	$17.2	$23.4	–$20.4	$3.0
California	$1,934.0	$210.0	$2,144.0	–$195.0	$1,949.00
Florida	$275.3	$102.0	$377.3	–$251.6	$125.7
Idaho	$38.9	$8.3	$47.2	–$25.8	$21.4
Indiana	$308.0	$29.5	$337.5	–$62.3	$275.2
Iowa	$33.6	$11.2	$44.8	–$20.0	$24.8
Maine	$45.7	$5.1	$50.8	–$15.3	$35.5
Michigan	$168.4	$43.5	$211.9	–$68.1	$143.8
Minnesota	$281.0	$13.6	$294.6	–$31.7	$262.9
Montana	$22.8	$7.0	$29.8	–$20.8	$9.0
Nebraska	$27.0	$8.6	$35.6	–$17.8	$17.8
North Carolina	$150.7	$58.6	$209.3	–$188.3	$21.0
Oregon	$116.0	$22.3	$138.3	–$59.3	$79.0
Pennsylvania	$171.8	$43.1	$214.9	–$149.7	$65.2
Vermont	$17.5	$3.3	$20.8	–$6.8	$14.0
Wyoming	$6.9	$4.5	$11.4	–$10.6	$0.8
Total	**$3,603.8**	**$587.8**	**$4,191.6**	**–$1,143.5**	**$3,048.1**

Source: White House Council of Economic Advisers, "The Impact of Health Insurance Reform on State and Local Government," September 15, 2009, www.whitehouse.gov/assets/documents/cea-statelocal-sept15-final.pdf.

a family of 4, and $45,960 for individuals) will receive a subsidy to help pay for the insurance plan (Title I, Sec. 1402).

We will discuss 6 interrelated subjects to elucidate the nature of the exchanges: (1) administration; (2) the tiers and premiums of the plans; (3) the types and levels of the subsidies in the exchange; (4) the essential benefits, including abortion; (5) the rules governing the insurance companies in the exchange; and (6) the individual and employer mandates.

Under the ACA, states were permitted to create 2 health insurance exchanges, one for individuals and one for small businesses of up to 100 employees (called SHOP exchanges). These SHOP exchanges could be opened to larger companies after 2017 (Title I, Sec. 1311–1312).

According to the law, the state agency administering the exchange could be a government or nonprofit entity responsible for enrollment procedures, including creating and maintaining the website, operating call centers for customer service, overseeing the qualified health plans that will sell in the exchange, and ensuring the insurance companies adhere to requirements for marketing, provider networks, cash reserves, and the like (Title I, Sec. 1311). One of the most important functions these agencies would fulfill is to reliably and confidentially link to the IRS to verify a customer's income and give them, in real time, the level of subsidy they would receive. Knowing the actual price you would pay for health insurance, rather than the higher sticker price, is key to informed and efficient shopping.

The ACA permits groups of several states to affiliate and form a regional exchange instead of each individual state operating its own exchange. In 2014 none have exercised this option. Beginning in 2016 states can also allow insurance companies from another state to offer plans in their state—not on the exchange—but to do so the benefits must be at least as good as those available in the exchange (Title I, Sec. 1333).

For the first year, 2014, 16 states and the District of Columbia have received approval from the Department of Health and Human Services (DHHS) to operate their own exchanges (see Figure 8.5). There are 27 federally facilitated exchanges in which the federal government operates exchanges for states that opted out of running their own entirely (Title I, Sec. 1321). In addition, there are 7 exchanges that are operated as a partnership between the federal and state governments (Title I, Sec. 1322).

FIGURE 8.5 State decisions on exchanges

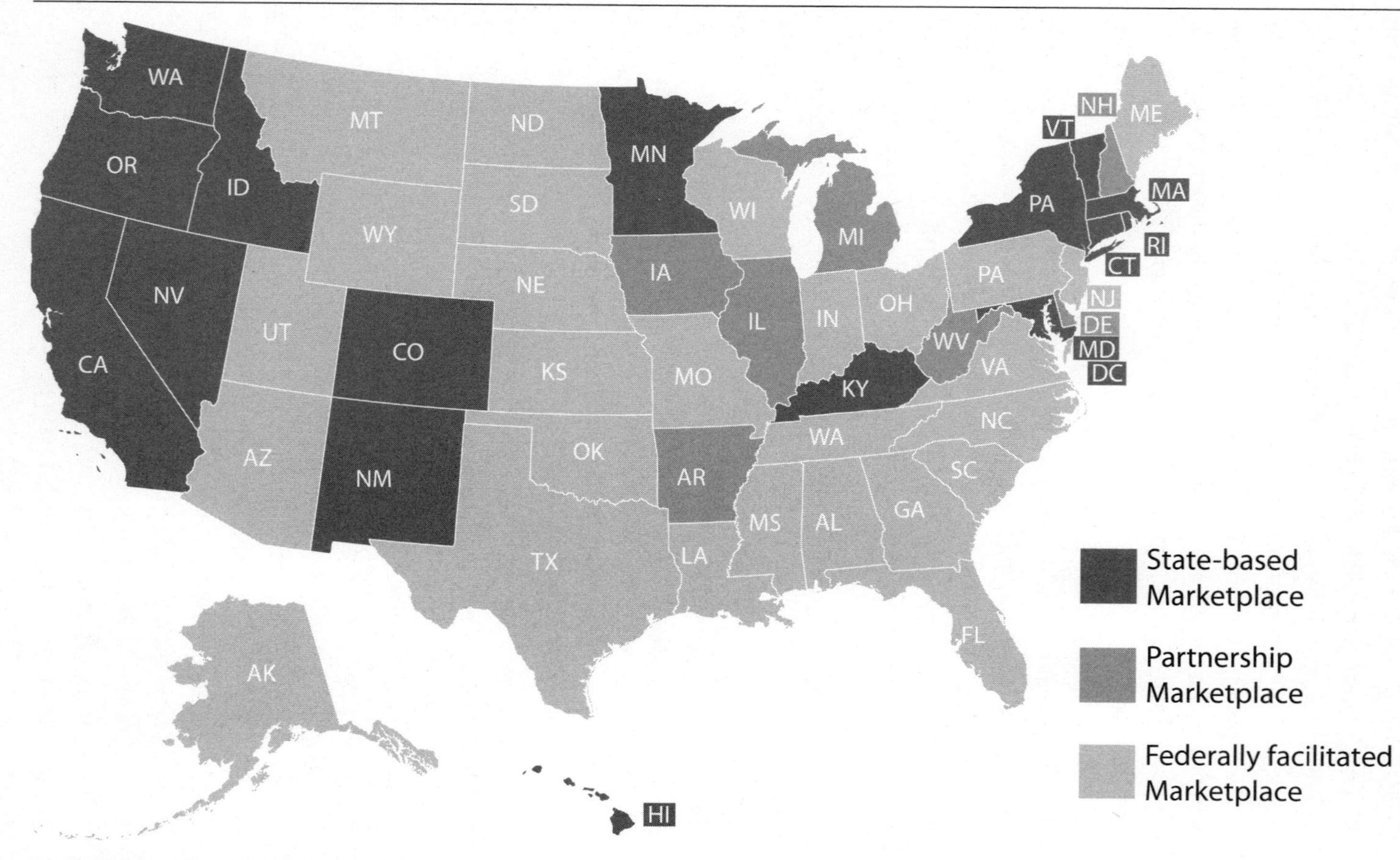

Source: The Henry J. Kaiser Family Foundation.

There are 2 potential types of exchanges. One is an open or passive exchange that places few restrictions on plans and lists all possible offerings for consumers to choose from. This is modeled on the Utah small-business exchange, avenueH (avenueh.com). The alternative is an active exchange that enacts stringent requirements for insurers and lists only select plans. These requirements could range from insisting the plans adopt alternatives to fee-for-service for paying physicians to creating lower-priced insurance products by limiting the choice of hospitals. The active exchanges are modeled on the Massachusetts Health Connector (mahealthconnector.org/portal/site/connector). Because of the complexity of simply getting the exchanges open and ensuring a wide variety of choices for consumers, most states are not instituting many additional requirements initially. However, as the exchanges become established, some states, such as California, anticipate that they will become increasingly active exchanges.

Health insurance policies in the exchange are to be offered in 4 different tiers: bronze, silver, gold, and platinum. These represent different levels of coverage and costs. Bronze plans cover about 60% of total predicted health care costs. They are like Erin's high-deductible plan, with a limit on out-of-pocket expenses that has been set by law: in 2013 $6,250 for individuals and $12,500 for families. If a patient reaches these limits, the insurance company must pay for all the remaining health care costs. These plans qualify as meeting the *minimum essential coverage* as set forth by the ACA. That means that bronze plans are the minimum that would satisfy the individual mandate, and having coverage that provides less than this—unless it is grandfathered in—violates the law. Silver plans are supposed to cover 70% of total predicted health care costs, gold plans 80%, and platinum plans 90% of predicted health care costs.

The ACA provides for a special catastrophic coverage option that is available only to people up to 30 years of age or those exempt from the mandate because they cannot afford their health insurance. Even these catastrophic plans must cover up to 3 primary care visits and preventive services, such as immunization and cancer screening tests, without any deductible. The catastrophic plans are much cheaper than even the bronze plans and satisfy the mandate for young adults.

Premiums for these different levels of plans will vary by state, the way the plans are designed, and the networks and the prices insurance

FIGURE 8.6 Number of options and premium estimates for 40-year-old nonsmokers, 2014

LOCATION	NUMBER OF INSURANCE CARRIERS TO CHOOSE FROM	NUMBER OF QUALIFIED HEALTH PLANS TO CHOOSE FROM	LOWEST UNSUBSIDIZED INDIVIDUAL MONTHLY PREMIUM FOR A BRONZE PLAN	LOWEST UNSUBSIDIZED INDIVIDUAL MONTHLY PREMIUM FOR A SILVER PLAN	LOWEST UNSUBSIDIZED INDIVIDUAL MONTHLY PREMIUM FOR A PLATINUM PLAN
Los Angeles, California	6	66	$188	$224	$285
Boulder, Colorado	5	54	$186	$245	None available
Baltimore, Maryland	5	37	$146	$229	$369
New York City, New York	8	106	$364	$460	$632
Atlantic City, New Jersey	3	28	$244	$268	$440
San Antonio, Texas	5	57	$169	$239	None available
Salt Lake City, Utah	5	85	$152	$173	$226

Note: Premiums are calculated for a 40-year-old nonsmoking individual in 2014.

companies have negotiated with hospitals and physicians. Figure 8.6 provides premium estimates for the lowest price bronze, silver, and platinum plans for a 40-year-old nonsmoker in various locations. It also shows the number of insurance carriers and plans that individuals in those locations would have to choose from. Although premiums cannot vary because of people's preexisting conditions, they can vary by age, with older people paying up to 3 times more than younger people, and by smoking status, with smokers paying up to 1.5 times more than a nonsmoker. Thus, a 60-year-old smoker could pay as much as 4.5 times the premium of a 30-year-old nonsmoker for the same plan. In California a 30-year-old nonsmoker would pay $732 and a 60-year-old smoker would pay $555 for the same silver plan.

However, the large majority of consumers, like Wayne and Baltazar, purchasing in the exchange will not pay these sticker-price premiums. In Pennsylvania someone like Wayne, earning $25,000, will receive an $88 subsidy each month. Indeed, the ACA provides for 2 kinds of subsi-

FIGURE 8.7 Premium subsidies

INCOME AS A PERCENT OF FEDERAL POVERTY LINE (2013)	PERCENT OF INCOME A FAMILY WOULD PAY FOR HEALTH INSURANCE AFTER SUBSIDY	MAXIMUM MONTHLY DOLLAR AMOUNT FAMILY WOULD PAY FOR HEALTH INSURANCE	FAMILY MONTHLY PREMIUM FOR SECOND LOWEST COST SILVER PLAN IN CALIFORNIA (STATEWIDE AVERAGE)	ACTUAL MONTHLY PREMIUM PAID BY FAMILY AFTER SUBSIDY	MONTHLY FEDERAL SUBSIDY
100% ($23,550)	2%	$39	$880	$39	$841
133% ($31,322)	3%	$78	$880	$78	$802
150% ($35,325)	4%	$118	$880	$118	$762
200% ($47,100)	6.3%	$247	$880	$247	$633
250% ($58,875)	8.05%	$395	$880	$395	$485
300% ($70,650)	9.5%	$559	$880	$559	$321
400% ($94,200)	9.5%	$746	$880	$746	$134

Note: Family is a 40-year-old couple, nonsmoking, with 2 children.

dies. The *premium subsidy* helps people pay for the insurance premium. The *cost-sharing subsidy* helps poorer individuals and families pay for the out-of-pocket expenses associated with insurance, such as deductibles and co-pays. Very importantly, these subsidies are only available if people purchase insurance in the exchanges; they do not cover insurance bought outside of the exchanges or for payments when employers offer health insurance to their workers.

The premium subsidies are determined by a sliding scale based on income (Figure 8.7). The amount of the subsidy is determined through a set maximum percent of annual income that a person pays for their health insurance, and the dollar amount of the subsidies is linked to the second-cheapest silver plan in the state. For instance, in California Baltazar receives a $177 per month subsidy to purchase insurance.

The subsidy is meant to achieve 2 desirable but opposing goals: (1) provide sufficient funds to ensure that people can afford their health insurance premiums and (2) provide a financial incentive for people to choose lower-cost plans.

Erin along with other individuals and families who earn more than 400% of the federal poverty line can also purchase health insurance in the exchange, but they receive no subsidy. They pay the full premium—the sticker price.

Premium subsidy levels increase each year based on inflation. The calculation for this increase is complex. Initially, the increase is tied to the increase in premiums over income growth in order to protect people from high health care inflation.

For Americans with incomes under 250% of the federal poverty line there also are cost-sharing subsidies that help them pay for deductibles and co-payments. For instance, for individuals and families at 150% of the poverty level the subsidy will ensure they will pay no more than 3% of their income in deductibles and co-pays.

The ACA also grants *small business subsidies* to encourage employers, such as Baltazar, with up to 25 low-wage employees to purchase insurance for their workers in the state exchanges. The value of the subsidy is on a sliding scale so that the biggest benefit goes to employers with 10 or fewer employees and average wages of $25,000 or less. The small business can obtain the subsidy only for 2 years.

The ACA established that a qualified health plan must provide benefits and services that meet the *minimum essential coverage*. Because in the past some insurers had eliminated coverage of basic services, such as maternity care, minimum essential coverage tries to ensure that health plans do not skimp on coverage. The 10 categories of services that have to be covered are:

1) ambulatory patient services
2) emergency services
3) hospitalization
4) maternity and newborn care
5) mental health and substance abuse services, including behavioral health treatment
6) prescription drugs
7) rehabilitative and habilitative services and devices
8) laboratory services

9) preventive and wellness services and chronic disease management; and
10) pediatric services, including oral and vision care.

Within these broad categories the ACA did not delineate what specific services must be covered but instead established a process for defining them. Heath Secretary Kathleen Sebelius ruled that for 2014 and 2015 each state would specify how insurance companies are to fulfill the 10 categories in order to satisfy the minimum essential benefits. They could do this by selecting a benchmark plan that satisfied the minimum essential benefits. The benchmark would be based on one of the following: (1) one of the 3 largest small group plans in the state; (2) one of the 3 largest state employee health plans; (3) one of the 3 largest federal employee health plan options; or (4) the largest HMO plan offered in the state's commercial market. Secretary Sebelius's move was viewed as an attempt to defuse the inevitable controversy and partisan attacks over whether a particular service would be deemed essential.

The one medical service the law was very clear on was abortion (Chapter 6, page 172). States can prohibit all insurers in the exchange from offering abortion coverage, in which no premium or cost-sharing subsidies can be used to purchase coverage for an abortion unless to save the life of a mother or for rape or incest. If a woman purchases a plan in an exchange that includes abortion coverage, then the subsidy funds must be segregated from her premium payments. It is a bureaucratic tangle to prevent any federal money from somehow contributing to an abortion.

The ACA only permits *qualified health plans* to be offered in the exchanges (Title I, Sec. 1311). To be qualified, a health plan must be accredited and be able to actually provide care to patients by having contracts with hospitals, physicians, and other providers as well as the financial resources to operate. In addition, qualified health plans must take all people who select their health plan, even if those people have a preexisting condition (Title I, Sec. 1201). This means that Erin cannot be excluded because she had cancer. This is called *guaranteed issue*. Further, in setting premiums, qualified health plans in the exchange cannot even take into account anyone's preexisting condition (Sec. 1201), which means that Erin's premium will not be higher than another 48-year-old female who does not have cancer. In addition, the health plans must guarantee *renewability* (Title I, Sec. 1201). In other words, if Baltazar were to have a heart attack, they must continue to cover him as long as he selects the insurance. Also, qualified health plans are not able to impose annual or lifetime limits on coverage (Sec. 1201); previously, many health insurance plans had a $1 million lifetime limit on coverage.

Additionally, the ACA contained a mechanism for a *consumer-operated and-oriented plan (CO-OP)*, a new, nonprofit, member-run health insurance company for the exchanges (Title I, Sec. 1322). CO-OPs were included to appease and appeal to those who wanted the public option but also for Plains states familiar with other types of cooperatives. In advancing this model it helped that the Group Health Cooperative of Puget Sound, a member-run cooperative headquartered in Seattle, is one of the best-performing medical plans in the country. As of July 2013 emerging CO-OPs in 24 states received $2 billion in federal loans or grants to get up and running.

Finally, there is the issue of the mandates. Because the long history of health insurance shows that a *voluntary* insurance system will inevitably collapse because of adverse selection (Chapter 2, page 41), mandates are necessary to ensure everyone, whether healthy or sick, purchase insurance.

Individuals who do not purchase insurance that meets the minimum essential benefits at the bronze level of coverage will face a penalty or, rather, as the Supreme Court ruled, a tax. The penalty is phased in. In 2014 it is $95. By 2016 the penalty is set at a minimum of $695 per year but up to 2.5% of a household income, with a maximum limit of $2,085. After 2016 it is adjusted with the cost of living.

There are exemptions to the mandate, such as for certain religious groups (e.g., Christian Scientists) and American Indians. In addition, individuals and families are exempt if they must pay more than 8% of their income to purchase even the lowest-cost health insurance option.

There is also an employer mandate that was central to the Clinton reform proposal (Chapter 5, page 149). The basic idea was to discourage employers from discontinuing their employees' health insurance when the individual exchanges provided an alternative. Small employers with 50 or fewer workers are exempt—they have no mandate and pay no penalty if they do not provide employer-sponsored insurance. However, employers with 51 or more employees are required to provide their workers with health insurance that satisfies the minimum essential cov-

FIGURE 8.8 Changes in insurance coverage because of the Affordable Care Act (CBO estimates, in millions)

EFFECTS ON INSURANCE COVERAGE	2020 WITHOUT ACA	2020 WITH ACA	CHANGE BECAUSE OF ACA
Total nonelderly population	284	284	
Medicaid and CHIP	34	47	+13
Employer	167	160	−7
Self-insured and nonelderly Medicare	27	22	−5
Exchange	0	24	+24
Uninsured	56	30	−26
Insured as a share of the nonelderly population	80%	89%	+9%

Source: Congressional Budget Office.

erage. Before the ACA, over 94% of these larger employers already did offer health insurance. Large employers that have even one employee who gets a subsidy in the exchange are assessed a penalty of $2,000 per full-time employee, after the first 30 employees. For instance, a company with 100 full-time employees that does not provide insurance would be assessed $140,000 penalty—$2,000 for 70 employees. This mandate was suspended for the first year largely because of confusion about what constitutes a full-time employee.

The Congressional Budget Office (CBO) estimates that in the first year, 2014, 7 million people will purchase health insurance in the exchanges. By 2020 CBO predicts that number will jump to 24 million. Figures 8.8 and 8.9 provide CBO's estimates of the ACA's impact on insurance coverage and cost. On average the subsidies will be $5,290 per enrollee.

COST CONTROL

An important motivation for enacting the ACA was to control rising health care costs or, as the director of OMB constantly put it, to bend the cost curve from growing at GDP+2% per person. The goal was to make health care costs increase at something closer to the growth in the economy, the GDP. The ACA incorporated 2 main cost-control approaches.

FIGURE 8.9 Budgetary effects of the ACA's insurance coverage provisions (in billions of dollars)

EFFECTS ON THE FEDERAL DEFICIT		2013	2014	2015	2016	2017	2018	2019	2020	2013–2020
Costs	New Medicaid and CHIP costs	1	21	41	62	70	76	80	83	434
	Exchange subsidy costs	4	26	51	87	108	118	123	129	646
	Small employer subsidies	1	1	2	1	1	1	1	1	9
	Gross cost of coverage provisions	**6**	**48**	**94**	**151**	**179**	**195**	**205**	**214**	**1,092**
Revenue	Individual penalty payments	0	0	-2	-4	-5	-5	-5	-5	-26
	Employer penalty payments	0	0	-10	-11	-14	-15	-16	-17	-83
	Cadillac tax	0	0	0	0	0	-5	-9	-11	-25
	Other revenue	0	1	1	-6	-14	-20	-23	-24	-85
Net cost of coverage provisions		**6**	**49**	**83**	**130**	**146**	**151**	**151**	**156**	**872**

Note: Numbers may not add up to totals because of rounding. Does not include savings from Medicare or Medicaid.

Source: Congressional Budget Office.

One was to cut prices paid for health care services, and the other, more challenging approach was to reduce the utilization of health care services—that is, to cut volume.

Cost Control Part 1. Reducing Health Care Prices

Substantial research had shown that the prices paid for health care services in the United States are high. American physicians and nurses earned much more than their counterparts in Europe, Australia, and other developed countries. Prices for brand-name drugs—although not generics—are much higher in the United States than they are in other countries. Prices for routine tests, such as MRIs and CT scans, are higher in the United States than they are in Japan and other countries. For instance, an MRI in Japan is $160, while in the United States it averages $1,700. Hence, one strategy to controlling costs is to reduce prices. This approach reduces the level of health care costs but does not significantly impact the annual rate of increase. In other words, it is a one-time "whack" at costs, not a bending of the rate of growth. Nonetheless, it does have an important though temporary impact on controlling spending.

The ACA contained many provisions targeted at reducing costs, in particular the prices the government pays with a few important efforts to reduce prices for the private side of health care. One important policy was to change the payment rates for Medicare Advantage plans, Medicare Part C (Chapter 2, page 58). It had long been argued that these plans cost more than traditional fee-for-service Medicare. One independent estimate reported that Part C plans were getting 10% more than what it would cost to cover similar patients in traditional Medicare.

The ACA implemented several different mechanisms to reduce the price Medicare pays to these Part C plans. For instance, the ACA reduced the basic benchmark payments for these plans but increased the bonus paid for achieving high-quality care from 1.5% of the basic benchmark premium to 5% in 2014. Overall, the CBO estimated that in 2014 these changes will save $8 billion but will grow to nearly $20 billion per year by the end of the decade.

Not surprisingly, because of lower prices, insurers threatened to stop offering Medicare Advantage plans and predicted that the number of elderly enrolling in these plans would decline. Both the CBO and Medicare's own actuaries agreed. Proving the experts wrong—and just how challenging it is to project what effects policy changes will produce—just the opposite occurred. In 2010 11.1 million seniors were in Medicare Advantage plans; by 2013 14.4 million were—a 30% increase, not decrease, despite the lower payments.

A second major price change relates to the annual increase in hospital payments. Each year Medicare updates its payment to hospitals to reflect the changes in the price of goods and services, such as the increase in labor costs. This is called the market-basket update factor. But many activities in hospitals are increasingly automated and occur more efficiently. For instance, blood tests are now performed in large batches by machines, not individually by humans, and CT scanners take their pictures faster, thus allowing more patients to be scanned per hour. Based on these increases in productivity, the ACA mandated that the market-basket update factor be reduced by a fixed amount each year. For 2014 the productivity reduction was 0.4%, and another ACA-based reduction was 0.3% of hospital costs. These changes will not eliminate the annual increase in prices paid to hospitals, but it does slow them down.

Another change for hospitals relates to the Disproportionate Share Hospital (DSH) payments Medicare pays hospitals for their care of uninsured Americans (Chapter 3, page 62). Because so many Americans would now be insured because of reform, the ACA reduced these DSH payments. Furthermore, the ACA adjusted the formula for distributing the DSH money, and it will now be based on how much uncompensated care each hospital actually delivers.

The ACA also puts price pressure on durable medical equipment (DME), that is, wheelchairs, walkers, hospital beds, oxygen equipment as well as prosthetics and other medical supplies. Medicare used to set prices for these items, but the Medicare Modernization Act of 2003 (MMA) replaced government-set prices with a bidding process in which manufacturers competed on lower prices, but only in some areas of the country. A CMS report showed that the competitive bidding process lowered prices by an average of 42% and was projected to save Medicare about $25 billion over a decade. Unfortunately, multiple attempts to expand this competitive bidding process failed because of political pressure from the manufacturers who lost money.

The ACA mandated expansion of this competitive bidding process in several steps so that by 2016 it would be nationwide. Why such a successful program should not have been expanded more rapidly and to more goods and services paid for by Medicare is unclear. Nevertheless, the ACA is going to substantially lower prices for DME, prosthetics, orthotics, and other supplies.

Another price cut relates to drugs. For seniors in Medicare who have enrolled in the drug plan Part D, there is the "donut hole," or coverage gap (Chapter 2, page 59). This means that after a person has spent $2,970 for drugs, most plans stop paying for drugs until spending exceeds $4,750—hence, there is a "hole." The ACA progressively eliminates the donut hole by 2020. Until then, drug manufacturers are required to provide Medicare beneficiaries a 50% reduction in the price of brand-name drugs when they are stuck in the donut hole. For biological agents, such as antibodies, which can often cost tens of thousands of dollars per month of treatment, the ACA authorizes the FDA to create a process by which to approve generic versions so as to put downward price pressure on these treatments.

There were a series of other price changes of smaller magnitude. Similar to the reduction in the market-basket update factor for hospitals, reductions were made for home health care, skilled nursing facilities, and hospices. In determining how much to pay for MRI and CT scans, CMS estimates how often these expensive scanners are used, also known as the utilization rates. For a long time the rate was 50%; however, the ACA increased the utilization rates, effectively lowering the payment per scan. In the context of health care, the savings was not much, less than $1 billion over 10 years.

The largest downward force on prices for private insurance arises from changes in the tax exclusion, also called the "Cadillac tax" (Chapter 6, page 153), which is really an excise tax. Beginning in 2018 there will be a 40% tax on the premium of private health insurance plans that exceed a threshold of $10,200 for an individual and $27,500 for a family. Thus, if in 2018 a family health insurance plan costs $30,000, there will be a $1,000 tax, or 40% of the $2,500 over the threshold. Insured individuals do not pay the tax; plan sponsors—that is, employers—do.

Unions won certain concessions with the Cadillac tax. There are higher limits for workers in high-risk professions, such as firefighters. Similarly, free-standing vision and dental plans are excluded from this limit. Conversely, those who think such a cap is important also had a victory: the threshold increases over time but does so at the rate of inflation, not the higher growth rate in health care costs.

Even though the Cadillac tax does not go into effect until 2018, it is already having an impact. Many employers are redesigning benefits, creating different care networks, experimenting with non-fee-for-service payment mechanisms, and changing deductible and co-payments in order to secure lower prices from hospitals, physicians, and other providers and to keep their premiums under the threshold.

Cost Control Part 2: Reducing Health Care Utilization of Services

Reducing the amount and kind of services used is an even more important cost-control measure than reducing prices. Yet this is harder for policymakers to bring about because, ultimately, physicians are the ones who determine the use of health care services by how frequently they see patients, how many and what kinds of diagnostic tests they order, which drugs they prescribe, which surgical and other procedures they perform, and at what facilities they perform these procedures. At best, influencing physician practices is indirect: no one can order them to do anything. All policymakers can do is alter incentives. To this end, the ACA implements several new policies.

Central to changing the delivery and utilization of services is changing payment away from the fee-for-service approach. A major initiative in the ACA for this change is through *accountable care organizations (ACOs)*, which are networks of physicians or physicians, hospitals, and other providers that take both clinical *and* financial responsibility for the care of patients. These providers are organized to coordinate patient care, especially for patients with chronic illness, who account for the vast majority of costs. An ACO is supposed to break down the silos between primary care physicians, specialists, hospitals, home health care agencies, hospices, pharmacies, and other providers. The idea is that by coordinating providers and care, focusing on high-quality and lower-cost interventions and not just on what services are paid for, the ACO will be able to reduce duplication and unnecessary interventions and still keep patients healthy, thereby reducing the need for treatments, referrals to specialists, emergency room visits, and hospitalizations. In some ways this is an attempt to encourage more physicians and hospitals to become integrated delivery systems like Kaiser Permanente and Group Health.

ACOs must do certain things to qualify. They must:

- Care for at least 5,000 Medicare beneficiaries
- Enter into an agreement with Medicare for at least 3 years
- Create a formal legal structure to receive and distribute payments as well as a process to distribute the shared savings among the providers
- Establish a physician-led governance process that includes at least one Medicare patient on the governing board
- Have mechanisms to promote evidence-based care and patient engagement
- Report to CMS on quality and cost performance

Changing how ACOs are paid is critical to their success. The ACA authorized the Medicare program to adopt the ACO model, and CMS went further and created 3 different ACO models because physician groups and hospital systems were at different stages along the road toward providing coordinated care and, thus, needed different incentive structures (see Figure 8.10).

FIGURE 8.10 Three different Medicare accountable care organizations (ACOs)

TYPE OF ACO	FINANCIAL ARRANGEMENTS	INCENTIVE
Shared Savings	Fee-for-service basis. Benchmark determined by previous 3 years of billings for Parts A and B	Two models: (1) One-sided shared savings—after 2% savings on benchmark, ACO receives 50% of the savings. (2) Two-sided shared savings—ACO receives a portion of savings if under the benchmark but also is at financial risk for spending over the benchmark.
Advanced Payment	Fee-for-service basis. Benchmark determined by previous 3 years of billings for Parts A and B	Same as shared savings, but receives an advanced payment up front from anticipated savings to finance capital investment for creating and operating the ACO.
Pioneer	Fee-for-service basis in years 1 and 2, with capitation—prospective per member per month payment—in year 3.	Facilitates transition to a population-based payment model that mitigates perverse incentives of fee-for-service payments.

The basic model is the Shared Savings ACO. This type of ACO retains the fee-for-service payment system but gives ACOs a share of the savings they realize if they meet certain quality metrics. It is meant to attract physicians and hospitals that are at the early stages of coordinating their care. In order to determine whether there are cost savings, CMS must calculate a benchmark, an estimate of what the Medicare patients would have paid for Part A and B services—hospital and physician care. CMS makes this determination by projecting out from the previous 3 years of utilization. Whether an ACO is saving money depends on next year's estimated cost of caring for patients. Actual costs vary depending on underlying inflation. They also vary based on utilization, which can vary substantially from year-to-year depending on the severity of the flu season or if a few patients happen to get diagnosed with expensive illnesses. Having more patients, such as 5,000, should reduce this random variation, but it means a great deal rests on the accuracy of the estimation of future health care costs. CMS created 2 options to determine how much of the savings the ACOs get. In one there is only shared savings. The ACO must reduce costs by at least 2% compared to the benchmark to share in the savings. (Medicare gets the first 2% in savings.) In the other the ACO also assumes some financial risk: if its costs go over the benchmark, it will be paid less. But its advantage is that it also shares in all the savings with no 2% threshold. ACOs will be monitored for their quality performance based on 33 different quality measures. For instance, there are a number of measures related to patient satisfaction and many related to prevention, such as whether patients have received vaccines for flu or pneumonia, whether they have been screened for obesity, and, if they are obese, whether there is a plan for weight reduction.

CMS also created the Advanced Payment ACO. This is essentially the Shared Savings model for rural and ACOs that lack capital. In this model ACOs receive upfront payments to provide them with capital to invest in electronic health records, care redesign, and other processes to transform how they deliver care.

Finally, CMS also created the most advanced ACO model: Pioneer ACOs. This model was designed specifically for 32 medical groups that already had significant experience with clinical, administrative, and financial integration. In the first 2 years of the ACO program these Pioneers will be in a Shared Savings arrangement. However, if they demonstrated savings during this initial period, in the 3rd year they will be able to move to more capitated payments—a single payment, per member per month, to cover most or all of the patients' costs instead of the fee-for-service billing for each service provided. One other significant advantage of these Pioneer ACOs is that Medicare patients are assigned prospectively, at the start of the year, so the ACO can know whom they are responsible for.

There are skeptics who worry about the rush to convert to ACOs. First, they are concerned that relying on a Shared Savings model means relying on fee-for-service payments, thereby making it hard for physicians to move away from ordering more tests, visits, and treatments so as to increase payments. Second, ACOs entail significant start-up costs for integrated electronic health records, disease registries, effective care management programs, telemedicine, and other monitoring mechanisms. Developing and deploying these effectively will take money, management skill, and time, and many are skeptical that ACOs will have the needed human and financial resources. A third worry is that by creating these big delivery groups, Medicare might be decreasing competition among physicians and hospitals. Although ACOs might lower costs for Medicare, a large ACO might have more leverage to negotiate higher rates with private insurers, thus eliminating any savings for the overall health care system.

Whatever the concerns, the ACO model has taken off. The ACA embrace of ACOs spurred additional use among private insurers. By May 2013 there were 287 Medicare ACOs in the 3 models, with over 4 million Medicare beneficiaries receiving care from ACOs. There were also more than 220 ACOs working with private insurers.

In addition to ACOs the ACA gave the Centers for Medicare and Medicaid Services (CMS) authority to conduct demonstration projects related to bundled payments (Chapter 6, page 181) (Figure 8.11). If these projects show either cost savings or quality improvement—or both—they can be spread to all of Medicare without the need for additional legislation.

Bundled payments empower physicians to determine how best to treat patients without government interference and without worrying

FIGURE 8.11 Four different Medicare bundled-payment models

BUNDLED-PAYMENT TYPE	DESCRIPTION OF PROGRAM	PAYMENT CHANGE
Acute-Care Hospital Stay Only	Medicare pays hospital a discounted amount based on the usual Medicare payment. Medicare continues to pay physicians separately.	Retrospective—payment is a discount from traditional Medicare payment.
Acute Care Hospital and Post-Acute Care	Unit of bundle includes both the stay in the hospital and care 30, 60, or 90 days after hospitalization. Covers skilled nursing and rehabilitation facilities as well as home health care.	Retrospective—payment is actual payments reconciled against a calculated target payment.
Post-Acute Care	Unit of bundle will focus on services 30, 60, or 90 days after hospital discharge.	Retrospective—payment is actual payments reconciled against a calculated target payment.
Acute-Care Hospital Stay Only	Single prospective payment that covers hospital and physicians as well as other care providers.	Prospective—Hospitals and physicians are given a lump sum payment for the entire amount of care.

about what tests or treatments will be paid for. Furthermore, they are the easiest way for physicians, hospitals, and other providers to begin the process of coordinating and redesigning care while also limiting physicians' and hospitals' financial risk.

Medicare has been criticized for not offering true bundled payments and for focusing so heavily on hospital-based bundles. Additionally, CMS has avoided deploying the bundled-payment model for chronic conditions, the very conditions that account for the majority of costs. Hopefully over time CMS will more fully embrace bundled payments and expand the situations and conditions that they are used for.

A third major initiative outlined in the ACA in order to transform the delivery of care tries to incentivize improvements in hospital quality that also save costs. Millions of patients experience hospital-acquired infections, falls, drug reactions, and other avoidable problems. These conditions cost billions. For instance, it was estimated that, on average, a bloodstream infection from central intravenous lines added $36,500 to a hospital stay, not to mention exposing patients to the risk of dying. The ACA (Section 3008) imposes a penalty on hospitals with high rates of hospital-acquired conditions (HACs) such as infections, falls, medication errors, surgical errors, pressure ulcers, and other preventable adverse events. Beginning in 2015 hospitals that rank in the top quarter of those causing hospital-acquired conditions will experience a 1% reduction in all of their Medicare DRG payments, excluding medical education and DSH add-ons. This may seem like a small percentage, but it has nonetheless focused the attention of hospital administrators.

A related ACA provision (Section 3025) penalizes hospitals that have a high preventable readmission rate. Under fee-for-service care, hospitals have a financial incentive to have patients readmitted frequently, as they collect more money for the second and subsequent hospitalizations. Research showed that approximately 20% of Medicare patients were readmitted within 30 days of discharge from a previous hospitalization. Beginning in October 2012 the ACA reduced payments to hospitals that had higher than expected readmissions. For these hospitals the ACA reduces DRG payments by 1% in 2013, 2% in 2014, and 3% in 2015 and subsequent years. Initially this policy applied to readmissions for 3 diseases: heart attacks, heart failure, and pneumonia. However, recently 3 other conditions—emphysema and hip and knee replacements—have been added. The secretary of Health and Human Services has the authority to expand the number of conditions considered. Some groups are calling for hospitals to be held accountable for all readmissions, regardless of the underlying disease. It seems likely this will be the measure in a few years.

Reducing readmissions will require hospitals to move outside their "four walls." This means that hospitals will have to provide more home visits after discharge and ensure there is an early follow-up visit with the patient's primary care physician. Although these additional services will cost money, presumably the money saved from reducing expensive hospitalizations will more than offset these costs. Already the ACA appears to be having an effect: within 18 months readmissions are down to 18.4%.

Through the ACA (Section 3021) Congress created the Center for Medicare and Medicaid Innovation (CMMI) and funded it with $10 billion to be spent over the first decade. CMMI's job is to design and test "innovative payment and service delivery models to reduce program expenditures . . . while preserving or enhancing the quality of care." And Congress granted the secretary of DHHS authority to expand these models nationwide—without having to seek additional congressional approval—if they save money and/or improve quality of care.

CMMI got off to a slow start. The projects it initially selected to pursue, such as the bundled-payment models, could be characterized as timid. However, changing payment away from fee for service, having physicians and other providers transform how they deliver care, and then evaluating these projects for their impacts on cost and quality takes time. A span of a few years is insufficient time for a fair evaluation of the impact of CMMI. Furthermore, there is the inherent problem of inducing physicians and hospitals to participate in demonstration projects that concern payment (Chapter 6, page 181). Given the significant investment needed to transform the delivery of care, having greater assurance that payment will really change beyond the demonstration time is vital when inducing physicians and hospitals to undertake the effort. Although the secretary's authority to expand successful projects is helpful and provides reassurance, it is clearly short of a guarantee that payment will be transformed. Inertia and this lack of assurance about payment change have led many physician groups and hospitals to be hesitant to make expensive investments in transforming the way they care for patients (see Chapter 12).

Cost Control Part 3: The Ultimate Cost-Control Backstop

Controlling increasing health care costs was such an important goal of the ACA that policymakers looked for a fail-safe procedure to ensure it. Two considerations motivated the development of this procedure. First, the independent Medicare Payment Advisory Commission (MedPAC) is an organization with a long history of insightful reports and recommendations to Congress about how to control Medicare costs. Because its recommendations are nonbinding, Congress routinely ignores them. Second, there is a precedent for an effective cost-control process: the Defense Department's Base Realignment and Closure Commission (BRAC). The Defense Department found it difficult to close unnecessary military bases because of the objections from Representatives and Senators whose districts and states financially benefited from those bases. To circumvent this political stalemate, in 1988 Congress created an independent, expert-based BRAC with the authority to close bases unless Congress voted to disapprove the entire list of bases for closing.

Thus, modeled on the BRAC, the ACA (Sections 3403 and 10320) created the Independent Payment Advisory Board (IPAB). IPAB is a 15-member independent board that will submit proposals for how to reduce the per capita growth of Medicare spending. The draft proposals will be submitted to the secretary of DHHS on September 1 and to Congress on the following January 15. Congress then has the power to remove any of the recommendations but only if it replaces them with alternatives that will save an equivalent amount. If Congress does not act by August 15, then the secretary of DHHS is empowered to implement the proposals.

The IPAB needs to recommend ways to cut health care spending only if health care inflation exceeds certain levels. The ACA specifies that beginning in 2013 the chief actuary of CMS, the office that estimates the official National Health Expenditures as well as projects Medicare's future spending, is required to estimate the per capita growth rate for Medicare. Between 2014 and 2018, if the growth rate exceeds the average consumer price index for urban consumers (CPI-U) and the consumer price index specific to medical care (CPU-M), then IPAB is supposed to issue recommendations for reigning in costs. Beginning in 2018 the target is GDP+1%. If per capita spending increases are below these levels, the IPAB does not need to make cost-cutting recommendations.

According to the ACA the IPAB's proposals "shall not include any recommendation to ration health care, raise revenues or Medicare beneficiary premiums, increase Medicare beneficiary cost sharing (including deductibles, coinsurance, and co-payments), or otherwise restrict benefits or modify eligibility criteria." Because of the various cost-cutting measures aimed at hospitals, they along with hospices are exempt from any IPAB recommendations until 2019.

The IPAB was supposed to make recommendations beginning in January 2014; however, the president has not nominated anyone to the IPAB. In part this is because Sarah Palin and other ACA opponents have identified the IPAB as the "death panel." Fortunately, there has been no need for IPAB recommendations, as per capita growth in Medicare has been well below the target.

QUALITY OF CARE

Hospital-Acquired Conditions and Readmissions

Many of the most important efforts toward cost control should also produce significant improvements in the quality of care. Clearly, the efforts to reduce readmissions and hospital-acquired infections, medication errors, falls, blood transfusion incompatibilities, pressure ulcers, surgical mistakes, and other preventable events will improve the quality of care. Similarly, in the ACO models, linking shared savings to adherence to quality standards will also improve quality of care. These are significant quality improvement efforts that are measurable, linked to financial incentives, and already have hospitals vigorously addressing these problems.

Electronic Health Records

Another change that will significantly impact quality of care over time was not actually in the ACA but rather in the Recovery Act, which pumped $787 billion into the economy to blunt the effects of the Great Recession. The relevant provision was known as the Health Information and Technology for Economic and Clinical Health (HITECH), and it offers physicians, hospitals, and other health care service providers financial incentives through Medicaid and Medicare to install and meaningfully use electronic health records (EHRs). Medicaid provides physicians who adopt EHRs and show meaningful use up to $63,750 over 6 years, and Medicare provides $44,000 over 5 years. In 2015 physicians who fail to achieve these standards will be penalized with lower Medicare payments, 1% less in 2015 and rising to 3% less in 2018.

As the Obama administration has repeatedly pointed out, the goal is not simply to adopt electronic health records but instead to ensure that their *meaningful use* improve the quality of care. By themselves electronic health records do not necessarily improve care, but they can be a foundational element of improving quality. This is especially true in the care of a whole population of patients. Electronic health records allow physicians and hospitals to track patients and determine who is getting appropriate care and who is not getting the care they need. They can warn of drug-drug and drug-allergy interactions, eliminate handwritten prescriptions and the mistakes they cause, and ensure that the right patient is getting the right medicine. Finally, EHRs allow the electronic submission, aggregation, and analysis of performance data to identify physicians who are failing to provide quality care and, then, help them improve. Figure 8.12 shows the standards for the first stage of meaningful use. The HITECH Act requires physicians adopt all 15 core measures and at least 5 of 10 of the menu requirements.

The early results of the HITECH Act are encouraging. In 2008 only 9% of hospitals had basic EHRs; in 2012 it was 44%. Nearly two-thirds of large hospitals have EHRs, and 72% of hospitals now have the capability to order medications electronically. The laggards appear to be for-profit hospitals. Among physicians, adoption of basic electronic health records has risen from 18% in 2009 to 40% in 2012, with younger physicians and those practicing in larger groups more likely to adopt. Importantly, 73% of physicians send prescriptions electronically, 67% have electronic warnings about drug interactions, and 50% have electronic reminders to alert them when they have not complied with practice guidelines.

The second stage of meaningful use, beginning in 2014, will significantly raise the bar in the exchange of information among providers and with patients. It also enforces standards to enhance interoperability, the exchange of data across different systems. In 2012 only 36% of hospitals could electronically provide information to hospitals outside their system, and just 51% could electronically provide information to ambulatory providers outside their system. Improvements in interoperability will be critical for reducing duplicate testing and facilitating research studies to determine what interventions work and for which patients in the real world. As the Office of National Coordinator, which has responsibility for overseeing the implementation of the HITECH Act, has stated, Stage 3 requirements for meaningful use will increasingly focus

FIGURE 8.12 Stage 1 requirement for meaningful use of electronic health records

CORE REQUIREMENTS	MENU REQUIREMENTS
1) Use computerized order entry for medication orders.	1) Implement drug-formulary checks.
2) Implement drug-drug, drug-allergy checks.	2) Incorporate clinical lab-test results into certified EHR as structured data.
3) Generate and transmit permissible prescriptions electronically.	3) Generate lists of patients by specific conditions to use for quality improvement, disparity reduction, research, and outreach.
4) Record demographics.	4) Send reminders to patients per patient preference for preventive/follow-up care.
5) Maintain an up-to-date problem list of current and active diagnoses.	5) Provide patients with timely electronic access to their health information (including lab results, problem list, medication lists, allergies).
6) Maintain active medication list.	6) Use certified EHR to identify patient-specific education resources and provide to patient if appropriate.
7) Maintain active medication allergy list.	7) Perform medication reconciliation as relevant.
8) Record and chart changes in vital signs.	8) Provide summary care record for transitions in care or referrals.
9) Record smoking status for patients thirteen years old or older.	9) Capability to submit electronic data to immunization registries and actual submission.
10) Implement one clinical decision support rule.	10) Capability to provide electronic syndromic surveillance data to public health agencies and actual transmission.
11) Report ambulatory quality measures to CMS or the states.	
12) Provide patients an electronic copy of their health information upon request.	
13) Provide clinical summaries to patients for each office visit.	
14) Capability to exchange key clinical information electronically among providers and patient-authorized entities.	
15) Protect electronic health information (privacy & security)	

not just on data exchange but also on using technology to improve patient outcomes.

Doubtless there are at least 2 big issues to work out before that is achieved. First, many physicians complain that the current systems are not user friendly and not customized to the needs of particular specialties. Secondly, the electronic exchange of information is still too limited, as manufacturers and providers having financial interests that do not align with the free flow of information. These are mainly technical problems, and as payment reforms that reward population health management and care coordination expand, there will be financial pressure to enhance the exchange of data.

Improving Quality Measurement and Reporting

Three other specific provisions of the ACA will improve quality of care. First, the ACA tries to address the significant gaps in the science of quality measurement and streamline quality reporting. Medicare has a multitude of programs requiring reporting on the quality of care, but their measures are lengthy and frequently duplicative and misaligned. Further, those for the Accountable Care Organization (ACO) program are not necessarily the same measures that the hospitals or physicians are required to report to Medicare for other programs, thereby increasing the burden on physicians and hospitals. In response, the ACA required the development of a national quality improvement strategy in part to align these measures not only across federal programs but also between the government and private insurance companies. In addition, the ACA provided a large grant for the development of additional quality measures that can be collected using electronic health records to minimize the costs of reporting data.

A second important advance of the ACA is to transform the Physician Quality Reporting System (PQRS). Since 2007 it has been a voluntary system in which Medicare paid physicians a 1.5% bonus of their regular payments just to report quality data regardless of their actual quality performance. With the ACA, the bonus payment instead becomes a penalty system for physicians who do *not* report quality data. In 2015, the penalty is a 1.5% drop in payment, rising to 2% in 2016. In addition, in 2014 the PQRS data are supposed to be publicly reported at Physician Compare on the Medicare website.

Third, for years hospitals have had to report on certain quality measures. The ACA now takes this experience and requires hospices, long-term care facilities, cancer centers, and rehabilitation hospitals to begin reporting on quality measures as well.

Value-Based Purchasing

Another major effort the ACA makes to improve quality of care relates to value-based purchasing (VBP) (section 3001). For years CMS has operated demonstration pay-for-performance programs. For instance, between 2003 and 2009 CMS ran a Premier Hospital Quality Incentive Demonstration project that provided financial bonuses for quality of care in certain health areas such as heart attacks and pneumonia. The ACA applied these programs not to a select group of hospitals participating in the demonstration but rather to all acute-care hospitals (section 3001(a)). The first program started in October 2012 and rewards acute-care hospitals for adhering to quality measures in 4 domains: (1) processes of care, (2) patient experience, (3) health outcomes, and (4) efficiency. For instance, in the processes of care domain, one measure is whether patients experiencing heart attacks receive a catheterization procedure to open up the blocked artery within 90 minutes of arriving at the hospital. Another quality measure is whether a patient undergoing surgery is started on antibiotics within 1 hour of surgery and stopped within 24 hours of the end of surgery. These various domains will be phased in from 2013 to 2015, starting with the first 2 and adding one domain each year. The inclusion of efficiency makes the program a focus on value, not just performance.

One of the important aspects of VBP for hospitals is that it rewards not only absolute quality but also improvement in quality so that those hospitals that initially are poor performers can be rewarded for taking steps to remedy their deficiencies. The pool of money for the rewards comes from a withholding of hospitals' DRG payment. The actual reward begins at 1% of the DRG payments in 2013 and increases by 0.25%

per year until it is 2% of payments in 2017 and beyond for hospitals that are high performers or have demonstrated real improvement. The ACA also requires that this VBP model be expanded beyond acute-care hospitals to ambulatory surgical centers, home health agencies, and other facilities.

Critics of the VBP program worry that too much emphasis is being placed on process measures rather than patient outcomes. Fortunately, there is a general push in the field to deploy more outcomes measures. They too will be part of the VBP program.

Patient-Centered Outcomes Research Institute

Many commentators have long complained that there is a lack of data about which medical interventions produce the best outcomes and for which types of patients. Although drugs are typically tested against a placebo to secure FDA approval, there are usually no data comparing the effectiveness of the various me-too drugs that act the same way to lower blood pressure. There has been a paucity of data comparing different treatment approaches, surgery, or medical management for the same condition, and many interventions have been introduced and used without any data about their effectiveness. For instance, whether use of ultrasound in a routine pregnancy makes any difference in ensuring healthy babies is unclear. These data are a public good: once produced, anyone can use them. Because of this lack of exclusivity, there is little incentive for drug companies, insurers, or others to generate the data. Many health policy experts have argued that this is the type of function best suited for the government.

Section 6301 of the ACA established the *Patient-Centered Outcomes Research Institute (PCORI)* as a nongovernmental organization with public and private funding, stating, "The purpose of the Institute is to assist patients, clinicians, purchasers, and policy makers in making informed health decisions by advancing the quality and relevance of evidence concerning the manner in which diseases, disorders, and other health conditions can effectively and appropriately be prevented, diagnosed, treated, monitored, and managed through research and evidence synthesis."

PRCORI is also responsible for disseminating and increasing use of the information it generates.

The ACA creates a 19-member board of governors that represents all stakeholders, from physicians, health systems, and patients to insurers, employers, and drug and device manufacturers. To reduce politicization, the comptroller general of the Government Accountability Office appoints the board. In addition, the heads of the Agency for Healthcare Research and Quality (AHRQ) and NIH are also on the board. Further, there is a technical methodology committee to ensure relevant and rigorous methods are used in comparative effectiveness studies funded by PCORI.

Funding for PCORI is unique. Based on the belief that the information to be generated is a public good, the ACA mandates that a common fee should be paid into a trust fund for every insured American, regardless whether that person has private health insurance or government-financed coverage. Patients are not responsible for paying the fee; the plan sponsor—the employer, insurance company, or government—is. The fee is very modest: $2 in 2014, and then rising, until 2019, by health care inflation. The legislation specifies that 20% of PCORI spending should promote information dissemination—that is, ensuring physicians and patients are aware of the findings.

Years ago Britain created a National Institute for Health and Care Excellence (NICE) that compared different treatments. It was entrusted not only with determining a treatment's effectiveness but also its cost effectiveness, usually measured as the dollars per quality adjusted life year (QALY). When NICE determined an intervention was cost-effective, it became part of the insurance package in Britain. Many people in the United States view NICE suspiciously if not negatively. The ACA explicitly distinguishes PCORI from NICE by prohibiting PCORI from determining the cost effectiveness of interventions based on "dollars per quality adjusted life year." Also unlike NICE, PCORI has no authority to determine coverage decisions for private insurers or government programs.

The PCORI board was appointed in September 2010. After multiple public hearings, in March 2012 the board announced its 5 focus areas for funding: (1) assessment of prevention, diagnosis, and treatment options; (2) improving health care systems; (3) communication and dissemination research; (4) addressing racial, gender, and other health disparities; and

(5) accelerating patient-centered outcomes research and methodological research.

The general reaction to PCORI may be best characterized as one of frustration. It is perceived to have had a very slow start and has been quite timid in the research projects it has funded. The big clinical questions in need of comparative effectiveness research—ones fraught with controversy, variations in care patterns, and high costs—are not the ones PCORI is tackling.

Overall Assessment on Quality

Overall, what will the impact of the ACA be on the quality of care in the American health care system? Although revolutionary, it still left some substantial deficits. Doubtless, over the next few years hospital quality, measured in terms of the reduction in infections, medication errors, falls, surgical mishaps, and other errors, will be much better. Furthermore, the ACA will induce better coordination between the hospital and primary physician regarding hospital discharge, better posthospital care at home, and fewer readmissions. There will also be a platform in electronic health records for monitoring the quality of care more carefully. Finally, there will be more quantitative information with which to compare the performance of hospitals, physicians, home health agencies, and other providers.

Maybe the most important impact of the ACA is psychological. It marks a point of no return on quality. The various provisions that improve the measures and require more reporting on quality shattered the idea that somehow physicians and hospitals could avoid objective assessment and public reporting on their quality of care. Although some physicians and hospitals still may be resistant, there is no longer any argument about the need for quality reporting; instead, the argument has become more technical—about how best to do it, how to make it reliable, and, most importantly, how to implement subsequent changes to improve quality. After the ACA physicians, hospitals, and health policy makers accept the need to develop objective, publicly reported, and actionable quality data.

That is important, but the ACA probably did not provide the absolutely optimal framework for quality improvement. Despite the emphasis in the ACA on developing a quality strategy, developing more measures, and requiring more quality reporting from physicians and other health care providers, there is a sense that there remains a deficiency in the overall structure that could make that a reality. In part the proliferation of measures without rigorous evaluation of their validity or the transparency of data has raised concerns that what is being measured is not necessarily a good reflection of quality. There is also concern that what is being measured may not readily translate into improved quality of care. Hospitals and physicians need more help when developing interventions and effectively implementing them to improve quality.

PREVENTION AND HEALTH PROMOTION

Many people complain that the ACA focused on access and cost of the health care system but did not do enough to prevent people from getting sick in the first place. The criticism might be characterized as too much focus on treating diabetes and lung cancer and not enough on preventing them.

The ACA was not the administration's only health reform effort. Just as the expansion of electronic health records was accomplished through the Recovery Act, many people in the administration view the ACA focus on prevention as synergistic with the First Lady's Let's Move initiative. What differentiated the ACA's approach was that it addressed prevention largely in the context of the health care system, whereas Let's Move is more of a health promotion campaign targeted at reversing the childhood obesity epidemic.

The ACA encourages 2 major health promotion activities to further the First Lady's initiative. First is menu labeling. Section 4205 of the ACA requires,

> restaurants and similar retail food establishments with 20 or more locations [to] list calorie content information for standard menu items on restaurant menus and menu boards, including drive-through menu

boards. Other nutrient information—total calories, fat, saturated fat, cholesterol, sodium, total carbohydrates, sugars, fiber and total protein—would have to be made available in writing upon request.

Many inside the White House were well aware of the data demonstrating that menu labeling in itself probably has little, at least, little immediate impact on people's food purchasing and consuming behavior. The behavioral economists knew that people must hear information multiple times before they absorb it, and absorbing information does not itself change behavior. Instead, most people working on the legislation expected that one impact would be to educate people over time about how many calories different food items have. The major impact, then, would be on manufacturers and food establishments, encouraging them to reformulate food items so as to reduce calories. When food labeling is required, no one wants a 1,000-calorie sandwich on their menu.

The ACA entrusts the FDA with developing the menu-labeling regulations and enforcement. Development has been slowed largely because of lobbying from major food establishments, particularly supermarkets selling prepared foods. Perhaps the intense lobbying can be interpreted to mean that food sellers think the menu labeling will have a real impact, forcing them to change their food products.

A second health promotion effort focused on wellness programs. The ACA permitted health plans to use rewards and penalties, such as lower premiums or deductibles, to motivate people to take steps toward living healthier, such as quitting smoking, losing weight, or meeting some other measure, and it also increased the amount that businesses could use for financial incentives for these so-called health-contingent wellness programs. In 1996 the Health Insurance Portability and Accountability Act (HIPAA) allowed companies to offer financial incentives worth up to 20% of the cost of health insurance. For a family plan worth $12,000, that would come to $2,400 in savings. Most employer wellness programs, however, offered savings well below that threshold, using incentives in the hundreds of dollars and finding no added return for higher incentives. Under intense public promotion, especially from Steve Burd, the CEO of Safeway, through the ACA, Congress increased the maximal incentive amount to 30% of the cost of health coverage, with a possibility of increasing to 50% for smoking prevention and treatment efforts.

This created controversy in part due to concerns that people might be penalized for poor health, precisely what the ACA was attempting to reverse, and might even be discriminated against or that these "incentives" may be used to encourage workers who were obese or smoked to leave an employer. In response, the Department of Labor has instituted safeguards, such as requiring that the programs be available to all "similarly situated individuals" and that workers who have medical conditions that make achieving these goals difficult or impossible can secure the rewards in other ways.

Again, the ACA, and the subsequent discussions of wellness programs it prompted, inspired many employers who were previously considering them to institute these programs and integrate financial incentives. According to a 2012 Health Research and Educational Trust (HRET) and Kaiser Family Foundation survey, 63% of all employers and 94% of employers with 200 or more employees offer some type of wellness program. Of those employers offering wellness programs, 80% now have some reward program.

The ACA also emphasizes prevention in the physician's office. In January 2011 Medicare beneficiaries could get a "wellness visit" with their physician for a health-risk assessment that would identify individuals' risks for injuries and diseases as well as modifiable risk factors, such as lack of exercise. For those who are obese, have high cholesterol, or some other condition identified, the physician and patient are supposed to draw up a personalized prevention plan.

The ACA also encourages greater use of preventive screening tests. A major reason people do not get recommended prevention services is cost. The ACA required Medicare, Medicaid, and health insurers to eliminate co-pays and deductibles for people getting preventive services. The preventive services covered were broad, including all those on the US Preventive Services Task Force A and B recommendations (based on the certainty of the evidence supporting health benefits), such as cancer screening tests—mammograms, Pap smears, and colonoscopies—and standard immunizations, including flu shots. Many other services were brought under the prevention rubric, including such things as screening for sexually transmitted diseases and high cholesterol. Much of the controversy with this latter provision centers on the coverage of women's birth control as a preventive service. However, birth control certainly prevents unwanted pregnancies and the potential complications that accompany them as well as, of course, the costs and risks of labor, delivery, and maternity services.

Finally, the ACA created grants to improve public health. The legislation created a $15 billion Prevention and Public Health Fund (PPHF) to award grants for various prevention activities. This amount was subsequently reduced by $5 billion, and some of the remainder is being used to inform people about the exchanges and coverage options. Nonetheless, what's left is funding a number of prevention programs. For instance, some money is funding nurses for home visitations for pregnant women and at-risk infants and toddlers in order to prevent problems such as injuries and improve school readiness. There are community transformation grants to support the development of infrastructure for healthier living, such as access to nutritious foods, playgrounds, and community-based smoking cessation programs.

Although the ACA may not have done everything people would want for prevention and health promotion, it did include significant programs for prevention both in public health and throughout the health care system. The claim that the act ignores the main underlying drivers of health care costs—diet, exercise, and smoking—is simply not true.

HEALTH CARE WORKFORCE

Many critics have voiced concern that the ACA would significantly increase waiting times. They argue that, by providing health insurance to 30 million more Americans, demand for health care services in general and physician services in particular will rise. With a limited supply of physicians, the increase in demand will lead to longer waiting times to see a primary care physician or a specialist. Indeed, the Association of American Medical Colleges predicts a shortfall of 90,000 physicians by 2020. In an attempt to address this concern, Title V of the ACA is devoted to workforce issues.

However, the concern may be misplaced and an overreaction. Before health reform waiting times in the United States were comparable to most other developed countries. Conservative critics like to say that, unlike citizens of European countries with more socialized medicine, Americans do not have to wait for health care. However, actual data may not bear out this assertion. It may be true that waiting times in Canada and Britain are longer than they are in the United States, but it is also true that more people in Britain can get next-day appointments and find it easier to get care at night or on weekends than in the United States. But the Commonwealth Fund, a private foundation devoted to improving performance in the health system, has done extensive cross-national studies that show the picture is more nuanced. Patients in other countries, such as the Netherlands, Germany, and New Zealand, experience consistently shorter wait times than those in the United States (see Figure 8.13).

Research from the Massachusetts Medical Society shows that when that state instituted its health care reform and 400,000 more people received health insurance coverage, average waiting times for both primary care and specialist physicians fluctuated, but did not become significantly longer. (Figure 8.14 shows the waiting time for internal medicine, family medicine, cardiology, and obstetrics and gynecology.) There are various explanations for the lack of increase in waiting times. One is that many services physicians provide do not require an M.D. degree and can be performed by nurses and health aides, thereby freeing up physician time.

Nevertheless, the ACA contains many provisions to address the anticipated physician and nurse undersupply. Ironically, probably the most important changes for the workforce are not in Title V but rather are in ACA provisions related to payment reform. The ACA increases the levels of Medicaid payment to primary care providers to Medicare rates for 2013 and 2014. It also provides a 10% bonus payment to primary care physicians serving Medicare patients from 2011 to 2015. These payment changes are temporary, however; some of the new payment models, such as ACOs and bundled payments, should improve the pay for primary care physicians over the longer term.

The specific workforce provisions of the ACA are usefully divided into 4 categories. One set of provisions provide for workforce analysis by creating a National Health Care Workforce Commission to assess the

FIGURE 8.13 Access to physician services, national comparisons

	USA	AUSTRALIA	CANADA	GERMANY	THE NETHERLANDS	NEW ZEALAND	UK
Last time needed medical care had to wait 6 or more days for an appointment	23%	18%	34%	26%	3%	8%	14%
Primary care practices where patients who request same or next-day appointments can get one	44%	36%	17%	57%	62%	45%	64%
Somewhat or very difficult to get care at nights or weekends	60%	62%	56%	35%	30%	39%	44%
Wait time of 4 months or more for elective surgery	8%	18%	27%	5%	7%	13%	30%

supply of health professionals and to make recommendations (Section 5101). It also provides grants to fund workforce planning and development programs at the state level (Section 5102).

A second set of provisions enhances the public health workforce. These provisions expand the Commission Corps of the US Public Health Service (5209) and create a new Ready Reserve Corp for serious health emergencies (Section 5210). In addition, there is a new student loan forgiveness program (Section 5204), granting up to $35,000 for people trained in public health who work at least 3 years in a government public health agency. Finally, there are a variety of programs to expand and fund public health training programs, such as preventive medicine training at medical and public health schools (Section 10501) or advanced

FIGURE 8.14 Waiting times for physicians in Massachusetts

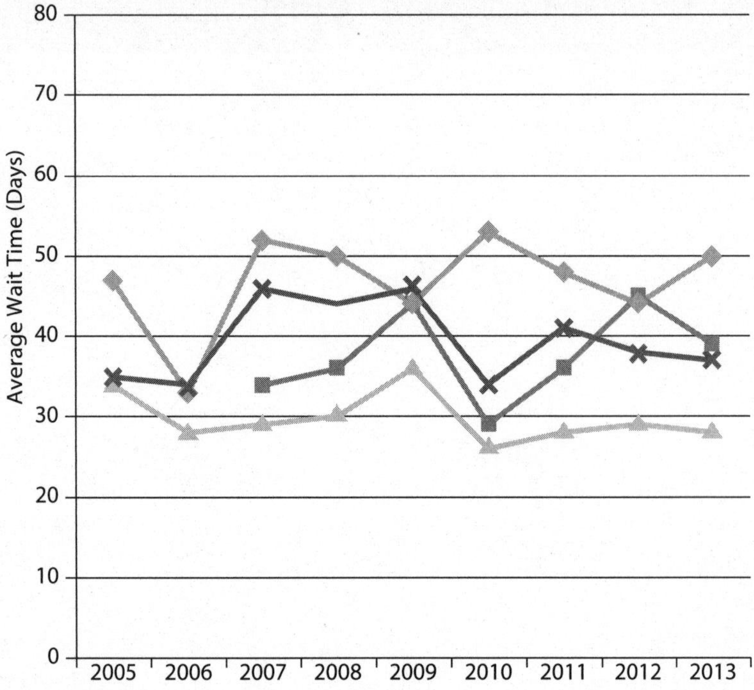

Source: Massachusetts Medical Society. Patient Access to Care Study, July 2013.

training of public health professionals working for government agencies (Section 5206).

A third set of provisions directly addresses physician shortage and training. Sections 5207, 5508, and 10503 expand the National Health Services Corps and provide scholarships and loan forgiveness to primary care physicians as well as dental and mental health providers who practice in underserved regions of the country. ACA increased loan forgiveness from $35,000 (the previous level) to $50,000 per student. It also allowed for part-time service so that physicians and nurses could take time off for having a family or doing research, teaching, or other care activities. Section 5405 funds extension workers to provide continuing education to practicing primary care physicians and others on matters related to preventive medicine, health promotion, and chronic disease management.

The fourth set of provisions relates to nursing and allied health professionals. A set of programs funds loans for nursing students, including grants to help minority students get nursing degrees (Sections 5202, 5308, 5309, and 5404). Another program tries to increase the number and retention of faculty at nursing schools by repaying the loans of nurses who elect to teach rather than practice nursing (Sections 5310 and 5311).

However, my overall assessment of the workforce issue is that it may be a bit overblown to begin with. There are clearly problems related to both the number of primary care physicians in the United States as well as the geographic distribution of physicians into rural and poor urban areas. But based on the Massachusetts experience, the prediction that health care reform will dramatically increase wait times for physicians may be incorrect.

If, however, this prediction comes to pass, it is true that the ACA did not entail a fundamental rethinking of the workforce problem with targeted solutions. Instead, it increased funding for the existing programs that hitherto had not really solved the workforce problems of primary care physician undersupply or their shortage in rural and poorer areas.

An alternative to the ACA approach would have been to address the 2 root causes of the undersupply of primary care physicians and nurses: (1) high educational debt and (2) low income, especially compared to specialists. This policy might have adapted the military's approach to hiring physicians—full loan forgiveness tied to an 8-year repayment period for physicians who go into primary care or work in truly underserved areas.

A cardiologist makes about twice that of a primary care physician. Even if most physicians are not primarily motivated by money and high incomes, this difference is persuasive. And a temporary 10% pay increase for primary care physicians is not likely to affect motivations significantly. An alternative would have been to change the way Medicare calculates payment significantly by changing how relative value units (RVUs) are determined and updated (Chapter 3, page 81) to reward more heavily primary care physicians' communication, coordination, and chronic disease management activities.

Overall, although the ACA does take steps to address health care workforce concerns, its approach of spreading money across existing programs may offer few added incentives over the long term to increase the number of physicians in primary care.

REVENUE

The basic philosophy guiding the funding of the ACA was to pay for half of it with savings and efficiencies from existing federal health programs, mainly Medicare and, to a lesser extent, Medicaid, and half of it through new revenues. The new revenues can be divided into 5 categories: (1) adjusting the tax treatment of health insurance, HSAs, and other health programs; (2) changing Medicare's payroll tax; (3) assessing tax penalties for not fulfilling the mandates; (4) assessing fees on health insurers, manufacturers, and others; and (5) levying new taxes.

In the long run the most important revenue source is probably the Cadillac tax. In part this is because it significantly contributes to cost control (Chapter 6, page 178). But if employers shift to paying less for health insurance and compensating people with additional wages, the effect will be to increase tax revenues through additional income and payroll taxes (see Figure 8.15a). Thus, in the decade of the 2020s it is expected to generate significant revenue both directly and indirectly through greater income and payroll taxes (see Figure 8.16).

Another revenue source, though much less important, is a change in the flexible spending accounts (FSAs) for medical expenses. The tax-exempt limit was decreased to $2,500 per year in 2013, with it increasing at the cost of living rate. In 2011 purchases of over-the-counter drugs were excluded from health savings accounts (HSAs) and FSAs. Also, beginning 2013 the tax on withdrawing funds from an HSA and using those funds to pay for things other than medical expenses was increased from 10% to 20%. For people taking itemized deductions for medical expenses, the threshold was increased from 7.5% to 10% of income. Also, as part of the Medicare Part D drug coverage program, some employers were double-dipping. President Bush had given both a subsidy as well as a tax deduction to employers so as to encourage them to continue to provide retirees with drug benefits; the ACA, however, eliminated the employers' tax deduction if they get a government subsidy for the drug benefit.

Second, beginning in 2013 the payroll tax previously used to pay for Medicare Part A was increased for high-income Americans. Individuals earning over $200,000 and married couples earning above $250,000 now have to pay an additional 0.9% of income that will go directly to Medicare Part A funding.

Third, the individual mandate means that, beginning in 2014, Americans who fail to purchase health insurance have to pay a tax penalty (page 218). Similarly, employers with more than 50 employees who do not provide health insurance must also pay a penalty, $2,000 per employee after 30 employees. This penalty has been delayed until 2015. CBO estimates these tax penalty payments will generate about $10 billion in 2015 and $17 billion in 2020.

Fourth, the ACA levied a variety of new taxes on health insurers and manufacturers, justified because they would be making more money as a result of the ACA (Chapter 6, page 170). Collectively, insurance companies are expected to pay about $8 billion in 2014, increasing to $14.3 billion in 2018, and increasing thereafter by the growth in the cost of premiums. A company's market share determines its portion of this total amount. The ACA's deal with the drug companies means that, beginning in 2011, manufacturers and importers of brand-name pharmaceuticals are taxed, initially $2.5 billion, rising to $4.1 billion in 2018, and then returning to $2.8 billion in 2019 and thereafter. Like the insurer tax, the drug company tax will be distributed among particular companies based on market share.

Probably the most contentious levy, certainly the one manufacturers have fought the hardest to try to repeal, is the 2.3% excise tax on the sale of medical devices, regardless of where they are manufactured. This began in 2013.

Finally, there were several other new taxes in the ACA. First, a 10% tax on indoor tanning salons started in 2010. Second, beginning in 2013 married couples earning over $250,000 will pay an additional 3.8% tax on any unearned income—that is, interest, dividends, royalties, annuities, and similar income. Basically, this applies the previously discussed Medicare payroll tax for earned income to unearned income, such as income from investments.

Many of these taxes, such as the drug and health insurance company taxes, were part of a negotiation and are considered a payment for their increased business that the ACA generates. Others, such as the tax on unearned income, are based on an idea of fairness. The general rationale is progressivity, namely that those who are better off should

FIGURE 8.15 New revenue source to pay for the Affordable Care Act

TYPE OF REVENUE	SPECIFIC TAX	LEVEL OF TAX	ESTIMATED CUMULATIVE REVENUE 2013–2022 (BILLIONS)
Change in existing health related taxes	Cadillac tax	40% excise tax on premiums over $27,500 per family and $10,200 per individual beginning 2018	$111.0
	Limit FSAs	Limit health flexible spending plans to $2,500; indexed to CPI	$24.0
	Change in FSAs, HSAs, Archer MSAs and other programs		$8.5
Violation of mandates	Individuals who do not buy health insurance	$695 per person or 2.5% of income—2016	$38.0
	Large employers who do not sponsor health insurance	$2,000 per employee after first 30	$120.0
Tax on insurers and manufacturers	Fee on pharmaceutical manufacturers	Annual fee on manufacturers and importers of branded drugs	$34.2
	Fee on device manufacturers	2.3% excise tax on manufacturers and importers of certain medical devices	$29.1
	Fee on health insurers	Annual fee on health insurance providers	$101.7
New taxes	Tanning salons	10% excise tax on services	$1.5
	Taxes on high earners	0.9% increase in Medicare payroll tax for individuals earning over $200,000 and couples over $250,000	$317.7
		3.8% tax on interest, dividends, annuities, royalties and other passive income for couples earning over $250,000. (Makes up for no assessment of Medicare tax on this income)	

Source: Joint Committee on Taxation, June 15, 2012.

FIGURE 8.16 ACA revenue

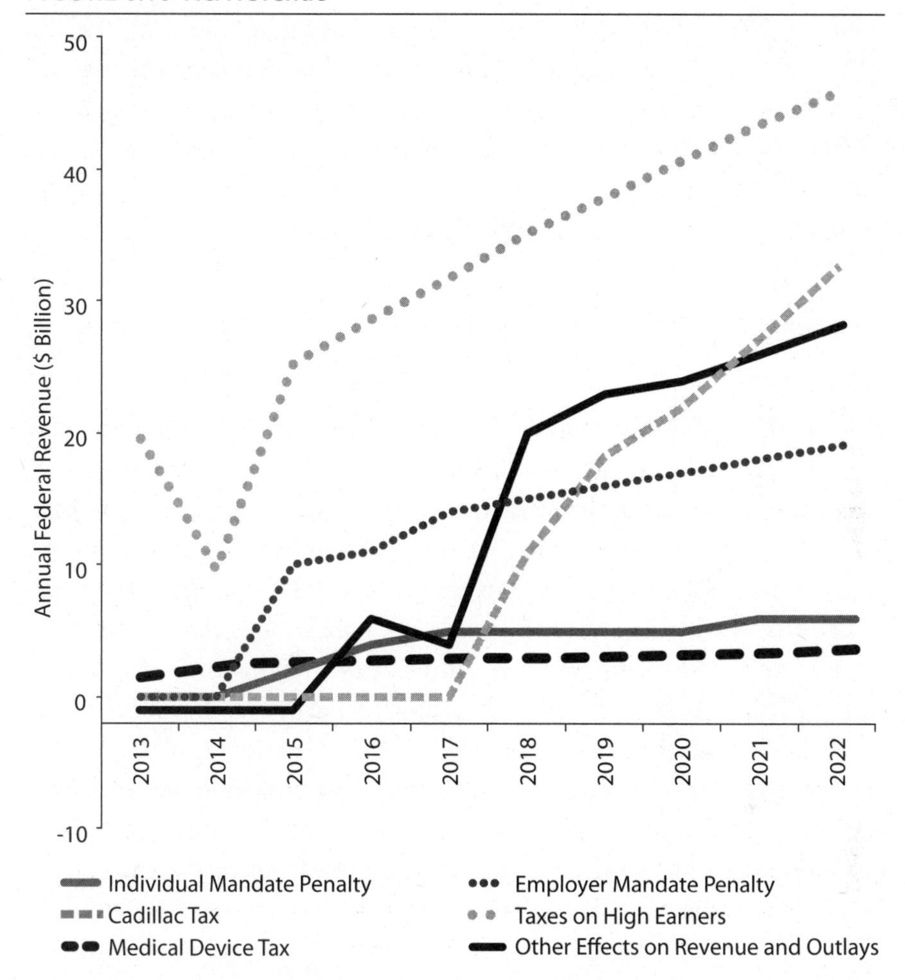

Source: Congressional Budget Office, Joint Committee on Taxation.

shoulder a greater proportion of payments for Medicare and that support for Medicare should not depend on whether income is earned as wages or unearned as the product of investments or capital gains. Other taxes, such as the increase in the Medicare tax for high-income individuals, also look to those with greater incomes to help those in need. The tanning salon tax is meant to discourage unhealthy behaviors. Finally, others are meant to avoid "double dipping," such as with employers who receive both Medicare Part D subsidies as well as tax deductions for extending drug benefits to their retirees.

Thus—and contrary to much rhetoric—the ACA does not add to the deficit or the national debt. The CBO estimates that after a decade the ACA will actually be generating revenue and, thus, reducing the nation's debt. Indeed, since the passage of the ACA the growth in health care expenditures has been less than predicted, leading the CBO to suggest that the cost of the subsidies will be lower than expected, thereby producing even greater debt reduction than initially predicted in 2010.

ODDS AND ENDS

It is worth highlighting 5 other changes in the ACA that do not easily fit into the previous categories. The first is administrative simplification. Almost everyone hates the amount of paperwork associated with insurance company bills. More than just frustrating, however, that paperwork is expensive. In a report by the American Medical Association, they estimated that the average cost of processing a physician's claim is $6.63 for a paper submission and $2.90 for an electronic submission. According to the company Endeon, which operates the largest administrative and clinical information exchange in the United States, moving all of the billing as well as other types of paperwork, such as physician credentialing, to a web-based system would save $30 billion every year. However, one problem with electronic administration comes from the fact that each insurance company has its own forms and electronic processing rules. In response, the ACA requires that the government, working with the insurers, physicians, hospitals, and others, develop uniform standards and operating rules for electronic processing of eligibility and claim status, transfer of funds, specialized attachments, and other processes related to claims.

If there is a problem with these provisions, it is that they do not go far enough. Although the ACA requires that insurers certify compliance with and implementation of the electronic standards and operating rules or face penalties, it does not impose the same requirements on physicians and hospitals. This means that physicians do not have to use the new simplified electronic systems once they are developed. Furthermore, the act did not include many other things that could be made electronic and, thus, simplified and made less costly, such as physician credentialing and prior authorization.

Second, the ACA imposes medical loss ratio (MLR) requirements on health insurers, and these went into effect in 2011 (Chapter 2, page 54). Basically, the MLR provisions require insurers to devote a minimum percentage of each dollar paid in premiums toward medical services and quality improvement activities rather than administrative costs and profits. If they fail to meet this minimum threshold, insurers need to refund their customers the difference. The level of this MLR threshold varies by types of insurance. For large groups the threshold is 85%: the insurance companies must spend 85 cents of every premium dollar on medical services and quality improvement. For individuals and small groups this amount is 80% because, the ACA recognizes, the administrative costs associated with marketing to, enrolling, and covering individuals are higher. In 2012 an estimated 8.5 million Americans received an average of a $100 rebate because of this provision, and many others paid lower insurance premiums.

Third, beginning in 2014 health insurers must cover the health care costs when their insurees are enrolled in an approved clinical trial. The medical research community has long fought to have insurance pay for the nonresearch health care costs associated with a research trial, such as routine laboratory tests or hospitalizations. Although most insurers did cover these expenses prior to the ACA, the act now requires every company to cover the health care costs associated with cancer or drug research as well as other trials seeking better treatments for life-threatening conditions. This will reduce the financial barriers Americans face when they seek to participate in medical research trials.

Fourth, in what are known as "sunshine provisions" (provisions to increase transparency regarding financial relationships), beginning in 2013 the ACA requires drug, device, and other companies to disclose their financial payments to physicians, pharmacists, hospitals, and others. Because many physicians consult for companies or give lectures promoting company products for fees, or accept free food and drink from company representatives, the ACA now requires transparency about these financial relationships. Beginning in 2014 CMS will post these relationships publicly on a website.

Finally, the ACA increases efforts to combat fraud and abuse. It has been estimated that for every $1 spent in fraud and abuse enforcement, the federal government saves $17—a great return every hedge fund manager would covet. Yet the federal government has been hesitant to be more vigorous in enforcing fraud statutes because, when dealing with a billion transactions, even very accurate enforcement strategies inevitably capture honest physicians, hospitals, and others, who then become offended. Nonetheless, the ACA devotes an additional $350 million over 10 years to combat fraud and abuse. More importantly, it changes some rules so as to reduce the number of fraudulent companies. For instance, the ACA permits more thorough screening and background checks for all providers seeking to participate in Medicare. It also increases some penalties and shares data on fraudulent health care providers across all federal health programs. The ACA also makes other special efforts to combat fraud, such as temporarily suspending new providers' ability to participate in the Medicare program in aspects of health care known to be especially prone to high levels of fraud, such as provisions of home health care, durable medical equipment, and nursing homes.

THE CLASS ACT

Title VIII of the ACA is the Community Living Assistance Services and Support Act, also called the CLASS Act. This act was meant to address the need for long-term care among the growing elderly population in the United States. The CLASS Act was structured as a voluntary, long-term public insurance program in which working adults pay premiums, and after a minimum of 5 years of contributions they could then access benefits. Americans would be eligible only if they were still working at the time of enrollment, and they could receive benefits only if they had functional or cognitive impairments. The benefit paid would be cash of at least $50 per day, depending upon the degree of impairment.

The CLASS Act had the advantage of having an initial net positive cash flow as people paid premiums but could not yet access benefits. Thus, the CBO estimated the act would generate over $70 billion in the first 10 years. By law the CLASS Act is required to be self-sustaining: "No taxpayer funds shall be used for payment of benefits under a CLASS Independent Benefit Plan." In October 2011, however, the Department of Health and Human Services (DHHS) ruled that the CLASS Act was not financially sustainable, and ultimately the act was repealed on January 1, 2013.

The problem was the *voluntary* nature of the program. Like health insurance, a voluntary program for long-term care will be subject to terrible adverse selection that will send it into a death spiral. People who need or have a high risk of needing long-term care are much more likely to enroll. A 30-year-old might need health insurance for preventive services, a pregnancy, an accident, or unexpected illness but can hardly believe he or she will need long-term care insurance and, thus, would be unwilling to voluntarily pay much for it. Because government subsidies are prohibited for this act, adverse selection would then force high premiums, which means that only people who *really* need the long-term care will buy it, but they will end up using more benefits than what they pay in.

Unless subsidized for almost 100% of costs or unless a program is needed at the time of purchase by 100% of people, no voluntary program for anything related to health care can be sustainable. It was ironic that the ACA included a mandatory health insurance program so as to address the adverse selection problem plaguing the nation's health care system but then created a voluntary long-term care insurance program that then was determined to be unsustainable because of the very same adverse selection problem.

Conclusion

This summary of the ACA reveals at least 5 conclusions. First, this 906-page piece of legislation is a comprehensive reform. It certainly addresses more than access, which is handled in just one of its 10 titles. The ACA also addresses cost, quality, prevention and health promotion, health care workforce issues, and many other matters.

Although reforming the whole system, the ACA does not do it all at once. The reforms roll out between 2010 and 2018 (see Figure 8.17).

FIGURE 8.17 Timeline for implementation of provisions of the Affordable Care Act

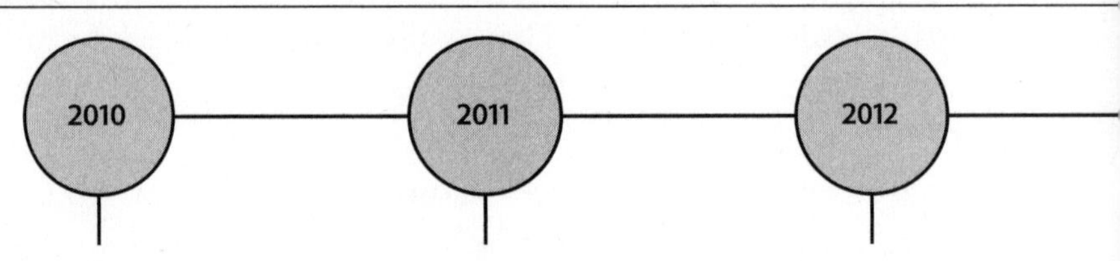

2010

- Patient Centered Outcomes Research Institute (PCORI)
- Prevention and Public Health Fund
- Donut Hole Rebates
- Generic Biologic Drugs
- Tax on Indoor Tanning Services
- Adult Dependent Coverage to Age 26
- Free Preventive Care
- Health Care Workforce Commission

2011

- Minimum MLR for Insurers
- Center for Medicare and Medicaid Innovation (CMMI)
- Medicare Advantage Payment Changes
- Medical Malpractice Grants

2012

- Accountable Care Organizations (ACOs)
- Annual Fees on Drug Manufacturers
- Medicare Value-Based Purchasing
- Reduced Medicare Payments for Hospital Readmissions

Source: The Henry J. Kaiser Family Foundation.

Some reforms, such as allowing young adults to stay on their parent's health insurance plan until age 26 and the Patient-Centered Outcomes Research Institute, started early, in 2010. Others, such as penalizing hospitals for high readmission rates, began in 2012. Still others, such as the insurance exchanges and Medicaid expansion, began in 2013 and 2014. (The exchanges opened for purchase on October 1, 2013, but the insurance did not become effective until January 1, 2014.) The last provision to take effect is the "Cadillac" tax in 2018. Even with the progressive rollout of provisions, the number and extent of changes required of everyone is significant.

The ACA is certainly more complex than the only other very large-scale health care reform ever attempted in the United States: Medicare

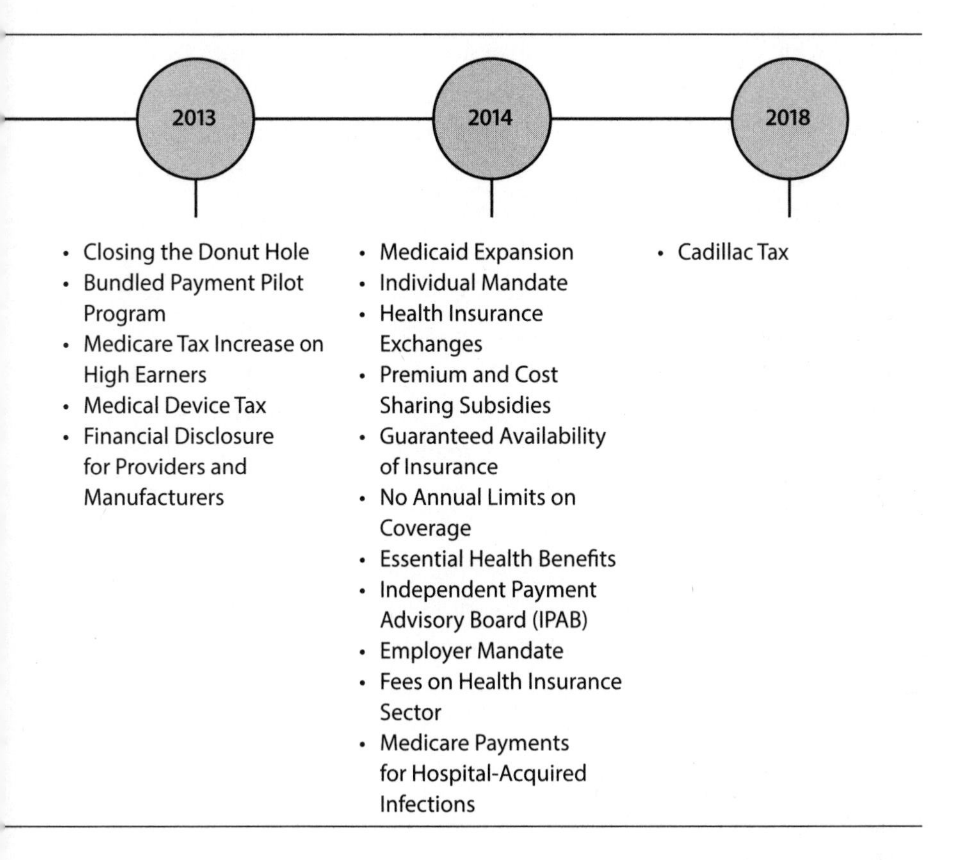

and Medicaid. Not only does it legislate for parts of the health care system that Medicare and Medicaid never did, even in its changes to access the ACA is more complex than the enrollment process in Medicare because it needs to work within and modify an existing system. By reforming what already existed and then adding new programs on top of that, the ACA became necessarily more complex than simply creating a new health insurance program *de novo*.

No piece of legislation is perfect, and particularly with the complexity of the American health care system, any change would necessarily involve tradeoffs, failures, and unintended consequences (Chapter 2, page 35), as improvements in one area may create unforeseen problems in other areas. Furthermore, not every reform will be a success. Just as venture capitalists and businesses expect some, maybe even most, of their new businesses and projects to fail, some parts of the ACA might not work or will not work as planned. Indeed, if there are not failures, then the act is probably not bold enough. Because the health care system is dynamic, there will need to be ongoing reforms, continual improvement, and maintenance. If the ACA is health care reform 1.0, we will need a 2.0 (see Chapter 12).There is no final reform.

Finally, this review of the ACA makes clear that this is not a government takeover of health care. Although the act does expand Medicaid, most of its spending on and method for expanding coverage are through insurance exchanges that are marketplaces for private insurance. And of course the providers of care—hospitals, physicians, home health agencies, and pharmacies—as well as the manufacturers—drug, device, and medical supply companies—all remain private; they are not employed by the government.

The ACA is an enormous and significant change that will structure the American health care system for the rest of our lives, even as it will need further modifications and revisions.

= CHAPTER NINE =

What Does the ACA Mean for Me?

For most people the details of any piece of legislation are overwhelming and largely irrelevant. Medicare beneficiaries do not understand or really care what the actual law says; they just want to know what benefits they have. Even if they have never heard of Medicare Parts A, B, and D, they understand which services are covered, how much drug insurance costs, and which drugs they can get and for how much. The same is true of the ACA. Most people will never understand the intricacies of the exchanges. But they will understand what directly affects them—their insurance options, monthly premiums, and choice of physicians and hospitals. So what does the ACA mean for you, whether you are a patient or a physician?

Patients

For the majority of Americans the ACA constitutes a big improvement. With all of the terrible news about the exchanges and cancellations and whatever else, it is easy for people to think the ACA is not going to be beneficial. It is easy to be nostalgic for the old days. But remember how much people hated the "old days," and remember that it was Wellpoint raising insurance premiums on some individuals by 39% in February 2010 that finally galvanized the House to enact the Senate's version of the ACA. So let's look past the immediate headlines—good or bad—and dissect the benefits of the law. Importantly, not all of the improvements will happen tomorrow, and not every single American will benefit from every change. Some people will lose on some things. No piece of legislation will have only winners. Those who are likely to pay more for their health care are mainly, though not only, people who are relatively well off and won't be eligible for ACA subsidies, or people who are relatively healthy and were formerly able to find very low premium coverage because sicker individuals could be charged exorbitant rates or excluded altogether. But here is a list of all the things that, over the next few years, are guaranteed to get better for all Americans because of the ACA. (The list is in chronological order, detailing the sequence in which they are likely to be fully available.)

- Security that whatever your age, employment, previous health problems, location, or other characteristics, you will be able to obtain affordable health coverage and so will your adult children and other family members..
- Free preventive services, such as 10 different immunizations, screening for cancers, high cholesterol, diabetes, depression, alcohol abuse, and many other services, all with no deductibles or co-payments. For American women this also includes free birth control.
- Safer hospitals with significantly lower chances of getting an infection, the wrong medication, or being on the wrong end of another mistake.
- Better follow-up care after a hospitalization to help the transition to home or other facility, ensuring you are improving, getting the right services, taking the right medications, and seeing your personal physician when you need to.
- An electronic medical record that any physician or hospital in the United States can get access to at any time.
- Hard data on the actual quality of hospitals for the performance of many specific tests and treatments.

These are standard improvements as a result of the ACA available to all Americans. The list does not include the many other advantages that people might not think of as part of health care reform because they do not involve health insurance and physicians, such as

- menu labeling,
- access to employer wellness programs to stop smoking and lose weight,

- less insurance paperwork, and
- greater transparency of price, quality, and physician conflicts of interest.

Beyond these changes, different groups of people with different characteristics will experience different improvements.

Young People Under 30 Years Old

For young adults the ACA has 3 big and distinct advantages. The first is that until they are 26, they can stay on their parents' health insurance plan. That frees them to take a job that lacks health insurance, knowing they can still be covered by their parents' plan. And even if their job offers health insurance, many younger people will get better insurance through their parents' plan: covering more services, hospitals, and physicians, and with lower deductibles and co-pays. According to the Commonwealth Fund, as of August 2013 there are roughly 4.5 million young adults between ages 23 and 25 covered under their parents' health plans who, before the ACA, likely would have been ineligible for dependent coverage.

For young adults whose parents might not have good health insurance from their employer or who do not want to rely on their parents, there are the insurance exchanges. The experience with shopping on the exchanges is all over the place, and it depends largely on your state of residence. In some states that run their own exchanges (Chapter 8, page 206), such as Kentucky, Connecticut, and California, the shopping experience is pretty good—many options, with good prices, and standardization, all of which makes it much easier to compare different options from before. In the states that opted not to operate their own exchanges and, therefore, the federal government is running them, the experience has gone from terrible to tolerable. In many there are good deals. Over time the shopping experience should improve. The federal website should get better, and there will be more apps and programs to help make comparison shopping even easier.

Up to age 30, for people whose jobs are not paying well or who feel as though they are healthy and only want to insure for the low likelihood of a "health disaster," they can purchase a catastrophic-only health plan.

After 30, however, they do have to grow up and buy regular insurance at least at the bronze level (Chapter 8, pages 213).

The most valuable thing is that these options will be affordable. For instance, in Los Angeles, California, a single 26-year-old earning $23,000 (twice the poverty line) will be able to buy a Blue Shield "Standard Silver" PPO insurance plan for as low as $86 per month, or one from Kaiser for $127 per month. A minimum coverage catastrophic plan, for which premium assistance cannot be used, would end up costing roughly $185 per month. In Utah the premium for the lowest-cost silver plan, without premium assistance, is $159, and the premium for the lowest-cost catastrophic plan is $108.

These are very, very good prices. True, some young people will have to pay more than what they paid before the ACA. But the coverage under the ACA will be significantly better. The insurers can no longer create plans that exclude things like hospitalizations, ambulance services, or maternity services, creating ridiculous arrangements they then call health insurance. For instance, before the ACA young adults working at McDonald's or other fast food restaurants who earned about $17,000 a year received pretty skimpy plans. At McDonald's they were paying $56 per month for just $2,000 total benefits (see Figure 9.1). As Baltazar's experience demonstrates, $2,000 in health care barely covers one emergency room visit for stiches and is totally overwhelmed if a person needs to be hospitalized for anything larger, such as a $25,000 appendectomy or cancer treatment. Under the ACA young adults get real health insurance.

FIGURE 9.1 Comparison of ACA health insurance with McDonald's and Ruby Tuesday's for young adults

	ACA SILVER PLAN (CALIF.)	ACA CATASTROPHIC PLAN (CALIF.)*	MCDONALD'S	RUBY TUESDAY'S
Monthly premium with subsidies	$41	$154	$56	$7**
Annual coverage limit	None	None	$2,000	$4,250

*Subsidies are not available for catastrophic plans.
**Premium after 6 months of working.
Source: Covered California, *The Wall Street Journal.*

These types of prices are good even compared with the low penalty payment for not buying insurance in 2014: $95 or 1% of income.

Self-Insured

Before the ACA about 15 million Americans were self-insured like Erin. They bought health insurance as individuals without any bargaining power. They often had to settle for plans with high deductibles or that excluded key types of coverage or that had caps that would not cover the most serious illnesses. Even worse, if they contracted a serious illness, the next year they would often find out they either could no longer get insurance or would see their premiums go up by 24%, like Erin did.

What would a 40-year-old woman like Erin, with 2 children but who earns $40,000 (200% of the poverty line) and lives in Denver, be able to buy in the Colorado exchange? A silver plan, after the subsidy, will cost her as little as $188 per month. And she gets that rate regardless of whether she or her children have had cancer, cystic fibrosis, or any other disease. With guaranteed renewability under the ACA, insurance can never be taken away from her and her children.

The Uninsured

What about Wayne, an uninsured American between 25 and 65? There are approximately 31.9 million people over 25 but under 65 who like him earn under 138% of the poverty line (in 2013, $15,856) and will thus receive Medicaid coverage; or they will in theory. Here, however, complications arise because of the Supreme Court ruling (Chapter 7, page 193). As of January 2014 there have been 26 states, mostly in the South and High Plains region, that balked and decided not to expand Medicaid for their residents. In these states nearly 5 million people will not be able to be covered. And the largest group excluded from Medicaid is childless adults, many of whom are working—the Waynes of the United States. Nonetheless, the ACA permits them to buy in the insurance exchanges with subsidies if they earn 100% of the poverty level ($11,490 for an individual in 2013) or more. But this also means that because of a quirk in the ACA—that those earning less than $11,490 per year cannot get subsidies—and these states' refusal to expand Medicaid, the most impoverished of all, adult Americans who earn under 100% of the poverty level, will remain uninsured. They will not be able to get Medicaid or buy with subsidies in the exchange. They will continue to receive the care as they had in the old system: through the emergency room with their costs being transferred to Americans who do have insurance.

Wayne and others who earn over $15,856 (138% of the poverty line), will be able to buy health insurance in the exchanges with subsidies. What will it cost? People earning $23,000 (200% of the poverty level) in Philadelphia, will be able to buy a silver plan at $76 per month after subsidies. They could even buy a bronze plan with more deductibles and copays for as low as $58 per month. Families who are uninsured but earn over $94,200 for a family of 4 (over 400% of the poverty line), who have been excluded perhaps because of a preexisting condition, are now guaranteed to get insurance. They can buy insurance without a subsidy but at premiums that are tied only to their age and smoking habits, not their health. For instance, in Philadelphia they would pay $256 per month for a silver plan.

The Silent Majority: Americans Between the Ages of 30 and 65 with Employer Insurance

The majority of Americans get their health insurance through their employer or a family member's employer. Over the next few years not much will change for them. Their children will be able to stay on their plans. Preventive care will be free. More wellness incentives have already begun at their workplace and may well expand.

One big difference is the security of knowing they can always get health insurance. And this will lead to a change that has not been discussed much: the end of job lock. Many people stay with an employer or do not start their own company because their employer offers good health insurance or they cannot get affordable coverage on their own. The ACA gives everyone freedom to quit because they know they can get affordable health insurance through the exchanges. This will allow people to take jobs they really want rather than stay at jobs they need because of the benefits. According to the members of the health committee in the Minnesota Senate, more than 31,000 people will start new businesses because they will be freed by being able to get their own insurance in the exchanges.

Employers are reacting to the ACA in different ways that will affect this large group. Some, like UPS, are responding by not covering workers' spouses who have insurance through their own employer. This is basically a form of "employer responsibility," in which one employer makes another employer take financial responsibility for providing insurance to their workers. It does not take anyone's insurance away. Other employers are redesigning their health insurance, often going to higher-deductible plans. This is part of a trend that pre-dated the ACA and is driven mostly by health care inflation. As we discuss in Chapter 13, other changes in employer-provided health insurance are likely to occur as the system evolves.

Seniors: The Impact on Medicare

Medicare was the ACA for seniors. They got guaranteed health insurance nearly 50 years before the rest of the country. The ACA makes important but minor adjustments that improve the Medicare system. First, like other Americans, seniors get free preventive services and a free annual prevention office visit. Medicare estimated that in 2012 more than 34 million seniors received one or more free preventive service. Second, seniors will also experience the progressive closing of the donut hole in the Medicare drug benefit—the crazy gap in drug coverage when spending for drugs is between $2,970 and $4,550 (Chapter 2, page 59). And while the donut hole is closing, over 7 million Medicare seniors and beneficiaries with disabilities have the advantage of drug company rebates on brand-name drugs when they are "in the hole."

The third advantage is the least visible but probably most important for sick Medicare patients: better care through the focus on reducing hospital-readmissions. Hospitals will be assuming responsibility for more care after a hospitalization so as to ensure that patients are getting needed services, taking their medications, seeing their primary care physician, and getting rehabilitation. This increased coordination among providers should lead to better health care and health.

Finally, the ACA has improved Medicare's financial outlook. Since passage of the ACA, health care inflation has been low. Some of this slowdown in costs is from the Great Recession, some pre-dates the ACA, but some is also directly from the impact of the ACA. On a per capita basis there was no health care inflation in Medicare in 2013. The CBO suggests the Medicare Trust Fund that pays for Part A will last an additional 12 years, until 2029, because of the cost-control elements in the ACA. This improvement is good not just for seniors but also for all taxpayers, as it will now be longer before general tax dollars are used to support this part of Medicare. More directly, for a senior this slowdown in costs means that premiums for Part B have actually remained relatively flat—almost unheard of—and for the lowest-cost prescription drug plan, they actually will decline from $15 per month in 2013 to $12.60 per month in 2014—truly unheard of.

Overall Service Changes

The care experience will also be different. This will not be immediate and not because of any specific provision in the ACA, but rather there will be an evolution to a different way of caring for patients because of the way the ACA changes incentives for physicians and hospitals. A major difference will be the digitalization of health care (Chapter 13). More services will be available outside of the physician's office and hospital. There will be more electronic connectivity. Health care has been slow to adopt e-mail, social media, and other electronic communications, but this will change over the decade. Physicians or their staff will be e-mailing with patients. More radically, there will be more frequent monitoring so that people in the health system will call you to provide suggestions and services related to prevention and health promotion.

The digitalization will go further. Already there are house calls by webcam. These will proliferate so you can be "seen" and get advice without ever leaving your home. And for situations that require in-person interaction, whether that is getting a vaccine, a physical exam, or a lab test, there will be many more convenient places to get them, from stores to pharmacies to storefront clinics.

Customer service will improve. The system will be waiting on you rather than you waiting on it. Over the next decade, because of the ACA, physicians' and hospitals' performance will increasingly be measured and publicly reported, including on customer service. Wasting your time sitting in a physician's waiting room for 30 minutes for your appointment or in the emergency room for 2 hours will end. It may never become Nordstrom's or the Four Seasons, but the health system will be much more patient centric, and different health plans will compete on the quality of their service, not just care. For more sick patients, hospitals and larger physician practices are likely to create navigator programs to help patients schedule their appointments, take them to appointments, and keep track of everything.

Overall, for patients on the insurance side there will be more affordable coverage, with guaranteed issue and renewability as well as no lifetime limits. And a very wide range of preventive services will be free. On the care side the system will become more customer-service oriented, with access in more locations, including your own home. Most importantly, going to the hospital will be significantly safer.

Physicians

Physicians are apprehensive about the ACA: the act is big, they are not trained to and do not regularly read legislation, and they know there is a lot of talk about cost control, electronic health records, and reporting. Uncertainty breeds fear and anxiety. What does health care reform mean for the average, non-hospital-based physician?

Physicians will have to go electronic. The Recovery Act of 2009 provided both incentives and penalties to encourage installation and use of electronic health records. For most physicians installing electronic health records, this is an essential first step, but it needs to be part of a process for transforming how they give care. Properly instituted, electronic health records combined with home sensors should allow physicians to track chronically ill patients better and intervene earlier before conditions escalate to the point that requires hospitalization; identify patients not receiving needed care; monitor how physicians, nurses, and others are performing their jobs; and facilitate reporting to insurers and Medicare on quality metrics. Adopting and incorporating electronic health records is a challenge for physicians and their offices and can be frustrating. It takes time to move information from paper to a computer and to figure out how to use electronic health records efficiently during a patient visit. But there is no avoiding it.

Physicians will also have to get used to being more accountable and transparent in their care. There will be more quality reporting, which will almost inevitably mean increasing transparency regarding their performance. And there will be increasing demands for price transparency. This transparency may be the aspect of reform they fear the most. Physicians have had Medicare incentive payments to just report data, but, increasingly, the data will be evaluated and publicly posted. For all physicians, figuring out what needs to be reported, how to do it efficiently, and, most importantly, how to improve on quality scores so they are best in class are the challenges. Again, this increase in accountability is inevitable, and physicians must get working on it now. The important first step is for physicians to get together and begin ensuring that their care for common conditions is at the very highest professional standards. The most important step in reaching this goal is standardization of care based on guidelines but with customization for unique patients. Instituting this process of standardization is critical to quality improvement, reporting, and probably increasing efficiency and revenue.

For the next few years many physicians will be caught in a misalignment with an outdated business model. Today, physicians are still largely paid on a fee-for-service model. Simultaneously, everyone, from their patients to insurers to the government, is expecting them to be more efficient and eliminate unnecessary services, often services on which they earn income. And they want them to report more data on everything. There is no doubt about it: these contradictory signals are enormously frustrating and counterproductive. In addition, as an adaptation to fee for service, most physicians' offices are structured to increase revenue. The business model is not one that targets increasing margin by delivering services more efficiently.

There are 4 things the average physician can do. One is to begin the process of transformation to more efficient practice, knowing that payment changes that move away from fee for service are inevitably coming. Unfortunately, there is no definitive timeline, and the timeline is likely to vary from region to region based on what private payers do. But payment change will come, and physicians who are ready will flourish in the long run.

Second, part of this transformation means that physicians will need to change their business model to increasing efficiency in their delivery of the services. Instituting electronic health records with electronic prescription ordering; shifting the duties of office staff that filed records and called in prescriptions to more productive jobs, such as monitoring sicker patients at home; assigning office nurses to manage common urgent-care problems can free up the physicians to do more productive work.

Third, physicians should engage insurers to try to modify contracts so that they have a financial reward for being more efficient. It isn't enough to leave this to insurers. Not all of them are innovative, but it is worth trying to negotiate contracts that reward saving money.

Finally, these impending changes confront many physicians with the major existential question of whether to sell their practice to a hospital system or remain independent. Selling to a hospital system is the easier thing to do, at least in the short term. The hospital system will be responsible for installing, maintaining, and updating the electronic health records system. If that hospital system is enlightened enough to understand the change coming, it will install the remote monitoring systems and other technologies needed to improve care. It will file all those quality reports. It will negotiate the new contracts to reward efficiency and value. It will assume responsibility for all the gyrations that will occur over the next decade, leaving the physicians to focus on patient care.

But to many physicians, selling their practices to a hospital system feels like selling out. They become employees in a large bureaucracy. They cease to be the captains of the ship and, increasingly, be just another, albeit relatively well-paid, deckhand.

To remain independent, physician practices will need some scale. Offices of 1, 2, or 3 physicians are unlikely to be viable in the long term unless they are somehow affiliated with other practices to share functions and costs. A private practice will probably need 10 or more physicians to have sufficient scale—financial resources, physician time and attention, and staff—to support the experimentation that will be part of the necessary transformation in care. In addition, physicians will have to act less like self-sufficient small businesses and more strategically. They will need to standardize their care processes. They may need to hire consultants to help them through the transformation process, especially when identifying high-cost patients who need more or different kinds of attention as well as high-cost services that can be preempted, avoided, or executed more efficiently. They may need help when negotiating different kinds of contracts with insurers and hospitals.

Physicians love autonomy, and selling out is not necessary; staying independent is definitely possible. That too will require changing practices, and to succeed physicians will have to learn skills they were not taught in medical school or residency. With some serious work they can remain captains of their ship, but such an entrepreneurial approach is not for everyone. Working for a larger organization where someone else assumes both risk and responsibility in choppy seas can be the right approach.

Insurers

The ACA will transform insurers in at least 3 important ways. First, insurers will have more customers. Even on the relatively conservative CBO estimates, by the end of 2020 they will have 25 million customers through the insurance exchanges, a net gain of 18 million people.

More importantly, the exchanges will transform how insurers sell insurance. Increasingly, they will sell directly to customers in a competitive marketplace. One of the big complaints of the pre-ACA world was that insurers sold through a business-to-business approach; the customer was the human resources department of a company, not the person being insured. Although businesses always said they were worried about health care costs, this was probably not their absolute highest concern. If all their competitors were faced with the same rate increases, then higher costs were not necessarily a competitive disadvantage; instead, one—if not the—major motivation of the human resources department was to minimize employees complaints by satisfying as many people as possible. Practically, this meant they bought insurance plans that covered many hospitals and physicians and had the fewest restrictions possible.

Such an approach gave "name-brand-must-have" hospitals and physicians, such as Memorial Sloan Kettering Cancer Center or the Massachusetts General Hospital, great bargaining power and, thus, kept insurance premiums high.

The exchanges turn this around. In the exchanges the customer is now the customer. Furthermore, the customer will be able to more easily compare insurance plans as they are standardized into 4 categories of benefits and premium levels. Everything we know indicates this will significantly increase competition, especially on price. Data from simulations run by consulting companies based on preliminary data from the state exchanges indicates that the vast majority of the people purchasing in the exchanges will focus predominantly on financial aspects of coverage: insurance premiums, deductibles, co-pays, and total out-of-pocket costs. They seem willing to sacrifice famous hospitals and expansive choices of physicians for lower prices, especially if they can be sure the lower insurance price still gets them access to "gold rated" coverage—that is, high-quality, if not name-plate, hospitals and physicians. (This will place much more importance on independent and reliable ratings of quality.)

In the near term this will have a significant impact. Insurers will need to differentiate themselves and cultivate customer loyalty—this could result in better customer service. To lower premiums, insurers will have incentives to create selective networks of efficient physicians and hospitals willing to accept lower prices. Insurers will also create tighter drug formularies that emphasize generics and mail-order drugs.

This shift to low-cost, high-quality selective networks will in turn put pressure on physicians and, especially, hospitals. It will make performance on the quality of care more important as a way to differentiate lower-cost plans. More importantly, expensive hospitals, especially academic hospitals, will feel pressure to lower their costs or show that they really do have measurably higher quality that justifies higher prices. The more people who get their insurance through the exchanges, the more this pressure to lower prices for insurance plans and, ultimately, for hospitals and physicians will play out.

Hospital systems are not waiting passively. To gain leverage so as to keep their prices higher, they are countering by acquiring many other

FIGURE 9.2 Insurance company profits and caring for sick patients

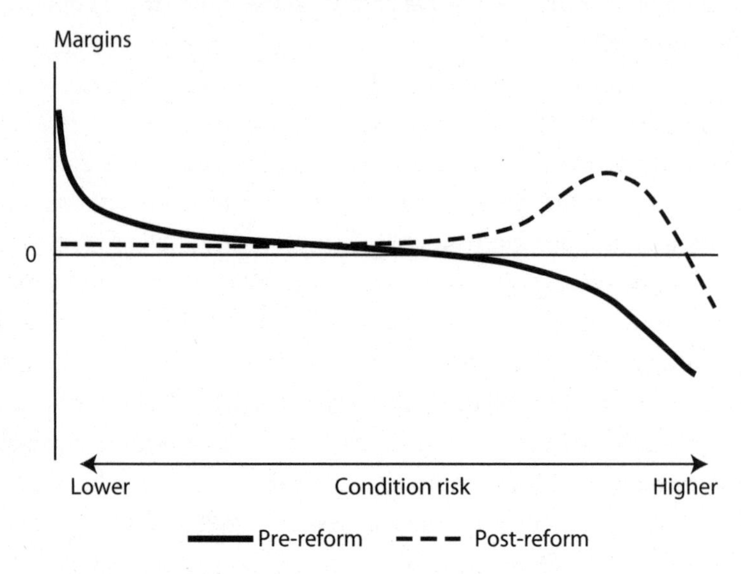

Source: McKinsey & Company.

hospitals in specific regions so they become "essential" and, thus, cannot be excluded in an insurance plan. The final wrinkle in this will be how vigorously the government's antitrust enforcers look into these mergers and, especially, the reach and pricing practices of hospital systems.

Thus, there will be a three-sided battle among insurers competing in the exchanges needing to lower prices to gain customers, a myriad of ever-expanding hospital systems trying to keep their prices up, and the antitrust police determining when to intervene. No one knows how it will evolve and be resolved. But no matter what happens, it will have a big influence on health care costs.

Finally, the ACA is changing how insurance companies make their profits. For years their profits depended on covering healthy young people, especially those highly profitable ones who paid premiums but ultimately rarely or never used any services (see the solid line in Figure 9.2 above). The ACA changes all of that. It requires insurers to guarantee issue—that is, provide for all people, regardless of health insurance status (Chapter 8, page 217). Furthermore, it excludes insurers from using preexisting conditions to set the insurance prices in the exchange. To prevent insurance companies from being financially disadvantaged and potentially going out of business when they happen to enroll sicker than average patients, the ACA risk-adjusts across insurance companies (see Chapter 2). This means it transfers money from companies that insure younger healthier customers to insurers that cover sicker patients.

Not only will insurance companies receive more money for enrolling chronically ill patients, but the companies will also find ways to make caring for these patients even more profitable. Chronically ill patients use a lot of health care services (Chapter 4, page 112), but a lot of these services are either avoidable or unnecessary. They result from poor preventive care, thus allowing patients to get sick when cheaper interventions could have preempted a hospital stay. This high cost of caring for these sicker patients and a lot of unnecessary services means there are more ways to save money—and more money to save—while still improving the quality of care.

For insurers, this suddenly means that profits are no longer in the young and healthy but rather, increasingly, in covering—and improving the care for—sicker patients. This change in incentives could lead to a real focus on improving the care for the 10% of patients with chronic illness who account for two-thirds of the spending (see Chapter 12, megatrend X). We may find insurers advertising how well they manage care for patients with diabetes or emphysema. What a change that would be!

Caveat

This view of the implications of the ACA for individuals, physicians, and insurers is optimistic. I am by nature an optimist, and I do think the ACA will galvanize significant improvement in the health care system. But there is a very real chance my view is overly positive. What could go wrong? First, if Americans really do focus only on the cost of their insurance and health care, it is possible that service and attention from both insurers and hospital systems could become like the customer service we associate with Internet providers, wireless carriers, and airlines—dreadful. If the vast majority of insurance-purchasing decisions really are driven by premium and deductible levels alone, and the quality of care a hospital provides really doesn't influence which insurance Americans select, then customer service and care won't be something that is deemed valuable and worth investing in. This could make health insurers and health care more unpleasant. Rather than having high-touch care, we might end up with high-aggravation care—which itself might be bad for our health.

Similarly, if people select insurance and hospitals mainly on price, the response might be simply cutting rather than improving value. We might get a return to the 1990s rather than a focus on keeping people healthy. That is, insurance companies might find it easier to reduce costs by "just saying no," and hospitals and physicians might just cut services. I would think insurance companies learned the lesson that too much "No" leads to backlash, but maybe they are also forgetful. I would also have thought that with increased monitoring on quality and penalties for readmissions and mistakes, hospitals and physicians would find meat-cleaver cuts in service counterproductive. But unless they develop care processes that keep patients healthy and out of the hospital, they may feel they have no other choice but to say "no" to reduce their operating costs.

Another potential black cloud could be dramatic increases in insurance premiums. Insurance premiums can rise for many reasons, such as changes in who buys insurance and greater costs either through the provision of higher-cost tests or treatments, or of prescribing more tests and treatments. In the next few years the real worry comes from a significant increase in sicker patients and fewer younger and healthier people buying insurance. This kind of adverse selection (Chapter 2, page 41) could occur in many ways. And the terrible rollout of the federal exchange website did not help. We will only know this when insurance companies have assessed enrollment for 2014 and have to provide their 2015 rates in the late spring of 2014. There are some policies that could mitigate this rate shock, such as re-insurance. But if rates go up significantly, there could be a bad, reinforcing cycle of people—especially young people—forgoing insurance and, thus, driving premiums ever higher. This could lead to an unraveling of the ACA.

This negative scenario is the less likely one. But it is possible.

Conclusion

There is a lot of anxiety about "What is health care going to mean for me?" And this anxiety has certainly increased as people received cancellation notices on their insurance, combined with the launch of a seriously flawed and buggy federal exchange website that made getting insurance very challenging. But these are short-term problems and will be resolved in months or a year or 2 at most. For the majority of Americans the ACA will lead to better health care: free preventive services, safer hospitals, and electronic health records; more affordable health care, with lower increases in insurance premiums; and more information about prices and quality. These changes will not happen immediately, but they are happening and will be fully in place by the middle to end of the decade.

You don't have to take my word for it that the ACA will make the health care system better for you. In the next section I outline dashboards on access, cost control, quality, and the overall health of American society by which we all can objectively assess whether the system is improving and whether the ACA is working. I also peer into the future to delineate the megatrends we can expect over the next 10 to 15 years.

Part III

THE FUTURE OF AMERICAN HEALTH CARE

= CHAPTER TEN =

ACA Implementation Problems

Are They Fatal?

Ask any venture capitalist (VC), private equity investor, or successful business leader what the most crucial element of a start-up venture is, and you will get one word: execution. Success is rarely determined by the quality or novelty of a new company's core idea or the technical specifics of a new product's design; rather, it is the capacity to implement that differentiates successful companies from failures.

Consequently, when investors or business leaders back a new venture or project, they spend lots of time recruiting the right people. It is what Jim Collins, author of *From Good to Great*, calls the top priority—getting the right people on the bus. And once the people are in place, VCs and business leaders spend countless hours setting up organizational structures that provide hands-on mentoring and decision support so that executives are equipped to succeed. The VC imperative is simple: execution and people are the key—more important than the product or idea to a successful business venture. Ignore this imperative at your peril.

As the disastrous launch of healthcare.gov laid bare, the execution of the ACA was seriously flawed. Three factors contributed to the rocky rollout: the nature of lawmaking, poor personnel decisions, and poisonous politics.

First, unlike business, lawmaking is not focused on execution, and its inflexibility makes the constant adjustments needed for effective implementation much more difficult. Laws in the United States are the progeny of a very large, diverse, and rarely unified Congress, whose members, if they are not actively trying to kill the laws just passed, are rarely focused on ensuring effective implementation. Political and financial considerations as well as the need for speed invariably trump execution-minded adjustments, and this often leads to unnecessarily complex and unwieldy policy. Furthermore, because enacting amendments is difficult even under the best of circumstances, the normal business practice of continually refining and adjusting a new product is frequently not possible—or it is seriously complicated and delayed by regulatory requirements. An existing bureaucracy with its own habits, patterns, and interests that may not align with effective execution further compound this morass. Thus, executing on legislation is actually more difficult than executing a new product launch in the private sector. In some ways, these challenges make it somewhat surprising when government programs, such as Medicare, the space program, or food stamps are implemented (moderately) successfully.

Second, in the case of the ACA there were personnel decisions that hampered effective execution. The people entrusted with implementation were skilled policy advisers, but they lacked managerial experience, particularly in e-commerce, health insurance, and related areas. And they had a culture that was not conducive to constant testing and learning through the process of building the website. This may be the place where business lessons most readily apply.

Third, these challenges were compounded by the need to implement in an intensely partisan atmosphere in which conservatives—politicians and the conservative media—were literally rooting for the ACA to crash and took every glitch as an opportunity to declare it a total failure. In such a context, short-term political calculations often overshadowed longer-term focus on effective execution.

Nonetheless, the fiasco of healthcare.gov was neither preordained nor inevitable. Today, the real question is not who is to blame for the failures and delays with the federal marketplace. Rather, the real question for the future of American health care is whether the poor launch of healthcare.gov and other delays will necessarily undermine the ACA's long-term positive impact. I do not think so.

The ACA is much more than the federally operated exchanges, which, in turn, are much more than healthcare.gov. Healthcare.gov's technical problems are remediable, and in the span of a few months a number of them have been resolved. Many state-based exchanges are operating well, and best practices will be shared with other states' exchanges. But like any e-commerce website, the exchange websites will need constant attention to ensure smooth eligibility determinations, premium payments, accurate enrollment data, development of applications to help consumers, and other enhancements of the user experience.

Beyond the website there is much more to do to operate the exchanges effectively, such as revising the rules for insurance companies participating in the exchanges. Making the exchanges an effective mechanism for transforming the health system is a constant work in progress. Yet healthcare.gov and the exchanges do not affect many of the act's important, system-changing reforms, such as reducing costs, changing systems of payment, and encouraging more coordination in the delivery of care. These are being implemented but could also use more work.

What went wrong?

The ACA Legislation and the Problems of Implementation

Effective implementation is rarely a top legislative priority in drafting a law. After all, legislators are politicians, and as such, they are acutely aware of the needs of constituents, the demands of interest groups and financial backers, and the need for credit. They are also well aware of the tyranny of the Congressional Budget Office (CBO) and the financing of any bill. And they understand the need for speed in the legislative process (see Chapter 5). Legislators, particularly good legislators, are consumed by the need to get bills passed as quickly as possible, warts and all. Otherwise nothing happens, which is often the worst of all outcomes. Consequently, if there is a conflict between execution-related concerns and political or budgetary-related concerns, inevitably it is execution that loses out. Legislators tend to underweight how various provisions might make implementation either easier or harder.

Congress is rarely held accountable for implementation. Once legislation is enacted, as far as Congress is concerned, the work is done. Execution is the job of the administration and bureaucracy. When laws are implemented well, Congress barely notices. Just as the news media rarely covers good news stories, there rarely are hearings trumpeting a well-functioning government program. Only problems sell. Thus, if, like healthcare.gov, implementation is filled with problems or failure, members of Congress can get attention by launching investigative hearings or other media events. And even these hearings tend to miss the point, as they are generally more concerned with finding scapegoats than uncovering deficiencies in a policy that may have hampered implementation.

This is not unique to the ACA; it is true of all legislation. Consider a few examples in which politics trumped execution in shaping the ACA. The employer mandate penalizes employers with 51 or more full-time employees who do not sponsor health insurance for their employees. The law defined a full-time employee as one who works 30 or more hours per week. This approach was hardly the most effective or administratively easiest way to implement the mandate and, along with complex reporting requirements, is part of the reason for postponing enforcement of the mandate. An alternative was to base the trigger for the mandate on payroll, not numbers of employees. This is much easier to enforce and much less liable to gaming by employers. It was considered but not enacted. Why?

Politics. Traditionally, large employers had opposed health care reform legislation. In the battle for the ACA, it was the small employers, through the Chamber of Commerce and the National Federation of Independent Businesses (NFIB), who vigorously opposed the law even though they were not subject to the mandate. But large employers, through the Business Roundtable, basically remained neutral on the ACA. Over 95% already provided health insurance, and most of the law's provisions were not going to require significant changes for them. But they opposed the payroll-based penalty, and this could have tipped their position. Easier execution was sacrificed to political considerations in order to keep the big employers passive.

Consider the SHOP exchanges. These exchanges are meant to provide a competitive marketplace for insurance in which small businesses can purchase coverage for their employees. The pooling of many small businesses in a competitive marketplace should drive down premiums to large-employer levels.

In theory, this is a good idea and something some senators had been advocating long before the ACA was a possibility. But anyone who was truly concerned with implementation would not have endorsed them. Trying to establish simultaneously 2 exchanges, one for individuals and another for small businesses, is a terrible idea. From a management perspective, the best approach would be to focus all the resources on getting one exchange up and running successfully then consider the need for a second. Trying to do too much undermines the chances of success.

Indeed, historically, small-business exchanges have proven almost impossible to implement in the real world. Despite having a very successful individual exchange, Massachusetts has tried for years to establish a small-business exchange to no avail. Similarly, many private small-business exchanges inevitably collapse because of the lack of a mandate and the consequent adverse selection. (Remember, businesses with fewer than 50 employees have no mandate.) And even a small-business exchange like the one in Utah has only attracted a few thousand participants. Given history and experience, the likelihood of successfully implementing a SHOP exchange is very low, so it is no surprise that the opening of the SHOP exchanges was postponed to 2015.

Why have SHOP exchanges in the ACA at all? Politics. It is a gesture to small businesses, and it also offers politicians who have been proposing SHOP exchange legislation for years a tangible policy victory they can showcase to their constituents. But in reality building separate small-business exchanges will divert human and other resources toward a dead-end project. The SHOP exchanges are very unlikely to work well, and even if they do, they will not have much impact. The CBO estimates that the SHOP exchanges will enroll just 1 million people total, less than 3% of the total number of people gaining coverage.

In the process of enacting the ACA Phil Schiliro, the White House director of legislative affairs, constantly and wisely emphasized that getting something passed by both houses of Congress was the most important imperative. After that, he promised, substantive policy issues, including issues that would affect implementation, would be addressed in conference (Chapter 6). Schiliro's push for speed was absolutely essential and right, even though I often chaffed at the time. Unpredictably and unfortunately, because of the Scott Brown victory in the Massachusetts Senate race to replace Ted Kennedy, the conference never happened. The House had to adopt the Senate version of the ACA, and there was no opportunity to fix provisions that might have facilitated effective execution. One short reconciliation bill enacted a few minor fixes to the ACA.

Thus, the nature of the legislative process—who is writing laws, the primacy of political and financial interests, the pressure of speed, the lack of congressional accountability for difficulties in execution—conspires to undermine the serious attention on how the law will be implemented. Like other major pieces of legislation, the ACA necessarily was going to be cumbersome in its execution.

But this structural problem with effective execution of the ACA did not have to lead to a failed rollout of healthcare.gov. Personnel and political issues compounded the challenges.

The People and Process Problems of Implementation

After passage of the ACA in March 2010 there was a sense of triumph—and exhaustion. Between the huge effort to enact and implement the Recovery Act to forestall a major depression along with the relentless fight for the ACA, the first 14 months of the Obama administration produced historic accomplishments, but they were draining.

That spring and summer there was a debate in the White House about the structure of the implementation effort. Some officials, mainly from the economic team, advocated following the VC imperative and hiring a CEO-type to lead the federal marketplace. Unlike the exiting staff, who were exhausted from an intense legislative push, such a person would be fresh and able to wake up every morning completely focused on overseeing and managing the federal health care reform. Coincidentally, David Cutler, a Harvard economist, sent an unsolicited memo recommending the hiring of person with management skills.

The intense political partisanship of the moment shaped the alternative view. Republicans were attacking the administration for having too many czars. Appointing a health implementation czar would potentially open the administration to even more criticism. Some believed the policy officials who helped enact the law were in the best position to implement it. Moreover, the Obama White House rarely brought in outside experts to manage important initiatives.

As this debate evolved, the advocates for a CEO-type—themselves independent experts—were leaving government. First, over the summer of 2010 several important staff members involved in the ACA efforts left. Jeff Liebman, chief economist at the Office of Management and Budget who built the model to predict ACA costs, returned to Harvard University. Bob Kocher, health adviser on the National Economic Council, returned to the private sector. Then in July 2010 Peter Orszag, head of OMB, left. Quickly thereafter the opportunity to run for mayor of Chicago prompted Rahm Emanuel's departure as chief of staff. And by the end of the year Larry Summers had returned to Harvard. The advocates for a health care CEO were gone.

Moreover, from the perspective of the White House, it made sense to appoint someone connected with the White House. Implementing the ACA was necessarily going to be organized at the White House level. Any major initiative that requires collaboration across major governmental agencies—Departments of HHS, Labor, and Homeland Security, the IRS, and more—can only be effectively managed under White House authority.

Nancy-Ann DeParle, head of the White House health reform effort, did not bask in the glory of a historic accomplishment—successfully shepherding passage of a health care reform law—and then rest; instead, she was selected to run implementation. Her White House implementation effort was staffed with policy advisers who had worked on the reform effort at HHS, including Jeanne Lambrew and Mark Childress. To ensure strong connections between the White House and HHS during implementation, Mike Hash, who served under DeParle both at Medicare and at the White House, was sent back to HHS to head the Office of Health Reform. After a few months, in early 2011, DeParle became deputy chief of staff, assuming broader responsibilities.

This emphasis on using policy advisers to implement the ACA contrasts with the approach adopted by states that have had successful exchanges. John Kingsdale was the executive director for the Massachusetts exchange from its inception in 2006 until 2010. Prior to being appointed by Governor Mitt Romney, Kingsdale had long experience as a senior manager in health care, doing strategic planning and reimbursement for Blue Cross and Blue Shield of Massachusetts and, then, for 20 years, serving as a senior executive at Tufts Health Plan, responsible for strategic planning, product development, and government relations.

Similarly, California has had a successful launch of its health insurance exchange. It is operated by an independent state agency overseen by a 5-person board with the authority to hire and fire the executive director and other top employees who are exempt from civil service pay and standards. In August 2011 the board hired Peter Lee as the first executive director. From 1995 to 2000 Lee was executive director of a consumer health care advocacy organization and, then, from 2000 to 2008, CEO of the Pacific Business Group on Health (PBGH) that operated a small-business exchange that ultimately failed because of adverse selection. For a few years he worked on the ACA as the director of Delivery System Reform for the Department of Health and Human Services' Office of Health Reform. He had years of experience with managing an exchange and working with private health insurers.

Here are 2 experienced CEOs with years of experience working with private insurers, and either of them could have been chosen to run the federal marketplace for the Obama administration. Lee was actually working on delivery system reform in HHS but was not hired to run the federally operated exchanges probably because of internal politics. DeParle offered Kingsdale a job, but he refused because it lacked CEO-level authority to actually execute on the exchange. In his words,

> To tell you the truth, it looked like it wasn't clear where and what I was supposed to be doing, but it was clear that I would be down under . . . in the bureaucracy. . . . [At the Massachusetts Health Connector] I was running something . . . [The federal job] looked much more like a staff role, one in which it would be very intense, a lot of work, a lot of commitment, but not necessarily a lot of authority.

We should not fall into the trap of thinking that empowering private-sector CEOs would necessarily have ensured a good rollout of healthcare.gov. After all, the executive director of the Maryland exchange was a former health insurance executive. The exchange has been a disaster, and she was fired in late 2013. And, of course, we all know that many private-sector websites, such as Amazon and Twitter, which are much less complex than the federal marketplace, have had rocky rollouts and buggy software. (Those events are now fading memories.)

Creating an effective health insurance exchange is difficult but eminently possible. A proven manger with private health insurance experience who is focused on execution is necessary but not sufficient. This person must be a collaborative team builder, goal driven, and someone who can get things done. And it helps to have an experienced board that can be called upon for regular advice and decision support, something both Massachusetts's and California's exchanges have. Even under the best circumstances, establishing a well-functioning exchange is hard, and success is by no means guaranteed.

Coincident with personnel changes at the beginning of health care implementation was an important change in the decision-making process. In the White House the Roosevelt room is the location for major strategy and decision-making meetings of senior officials. All through the effort to craft and pass the ACA the White House chief of staff, along with the secretaries of Treasury and Health and Human Services, the heads of the National Economic Council, Domestic Policy Council, Office of Management and Budget, Office of Information and Regulatory Affairs, political and communications officials, and others met in the Roosevelt room on an almost weekly basis. Over the summer of 2010 the meetings stopped focusing on strategy. Instead of serving as a place to thrash out issues and settle strategic matters, they largely became information transfer sessions. Senior officials gradually stopped making attendance a priority, and the meetings fizzled out.

Instead, implementation discussions shifted to a biweekly intergovernmental meeting chaired by Nancy-Ann DeParle and focused on considering impending regulations regarding the implementation of the ACA. Serious mid-level staff from the White House, CMS, HHS, Labor, Treasury, and other agencies attended. Though substantive, these meetings almost never attracted the most senior officials with internal political authority. But after a few months the debates about substantive issues seemed less important, as staffers recognized that the smaller group of implementation officials, outside of these meetings, was actually making the key decisions. Consequently, attendance also trailed off.

Ultimately, official responsibility of healthcare.gov and other exchange issues shifted to smaller offices within CMS, such as its Office of Information Services and Health Reform, with real authority resting with the small group of White House policy advisers running health care implementation. Here there were other management mistakes, such as contracting with CGI, who had a poor track record on IT projects, rather than an IBM lead consortium, rather than hiring an integrator to oversee and combine the various components relegating that activity to CMS itself, with almost no experience for the job, and, finally, having a top-down management style that was focused on what one commentator called, "the waterfall method, because on a timeline the project cascades from planning, at the top left of the chart, down to implementation, on the bottom right." This is the opposite of lean start-up philosophy and how new technology is developed through an iterative process of testing—refinement—more testing—more refinement—more testing—more refinement to learn what is working and what is not and then to constantly change the product to ensure the overall objectives are being met effectively. The health policy advisers running the implementation did not understand how to develop or manage for a new web start-up, and yet that is what they were doing.

Execution on a start-up is hard even with an experienced CEO. With exhausted policy advisers and low-level CMS bureaucrats directing implementation, lacking both the management and technology expertise as well as participation of senior leaders that had characterized the push for passage of the ACA, successful implementation was going to be even harder. And then the Republicans and their allies made it even harder.

The Politics and Problems of Implementation

A political environment more poisonous than any since the Civil War further hampered efforts by the White House team to implement the ACA effectively. First, Republicans were determined to delegitimize and undermine everything related to the ACA. This is one of the reasons the White House was hesitant to appoint a CEO to run healthcare.gov and the federal health insurance marketplace.

Second, no one could anticipate the very large number of states that would not opt to operate their own health insurance exchanges. Republicans perennially lament federally operated programs, preferring instead federally financed programs entrusted to the states for administration. As Medicaid shows, these federally financed but state-administered programs tend to be of uneven quality and much more complex. Nevertheless, when it came to the exchanges, Republicans got their wish—and more. The ACA contained significant financial support for states that opted to establish and operate their own exchanges. And yet to demonstrate their anti-ACA credentials, more than half the states, predominantly Republican-controlled ones, rejected the opportunity and the money. This was completely unexpected given Republicans' professed preferences, and it dumped a significant workload on the federal government, much of it very late in the implementation process. Not only did HHS have to set up the various state websites and contract for larger-than-expected call centers, but it had to solicit bids, certify qualified health plans, interface with state Medicaid agencies, and perform many other exchange-related functions. This landed an even larger burden on the already small, overworked implementation staff at federal agencies without much time before open enrollment.

Third, although the ACA contained some funds for the federal part of the implementation, Republicans made repeated efforts to deprive the government of necessary resources. Congress appropriated insufficient funds, so all sectors of the government, from HHS to the IRS, were operating with too little for an effective implementation. True, the government spent hundreds of millions for a website that could have been developed for less. Part of this was the nature of federal IT procurement, and part was the structure of ACA implementation. But because of how federal budgeting works, which is different from private-sector financing, even as one part of the implementation effort had too much money, lack of funds hampered other parts.

Fourth, the politicized environment overshadowed every major implementation decision. In Washington short-term political calculations tend to be favored over a longer-term perspective, especially in an election year like 2012. And the policy advisers running the implementation, all of whom were experienced in legislative battles over the ACA, were more likely to stress political calculations in their decisions. They were not inclined to adopt a view that the best political choice was to sacrifice short-term gains to ensure a successful healthcare.gov rollout. This thinking is in contrast to what an exchange CEO would have done. For instance, publishing "concept of operations" diagrams for the websites would have been good so as to get feedback and to share plans with the states. But the administration was worried that Republicans would seize on these diagrams and resurrect the attacks against the Clinton reform pioneered by Senator Specter's chart (Chapter 5). So the White House implementation team dodged the issue and refused to publish the charts. Similarly, publicizing a draft request for proposals for the website design would have been helpful so as to elicit feedback from the public, patient advocates, and health insurers before soliciting actual bids. California did this to improve its website contracting and design. But opponents of the ACA would have exploited this as well. There were many regulations necessary for the functioning of the federal health insurance marketplace, such as those for the essential health benefits, the risk adjustment and risk corridors, and standards for network adequacy that allow insurers to prepare their exchange offerings and set premiums. The policy advisers running implementation frequently delayed issuing these regulations so as to minimize political controversy and take them out of the 2012 election campaign. Then, in the spring of 2013, negative evaluations of progress on the website were delivered to key members of the administration. Six months before launch soliciting external assistance or even developing a strategy to phase in the website's launch might have addressed many of these problems. After all, the "tech surge" effort led by Jeff Zients dramatically improved the website in about 6 weeks. But the administration feared that acknowledging problems and obtaining tech assistance would open them up to severe attacks. As one report noted, "Former government officials say the White House, which was calling the shots [on healthcare.gov], feared that any backtracking would further embolden Republican critics who were trying to repeal the health care law." And so the bad news did not lead to a change in the implementation plan such as a phased rollout.

In the heated political environment surrounding the ACA and the hotly contested election of 2012, sacrificing effective execution to shorter-term political insulation was all too easy. Ironically, these short-term political calculations contributed to the website's rollout problems, which proved much more politically damaging than an approach that emphasized the effective execution of the federal marketplace, no matter the immediate political controversy.

The Ultimate Impact of Implementation Problems

The problem with the rollout was not a fundamentally flawed ACA, nor was it primarily technical. Instead, it was fundamentally managerial. Despite execution challenges posed in any legislation as complex as the ACA and despite the unremitting attacks from conservatives, there was no inherent reason why the launch of the federally operated exchanges had to be such a fiasco. Exchanges in Kentucky, Connecticut, California, Minnesota, and other states as well as the quick repairs to healthcare.gov overseen by Jeff Zients both demonstrate a successful launch of healthcare.gov was eminently possible.

The disastrous rollout of healthcare.gov had real consequences. It significantly reduced enrollment and may alter the risk pool, contributing to more older and sicker enrollees. It shook the confidence of health insurers in the exchanges. It certainly caused a branding problem for the website. It gave the ACA's critics an opening to cast doubt on everything related to reform, even things that have not been problems, such as the security of the website. At least temporarily, the bad rollout reduced support for health care reform not only among the public but also many in the health sector. And it might further undermine Americans' view of government's competence.

Ultimately, however, health care reform is a long-term proposition. Although the media and politicians are focused on the day-to-day battles, success of the ACA will be measured by what happens over the course of the decade. Reforming the equivalent of the 5th largest economy in the world cannot occur in just a year or 2 or even 3; rather, it requires a long-term perspective and needs to be assessed by how the health care sector is performing in 2020 and beyond.

By this metric the problems with healthcare.gov are ephemeral. There is no reason to despair or give up on health care reform itself. As many high-technology companies have shown, it is possible to bounce back from flawed website rollouts. But this is only possible if relentless focus on execution becomes a reality. Here are 4 key items that ought to be on an implementer's to-do list who wants to ensure the success not only of the federal marketplace but also of the ACA and the transformation of American health care.

First, although healthcare.gov is working much better, the website must be the focus for continuous improvement. Just as Amazon, Google, and every other successful Internet company is continuously installing upgrades and changes to the user experience, healthcare.gov always needs to be a work in progress. The updates need to prioritize the customer experience as well as the link between the website and insurers. This will facilitate comparison shopping, registration, enrollment, and purchase. For instance, there should be testing of new web page designs to make them easier to navigate and read. There should be development of new functions to help customers calculate which combination of premiums and deductibles is likely to be the best bargain for them. In December 2013 the administration hired an experienced technology executive from Microsoft to work on healthcare.gov—a welcome development. But this is not just a 6-month job. There needs to be an experienced tech manager who will run healthcare.gov for the long haul.

Second, the administration needs to regain health insurers' confidence. Both 2014 and 2015 are critical for the exchanges' success. Shortly after the open-enrollment period ends in March 2014 the insurers will decide whether to continue—or even expand—in the exchanges and determine their 2015 premiums. If they leave the exchanges or significantly raise their premiums, the federally operated exchanges could be permanently undermined.

Much will depend on the health insurance companies. In the matter of the exchanges insurers are allies, rooting for the success of the federal marketplace. But they are also businesses. And their perception of the market environment will shape their decisions for 2015. Chief among these is how they perceive the quality of the federally operated exchanges' management. If they have confidence the operations will significantly improve and enrollment of a well-balanced risk will occur, they are likely to continue in the exchanges and propose competitive premiums. This is more psychological than anything else, but it is nonetheless vital to the future of the federal marketplace.

The administration needs to clearly communicate to these private insurance companies that the exchanges' management will improve. There is probably no better way to do this than to hire a CEO for the federally operated exchanges and pair this person with a strong independent board. As noted, this cannot guarantee success, but the right person can significantly raise the chances by reassuring insurers. Hiring a CEO is not the administration's usual modus operandi, but this is not a usual moment—the success of the ACA is at stake. The fall of 2014 cannot have insurers exiting from the exchanges or generating rate shock.

Third, there is an important implementation decision that is deep in the weeds but can have a profound impact on both healthcare.gov and the efficient operation of the exchanges: more standardization. One thing the California exchange did very well was to standardize their benefit designs well beyond just 4 levels of benefits—bronze, silver, gold, and platinum. It also required participating insurers to adhere to very specific deductible, co-payment, and other standards in the plans they offered. This meant that there were 400 different plan offerings in the California exchange rather than thousands. This streamlined operations by reducing the complexity of the website, thereby making customer comparisons easier and facilitating transactions with insurers. Standardization of the federally operated exchanges would greatly facilitate efficient operations.

Fourth, contrary to conservative claims, the ACA is more than the website. There are other programs necessary to the ACA's success that will shape the public's attitude toward health care reform more generally. These programs need to be emphasized and vigorously executed. At the top of these efforts are the ACA's cost-control measures. If successful, the public and businesses will experience stable premiums, co-payments, drug costs, and other health-related expenses and then will grasp the ACA's personal benefits. Many of the ACA's cost-control measures are working well. For instance, the policies to reduce hospital readmissions seem to be having an effect. The program has already been expanded from applying to 3 diseases to 6, and it could be further expanded to all readmissions.

Another critical cost-control measure would be a vigorous push to change the way payments to physicians and hospitals are calculated.

This entails changing incentives so as to encourage providers to move away from fee-for-service payments. The government needs to accelerate this change; Chapter 12 provides a variety of concrete suggestions. Similarly, more price transparency and competition to lower prices for medical goods and services is vital. Annually, Medicare should disseminate the charges it receives from hospitals, and the federal government should pursue various efforts to publish and rein in prices, such as deploying competitive bidding more widely. Another important measure is vigorous enforcement of antitrust laws concerning hospital mergers. With the push for ACOs and other incentives driving hospital consolidation, there is a strong worry that hospitals will form local market monopolies that drive up private insurance prices. The government needs to be vigilant so as to preempt excessive consolidation and instead foster competition. A strong push on cost control that lowers the rate of health care inflation would be visible and widely celebrated.

Another place the public has a negative experience of the health care system is paperwork. Accelerating and expanding efforts to reduce paperwork and improve the transfer of electronic health records so that excessive paperwork disappears would be a noticeable change in people's lives and, thus, would be positively received.

The disastrous rollout of healthcare.gov has many people worried about the fate of health care reform. Part of this worry stems—rightly—from the fact that the rollout did not have to be a disaster. There was a failure of execution. And a large measure of that was a failure to follow the VC imperative compounded with a fear of political attacks in the short term.

Fortunately, the website is improved. But the success of health care reform is made up of much more than a well-functioning website. Implementation is a long-term endeavor, and a great deal of work remains. There is no reason it cannot be a success. And if long-term execution becomes the top priority, the ACA will transform American health care for the better. It will take time, but it will be worth it.

How will we know if the transformation is happening? What metrics can we follow to assess success or failure of health care reform?

= CHAPTER ELEVEN =

The ACA Dashboards

How to Tell If Health Care Reform Is Working

In the debate over health care reform it frequently seems like there are 2 alternate versions of reality. Conservatives, resentful of the ACA, never tire of attacking Obamacare as a failure and a threat not only to the health care system and the federal government's fiscal health but also to the American way of life. Liberals, politically invested in the ACA's success, minimize any glitches in its implementation and paint a rosy picture of the future once reform has taken hold.

How can the impartial American know whether the ACA is succeeding? How are we supposed to tell whether the law is really expanding coverage, whether it is "bending the cost curve" and improving the quality of care and the nation's overall health and well-being? What data should we monitor to assess the success or failure of the ACA objectively? Here are my 4 health care reform dashboards.

On expanding coverage and the success of the exchanges, Figure 11.1 highlights the key data points.

Right now the Medicaid expansion is tied up in politics. As of January 2014, 23 states have chosen to not expand Medicaid. With the hefty federal aid provided by the ACA, it makes total economic sense for states to expand Medicaid, but in some states ideology and politics have gotten in the way. Much of the 2014 election will be fought over the ACA. Once that election passes, some states are likely to expand Medicaid rather than forgo all the federal Medicaid money. My prediction is that by the end of 2015, at least 7 more states will expand Medicaid. And then, after the 2016 election, I believe all the rest will come on board, probably in 2 waves, with the last of the states—probably Texas—coming on closer to the end

FIGURE 11.1 The coverage dashboard

AREA	SPECIFIC MEASURE	QUANTITATIVE METRIC (CBO PREDICTION)	ZEKE'S PREDICTIONS
Medicaid expansion	States expanding Medicaid by the end of 2015	N/A	7 of the 22 states that refused to expand initially will expand Medicaid
	States expanding Medicaid by the end of 2020		All States
Exchanges	Number of Americans purchasing insurance through exchanges—April 1, 2014	7 million	Over 7 million
	Number of Americans purchasing insurance through exchanges—January 1, 2016	22 million	Over 30 million
	Number of Americans purchasing insurance through exchanges—January 1, 2020	25 million	Over 50 million
Employer-sponsored insurance	Number of Americans who no longer receive employer-sponsored insurance but are covered in the exchange—January 1, 2016	5 million	10 million
	Number of Americans who no longer receive employer-sponsored insurance but are covered in the exchange—January 1, 2020	11 million	25 million
	Proportion of private-sector workers with employer-sponsored insurance—January 1, 2025	61% of workers in private sector companies (2013)	Less than 20% of workers in private-sector companies

of 2020. After the presidential election in 2020, I believe all states will have expanded their Medicaid programs. Remember that the last state to implement Medicaid did it 17 years after the program was enacted.

The initial rollout of the federally operated exchanges was nothing short of a real disaster. It was a spectacular failure. The design and operation of the website, healthcare.gov, was deeply flawed. Americans were understandably frustrated and mad as hell because they were unable to see coverage options and premiums available to them without registering. And the registration process was filled with technical problems and invasive security questions that made signing up at the outset practically impossible. It ended up taking about 2 months to get the site to work well enough for 80% of the people to get through the process. At the federal level this was a failure no matter how you slice it.

But although healthcare.gov floundered, several state exchanges fared much better. Kentucky and Connecticut were among the best. Washington state and California were pretty good as well. Successes at the state level showed that building a functioning online health exchange website was not an impossible task. They showed that, with renewed focus and proper management, the federally facilitated exchange websites could improve and that they will continue to improve as time goes on. By fall 2014, open-enrollment period at healthcare.gov will offer an easy shopping experience. There will be more choices among insurance products and better tools for comparison shopping. And if you want to keep an eye on the exchanges' progress, there are 4 key data points to monitor.

First, how many people will sign up for the exchanges by March 31, 2014? This is the date that the first open-enrollment period ends. The CBO predicts that in the first year 7 million Americans will sign up for health insurance through the exchanges. If the total number is at 7 million or higher, the ACA will be declared a victory.

Second, how many will have signed up by the end of the 2016 open-enrollment period? This will be the beginning of the 3rd year of the exchanges, and the glitches should be a distant memory. The CBO predicts that by this time a total of 22 million people will have signed up for insurance through the exchanges.

Third, what are enrollment levels at the end of the 2020 open-enrollment period? The CBO estimates 24 million Americans buying through the exchange. My own view is that, because of the botched rollout of the federal exchanges, the 7 million figure for the end of the first open enrollment period is likely to be accurate and it might be high, but the longer-range predictions, 2016 and 2020, are too conservative. By the end of the decade the numbers will begin to soar past 50 million Americans buying health insurance through the exchanges.

Fourth, how many employers will drop their own health insurance and instead ask their employees to shop for insurance through the exchanges either with an employer contribution toward the premium or with the employer just paying the penalty for not providing coverage (Chapter 8, page 219) and increasing cash wages? By 2016 the CBO expects that a 6 million people will *gain* employment-based coverage as they demand their employer offer coverage, with about 5 million people *losing* employer-based coverage compared to what would have happened without the ACA. And by 2020 the CBO predicts 12 million people losing employment-based coverage and 7 million gaining employer-sponsored insurance.

My own view is that by 2016 many more employers will determine that the insurance exchanges provide a good variety of health options at competitive premiums. Simultaneously, many workers will find the options in the exchanges appealing and request that their employers allow them to buy coverage in the exchange. Thus, employers will gradually decrease their involvement in their employees' choice of health insurance, opting instead to direct their employees to the exchanges, in many cases with financial contributions to help defray the costs. My prediction is that by 2016 over 10 million people who had employer-based insurance will be purchasing in the exchanges, and by 2020 more than 25 million Americans who once got insurance though their employer will get their coverage through the exchanges. Today 60% of workers in the private sector receive their insurance through their employer. I believe that by 2025 fewer than 20% of workers at private companies will continue to receive their health insurance through an employer-sponsored program. Nevertheless many will still receive an employer contribution, a so-called defined contribution toward the purchase of health insurance in the exchange. I believe the majority of private-sector workers will get their coverage through the exchanges.

Finally, there is an interesting experiment underway in Arkansas and Iowa. The ACA requires people earning under 138% of the federal poverty level to receive Medicaid. However, Arkansas and Iowa have taken a different approach. Rather than enroll these people in traditional Medicaid, they are allowing them to purchase private insurance through the exchange with subsidies that cover almost the whole cost of the insurance. This will provide an important comparison of traditional Medicaid coverage versus private insurance coverage. Traditional Medicaid has more comprehensive benefits on paper with no deductibles and nominal co-payments, whereas private insurance has better reimbursement and access to more specialists. Evaluating how the 2 groups compare in terms of health status and satisfaction will be important when guiding future reforms of the Medicaid system.

Another main goal of the ACA is reining in the growth of health care spending, which has ballooned since the 1960s (see Chapter 4, pages 101–103). Continuously evaluating the ACA's impact on health spending will be crucial for health policy analysts and lawmakers because unchecked cost growth is a serious threat to long-term economic prosperity. In my view there are 3 key metrics as well as several secondary metrics that experts and the public should use to assess the ACA's success in curbing health care spending (see Figure 11.2).

The Independent Payment Advisory Board (IPAB) (Chapter 8, page 231) is the ultimate cost-control backstop. It has authority to make

FIGURE 11.2 The cost-control dashboard

AREA	SPECIFIC MEASURE	QUANTITATIVE METRIC (CBO PREDICTION)	ZEKE'S PREDICTIONS
IPAB role	No need for IPAB recommendations on cutting Medicare costs	NA	IPAB will not have to make recommendations to control inflation through 2020
Federal Medicare and Medicaid spending	Exceeds $1.0 trillion	2016	2018
	Exceeds $1.5 trillion	2024	2025
Overall per capita health care inflation	GDP +0%	GDP +	2020

changes to Medicare—which Congress can overrule—if the per person spending exceeds specific targets. From 2015 through 2019 that target is linked to inflation in a complex way (mixing consumer price index and medical inflation), whereas beginning in 2020 the target is GDP +1%. The first key cost-control dashboard measure is whether the IPAB is superfluous. If health care cost control is effective, there should be no need for the IPAB and its recommendations through the end of 2020. That would constitute a real victory.

Another major cost-control metric is linked to federal spending on Medicare and Medicaid. In 2012 federal spending on these programs was $802 billion. (This excludes the states' contributions to Medicaid.) In its November 2013 report the CBO predicted federal spending for these 2 programs will exceed $1 trillion in 2016 and $1.5 trillion in 2022. If health care costs are reduced, these thresholds should be surpassed several years later. My own predictions are that Medicare and Medicaid will pass $1 trillion by 2018 and $1.5 trillion by 2025, thus saving the federal government hundreds of billions of dollars.

Finally, perhaps the most telling measure is the per capita rate of growth of national health expenditures compared to the rate of growth of the overall economy. Historically, over the last 40 years national health expenditures have exceeded GDP growth by roughly 2%. In my boldest and perhaps most ambitious prediction, I believe that by 2020 overall per capita health care inflation will actually decline to GDP+0%. Achieving this metric would have a truly profound impact on the health care system. If we hit GDP+0%, we will have unequivocally succeeded in "bending the cost curve."

There are other important cost-control metrics that should be monitored as well. These include the premiums of the second-lowest silver plan in the exchanges (Chapter 8, page 215). The level of these premiums is a good indication of overall health care cost control in the private sector, but they also determine the per capita level of federal subsidies. (I do not consider either the premiums or total level of federal subsidies to be key cost-control metrics because they are influenced by both the number and health characteristics of the Americans who enroll in the exchanges, both of which can change.) If, between now and 2018, the annual growth in the average premium for the second-lowest silver plan is low—lower than GDP +1%—that will be a very good thing.

Finally, I would follow average national expenditures for certain medical devices and procedures. Variable and excessive prices for medical goods and services contribute to the high level of US health care spending and to about half of the cost growth in the American health care system. If reform is successful, there should be serious and persistent downward price pressure, primarily through pricing transparency, expanded competitive bidding, and alternative methods of paying physicians and hospitals. This should translate into lower actual prices for certain devices and procedures. I would follow the average prices paid for devices such as artificial hip implants, spine implants, and cardiac stents as leading indicators of cost control. Another way of monitoring this is to examine the profit margins of the leading device companies, which should decline if prices decline substantially. I would also follow prices the big private insurance companies pay for imaging, especially tests such as CTs and MRIs. Transparency and shifts to bundled payments and capitation should force down the average prices for these tests. Indeed, the actual prices the commercial insurers pay for these imaging tests should decline by 25% to 50% by 2020.

The third important dashboard is related to quality, for which there are 4 clear metrics to follow. The first relates to reductions in hospital readmissions (Chapter 9, page 265). Beginning in 2013 the ACA penalizes hospitals that fail to reduce preventable hospital readmissions, and these financial penalties increase over time. There has already been a significant impact. Readmissions declined from 19.5% before the ACA to 18.4% at the end of 2012 (the last time data were available). In addition, Medicare has expanded the number of conditions it will include in the determination of readmission rates to include emphysema and elective hip and knee replacement surgery. A key metric is when preventable readmissions are lower than 15%. My prediction is we should see a steady decline and a drop below 15% no later than 2018. By 2022 preventable readmissions should be below 12%.

Another quality metric relates to declines in hospital-acquired complications, such as hospital infections and medication errors. Beginning in 2015 the ACA requires penalizing hospitals that have high levels of complications. According to studies by the CDC, approximately one in every 20 hospital admissions, about 1.7 million Americans, suffers a hospital-acquired infection each year. In 2010 the government made a

FIGURE 11.3 The quality dashboard

AREA	SPECIFIC MEASURE	CURRENT LEVELS	ZEKE'S GOALS
Hospital readmissions	All cause hospital-wide readmission rate for Medicare	18.6%	15.0% by 2018 12.0% by 2022
Hospital-acquired infections	Overall hospital-acquired infections	1 in 20 patients	Lower than 1 in 40 patients by 2016
	Central line–associated infections	41,000 annually	10,000 by 2016
Electronic health records	All patients obtain their complete medical records electronically		2018

commitment to reduce many of these infections. There was an effort to reduce central-line bloodstream infections by 50% and urinary catheter–associated infections and surgical-site infections by 25% over 3 years. And these goals appear to have been met. A key metric would be to decrease overall hospital-associated infections by 50% (to 1 in every 40 patients) by 2016 (see Figure 11.3 for goals).

Third, it is worth noting that most health care occurs outside of hospitals. We have very little data on the safety of outpatient care. One place to start is the safety of surgical centers, imaging facilities, and the like. Another is physician office visits. Simply having a regular—say every 3-year—estimate by the CDC or AHRQ of preventable deaths in the outpatient setting, stratified by location, would be a big advance. Because we do not know how many preventable deaths there are in the outpatient setting, just getting the first estimate would be a key—and, like the Institute of Medicine's first estimate of preventable hospital deaths in 1998, likely shocking—data point. We need to develop an outpatient measure of preventable outpatient deaths.

The measure of hospital-acquired infections requires an important change in culture, one that focuses on improving safety, that can have an important ripple effect.

A fourth key metric relates to the spread and meaningful use of electronic health records. The American Recovery and Reinvestment Act spurred a huge expansion in the number of physicians and hospitals using electronic health records. A key target would be for every patient to be able to get an electronic copy of their entire medical record. If patients can get their EHR, then we would know that the electronic health record contains all the relevant health information and that it can be transmitted to any electronically linked physician, hospital, or other health care provider. If this can be accomplished by 2018, it would mark a major improvement in health system efficiency.

In some sense there are an unlimited number of quality metrics, one for every test and procedure the health care system provides. But it would not be helpful to follow each. Here are a few that might be good, broad measures of quality.

- Elective cesarean sections: Fully 33% of all births in the United States are done by C-section. Everyone agrees this is way too high. Another important goal might be to have this cut in half by the end of the decade.
- Diabetes: A sign of poor care for diabetics is the amputation rate of toes and legs. This happens because their blood sugars are not well controlled and small infections on the toes and legs are not carefully treated. Having the amputation rates halved would be another measure of overall quality for diabetics.
- End-of-life care: Everyone agrees this is an area that could be done better. Most Americans want to die at home in the comfort of their family. And yet many end up going to the emergency room and being admitted to the hospital in the last few months of life. One metric might be to cut in half the number of emergency room visits and hospitalizations in the last 2 months of life. This would spur increased use of palliative care and hospice services.

A 4th dashboard to follow relates to the nation's overall health (see Figure 11.4). After all, the point of a well-functioning health care system is to keep people healthy and to not need the health care system. Here are 3 key metrics of the nation's health that matter. One is the overweight and obesity of the country. Today 69.2% of adults and 28.2% of children

FIGURE 11.4 The overall health status dashboard.

AREA	SPECIFIC MEASURE	CURRENT LEVELS	ZEKE'S GOALS
Obesity	Proportion of adults who are overweight or obese	69.2%	59% by 2025
	Proportion of children who are overweight or obese	31.8%	22% by 2025
Infant mortality	Infant mortality rate	5.9 per 1,000 live births	4.0 per 1,000 by 2025
Adolescent mortality	Deaths of adolescents ages 10 to 24	60 per 100,000	40 per 100,000 by 2025

are overweight or obese. We want—really, *need*—these metrics to decline. A modest but important measure is whether they can go down to the 1990 levels—59% for adults and 22% for children—by 2025.

A 2nd overall health metric is infant mortality. The infant mortality rate in the United States would be an embarrassment were it not so deadly. In 2012 our infant mortality was 5.9 per 1,000 live births—we rank 50th in the world. By comparison, Japan, ranked 2nd, had a rate of 2.2 per 1,000 live births. Sweden, ranked 5th, had a rate of 2.7 per 1,000. France's rate, 3.3 per 1,000 live births, was good for 10th. The United States lags well behind countries like Belarus, Slovenia, and even Cuba. We must do better. We should at least try to catch Cuba, at 4.8 per 1,000 live births, by 2025.

A 3rd overall health metric relates to adolescent deaths. Nearly 60 out of every 100,000 American kids between the ages of 10 and 24 died in 2009 (see Figure 11.5). That's more than double the mortality rate for the same age group in Japan, Germany, Italy, and France. Americans love to say that our children are our most precious resource, but the fact is we are not doing a very good job of caring for them. Our goal should be to reach the level of Canada and Finland, at 40 deaths per 100,000, by 2025.

These 4 health reform dashboards provide specific, quantitative, and objective measures of how the ACA and the American health care system are working. Not only do they provide a simple and handy way to determine whether the system is getting better; they also provide a way

FIGURE 11.5 Adolescent death rates

Deaths of 10- to 24-year-olds per 100,000 population, 2009*

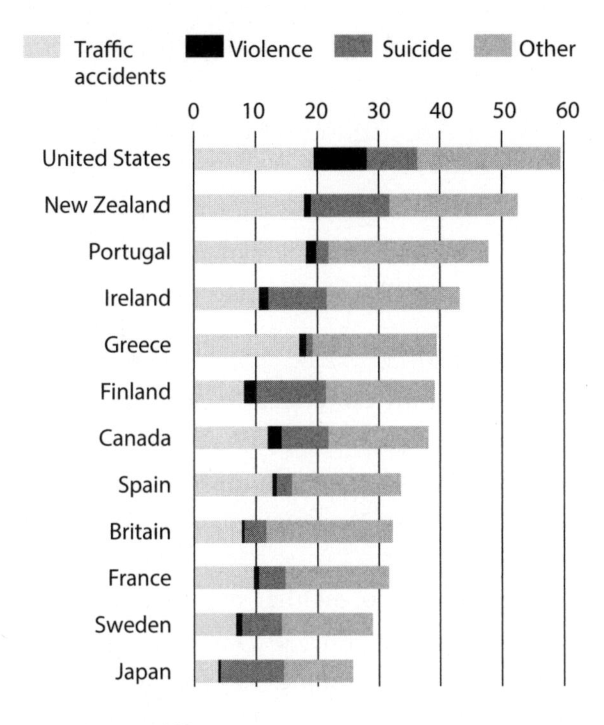

*Or latest available.

Source: The Lancet, George Patton, University of Melbourne in *The Economist.*

to hold physicians, hospitals, and others accountable. If we achieve these goals—even half of them—the system and the health of Americans will be much better than it is today.

Recognizing that the ACA was far from a perfect piece of legislation, what can we do to make reform better? What are a few of the practical things that can be enacted to improve the American health care system?

= CHAPTER TWELVE =

Health Care Reform 2.0

What Are the Post-ACA Reforms?

The Affordable Care Act was passed in 2010. However many changes it introduced to improve the American health care system, it was far from perfect. Everyone recognizes there were some things left out, some things done poorly, and some things that need further modification. There are many additional changes that could be implemented to improve the system.

There are 4 important reforms that build on the ACA to advance health promotion and prevention, cost control, and quality improvement that are "shovel ready," meaning they can be initiated quickly and with lasting impact.

Raise Cigarette Taxes

A quick and easy way to prevent serious illness is to raise cigarette taxes. Cigarettes and small cigars represent the single-greatest preventable cause of death in the country. Over the last 50 years or so, the United States has reduced adult smoking rates by half—a great public health triumph. According to most experts a combination of factors, from eliminating advertising and adding graphic package warnings to forcing smokers out of restaurants and office buildings and raising cigarette taxes, have contributed to positive outcomes. The reduction in smoking rates has tapered off, however. Today about 20% of adults smoke, and it has remained at about that level for the last 5 years.

One effective way to further reduce smoking is to raise its cost. In 1862, during the Civil War, the federal government imposed an excise tax on tobacco. By 1969 all states had their own additional excise tax on tobacco. In 2009 the federal excise tax on cigarettes was raised from 39 cents to $1.01. If we raised the federal excise tax by 50 cents, the Congressional Budget Office estimates smoking rates would drop by about 3%, mainly by persuading younger people not to take up smoking. Because most people who smoke start as teenagers, this would lead to a prolonged decline in the smoking rates as well as declines in emphysema, lung cancer, heart disease, and the many tobacco-related illnesses—an important long-term preventive measure. Furthermore, this tax will reduce the disparity in smoking. Lower-income Americans are more likely to smoke and are more price sensitive. Raising the cigarette tax will disproportionately reduce smoking among Americans with lower incomes—a very good thing.

Not only would this policy improve health, it would also generate $37 billion over the next 10 years. That money could be used either to reduce the deficit or even to further improve the health of American children by investing in early childhood interventions.

More Competitive Bidding

Ever wonder how much a wheelchair costs? Or, more importantly, ever wonder who decides how much a wheelchair costs? You probably aren't that concerned about the price of a wheelchair because in all likelihood you don't think you'll ever need one. You may feel that medical prices are too high but think you don't have much bargaining power to influence them. Private insurance companies and public payers like Medicare have the power to ensure the prices are low.

The problem is that our system for setting prices and paying for medical devices, equipment, and procedures is broken—and we need to fix it. Before the ACA, the government effectively set the price of a wheelchair. Medicare determined what it paid manufacturers for their wheelchairs. However, few Americans believe government price setting is the best way to ensure low-cost, high-quality wheelchairs; instead, most Americans believe the market is the best way to set prices.

The ACA contains provisions designed to change the system, to move from a government-price setting to market-price setting. One of these provisions is competitive bidding in Medicare (Chapter 8, page 222), requiring competitive bidding mainly for wheelchairs, hospital beds, oxygen equipment, artificial limbs, and a few other things—what are technically called durable medical equipment, prosthetics, and orthotics. The program began in 9 geographic areas in January 2011. Instead of the government setting prices, the companies bid on how much equipment they would supply and at what price. The program has succeeded remarkably. Overall, prices for wheelchairs, hospital beds, walkers, oxygen equipment, and other goods dropped more than 40% in 3 years. The ACA requires this competitive bidding program expand nationwide by 2016. The CBO projects that over the next 10 years it will save the government nearly $26 billion and Medicare beneficiaries, through reduced co-payments, $17 billion.

Behind the scenes, however, private companies that typically champion the free market in their public remarks are trying to modify and weaken the law. They have profited from the old government price-setting arrangement and, despite their rhetoric, don't really like the competitive market as much. Using claims of artificially low prices, limited supply, and shoddy quality, they are suggesting ways to keep prices up.

What should the government do? Resist these company entreaties and expand competitive bidding. First, given the success of the program thus far, there is no compelling reason to wait until 2016 to expand it nationwide. Why not expand it nationwide by 2015 and reap billions in additional savings not just for the government but also for seniors?

Second, to help CMS run this process even better, we might establish an independent advisory board composed of business and academic experts in the competitive bidding process. For instance, wouldn't you want Walmart's or GE's experts to help run the government's competitive bidding process? There are economists who study successful and unsuccessful competitive bidding processes that can also help to improve the operations. Adjustments in how the competitive bidding process is run can help ensure low prices, a diversity of suppliers, and high-quality equipment.

Finally, there is no reason competitive bidding should be limited to hospital beds, wheelchairs, walkers, and oxygen tanks. There are many other medical goods and services that could be subject to competitive bidding to save money. What about all those disposable supplies, such as gauze pads, tape, sutures, and tubes? What about pacemakers and stents? What about forcing the manufacturers of artificial hip, knee, and spine implants to compete on price? Right now spine implants cost about $50 to produce and frequently sell for $5,000. Moreover, the prices hospitals charge for the same procedure vary by three- or fivefold. Competitive bidding could easily drive those prices down. And it is not just devices that are pretty standardized and could be competitively bid; so too are simple but common laboratory blood and chemistry tests. What about the taking—not the interpretation—of X-rays, CT, and MRI scans? Because these tests are largely standardized and automated, driving efficiency up and prices down through competitive bidding should be possible. The independent advisory board could be entrusted with finding other areas of the health system appropriate for competitive bidding without lowering—and perhaps even improving—quality. Lower prices could be publicized and applied to Medicaid and all the private health plans in the exchanges. After all, because taxpayer money subsidizes purchases in the exchanges, we all have an interest in ensuring prices are as low as possible.

Government price fixing rarely works, and it isn't American. Competitive bidding in a competitive market is one of the things both the left and right agree on. Expanding competition to lower prices and save money is the right thing to do. The ACA made a good start and showed that competitive bidding can work to dramatically lower prices. So let's do more of it—much more.

More Administrative Simplification

Everyone hates the paperwork involved in the health care system. Filling out all those forms when you go to the physicians' office and then filling them out again when you go back to the same physician or to another one. Getting those incomprehensible—and invariably wrong—medical bills that aren't really medical bills. All that paper costs a huge amount. The Institute of Medicine estimated that as much as $190 billion a year is wasted on excessive administrative costs.

The ACA contains provisions that should reduce the paperwork, but much more could be done. The goal is clear: there should be seamless electronic transmission of both administrative and clinical health care information among all stakeholders—patients, physicians, hospitals, home health care agencies, pharmacies, insurance companies, and those behind the scenes, such as vendors and billing clearinghouses. Here are 5 specific steps to reduce the ridiculous amount of paperwork, achieve this important goal, and save money.

First, the federal government should ensure that any requirement for electronic transmission of health care information applies to all stakeholders. That means everyone—insurers, patients, *and* providers. One of the deficiencies of the ACA requirements is that they only require insurers to provide information electronically on patient eligibility and claims status and to transfer funds; the ACA did not require physicians, hospitals, and organizations that manage the provider's billing operations to share such information electronically. This means the physicians and hospitals can still conduct most of their business on paper.

This makes no sense. The government should require that, by 2016, all stakeholders, including physicians, hospitals, and all other organizations that conduct and manage administrative transactions on behalf of providers, perform electronically all the administrative functions insurers are mandated to do electronically. This would ensure that when insurers comply with the new operating rules for electronic transactions under the ACA, they will have a partner that also responds electronically. They won't have to spend valuable time and man hours processing information from a paper form and entering it into a computer program.

Second, the government could modify its quality reporting from physicians and hospitals to establish a core set of quality measures that can be reported directly from electronic health records (EHRs). The ACA requires hospitals and physicians to report on quality—this is good. Unfortunately, different Medicare and Medicaid programs require different measures, and the differences often impose significant administrative burdens—and costs. The government should streamline and unify the quality measures across programs and require vendors producing EHRs to ensure they can report on these core measures electronically and directly without additional add-on interfaces.

Third, the government should encourage providers to merge the administrative and clinical functions in electronic health records into one system. Today physicians and hospitals typically operate an electronic health record system, if they have one, and a separate billing system. And when clinical information is needed for billing, such as for prior authorization, someone must retrieve it from the EHR and enter it into the billing system manually. This process is time consuming, error prone, and costly. The government should expand the requirements for physicians and hospitals to receive federal payments for installing new electronic health records (Chapter 8, page 232) to ensure that both the billing and clinical functions are integrated into the electronic health records.

Fourth, the physician credentialing process should be streamlined to resemble the common college application. Currently, physicians must apply separately to each health plan and hospital they work with, providing vast quantities of information on their medical school courses and graduation, various licensure tests, malpractice history, and the like. It is estimated they fill out an average of 15 to 20 credentialing applications each year. This could be simplified if everyone—all physicians and hospitals as well as Medicare, Medicaid, and private payers—were required to use the Universal Provider Datasource (UPD). Physicians would provide their information once, and hospitals or payers who needed it could get it from the UPD source. Physicians would welcome the reduction in superfluous paperwork.

Finally, the whole process of reducing paperwork needs a system of accountability. There is no annual progress report nor anyone who wakes up every morning dedicated and empowered to squeezing out the paperwork from the system. Hence, progress on administrative simplification has been slow and irregular. The Department of Health and Human Services should empower its chief information officer to focus on administrative simplification, develop measures to assess progress on administrative simplification, and report on that progress. Putting the CIO in charge and requiring annual reporting would focus attention on this annoying, mistake-prone, and costly problem and, hopefully, encourage more electronic transmission of data. It is time to bring the medical system into the 21st century when it comes to computerization.

More on Payment Reform

What I regret most about composing the ACA is that it should have done more on payment reform. One important consequence is that today there is a serious misalignment between what we want physicians and hospitals to do in terms of improving value, efficiency, and reducing unnecessary care and how insurance companies, Medicare, Medicaid, and others pay them. About 85% of payment remains fee for service that encourages more office visits, hospital admissions, emergency room visits, and more tests and procedures. This dissonance makes it hard for physicians and hospitals to transform how they deliver care because we are effectively asking them, in some cases, to act against their own financial interest: if they emphasize value, they are likely to lose money.

What is the solution? The government needs to clearly delineate a specific timeline for switching off payment for fee for service to alternatives, such as bundled payments, capitation, or other payment systems. The federal government should declare a timeline; for instance, by 2022 75% of Medicare payments will be non-fee-for-service payments. To ensure this ambitious but necessary goal is realized, the government should specify 3 important milestones.

First, the federal government should rapidly implement its successful bundled payment program that compensates providers with one fixed payment for an entire episode of care. Consequently, physicians aren't incentivized to prescribe more tests and treatments just to increase revenue. Before the ACA was passed, Medicare launched an experiment called the ACE (Acute Care Episodes) demonstration project that paid one, fixed bundled payment for cardiac and orthopedic procedures, such as cardiac bypass surgery, valve surgery, defibrillator placements, stents, and hip and knee replacements. After 3 years an independent study of the program showed the bundles reduced costs without cherry picking patients or stinting on care. There is a provision in the ACA that allows the secretary of DHHS to apply successful demonstration projects like ACE that save money and/or improve quality to the entire country without the need for additional legislation.

Thus, one important step to moving away from fee for service would require the secretary of DHHS to announce that she will institute ACE for all hospitals and surgical centers in the country beginning in 2015. This will both inform and assure hospitals and physicians that the payment reform timeline is real, not empty rhetoric. It will change the payment for surgeons, cardiologists, anesthesiologists, and radiologists as well as hospitals. It will also reward hospitals and physicians who are changing their delivery of care and strengthen the voice of those in the medical community who are advocating for more rapid change in delivery. And we can be reasonably certain that just as they adopted Medicare's DRG payment system for hospitals, many private insurers will adopt the same bundled payment for these procedures. This will make life a lot easier for physicians and hospitals.

Second, ACE was innovative but it was not exactly the ideal bundled payment approach. It did not include rehabilitation and other postoperative services. A recent Institute of Medicine study showed that these so-called post-acute-care services, such as rehabilitation, are quite variable, accounting for 73% of the differences in the use of services and costs for the same procedures. An important follow-up demonstration project would be to expand the ACE bundles to include 90 days of care after the procedures and a guarantee that the physician and hospital will cover anything that goes wrong, without additional cost. Geisinger Clinic in Pennsylvania provides such guarantees for surgical operations such as cardiac bypass surgery. Many hospitals and health systems would find such an expanded bundled payment attractive because where there is variability in care there are also tremendous opportunities for improving care and reducing costs. This could be a big win-win-win, saving money for Medicare while also providing incentives for hospitals to transform how they care for patients as well as giving patients a 90-day guarantee on their care.

The DHHS secretary should also add one more thing to the expansion of the ACE demonstration project: shared decision making. For many conditions, such as stents and knee replacements, there are several therapeutically equivalent options. For instance, stable single-vessel coronary disease that causes intermittent chest pain can be treated either by placing a stent or by management with medications. Research suggests that there is no significant difference in survival, number of heart attacks, number of hospitalizations, or long-term pain control between these 2 options. The decision whether to undergo a stent procedure is a personal choice based on risk tolerance. There are similar findings regarding knee replacements and other procedures.

In cases in which there are different treatments that are clinically equivalent, shared decision making should be the standard. It entails providing patients with written, computer, or video-based objective information about the various treatment approaches; their comparative risks and benefits, costs, and rehabilitation processes; and then letting the patients decide what they want. Typically, when given this kind of information, between 10% and 33% of people opt for the noninvasive approach. Hence, in rolling out the ACE bundles, CMS should also require physicians and hospitals use shared decision making so patients receive the treatment they actually want. To ensure shared decision-making actually occurs, physicians and hospitals should have to report on the number of patients who participated in the shared decision-making process for each type of procedure, the number undergoing the various procedures, and produce signed consent forms from patients attesting that they participated in the shared decision-making process.

Another potential improvement would be to develop bundled payments for a chronic disease, such as cancer. Patients with chronic diseases account for more than three-quarters of health care spending (Chapter 4, page 109). Unfortunately, there have not been many demonstration projects using alternative payment structures for chronic conditions. Nonetheless, cancer is a good place to start. Why? Unlike knee or back pain, the diagnosis is not subjective. There is a totally objective way of determining whether a patient has cancer and needs treatment. Second, there are many professionally developed guidelines for how to treat cancers that go into extensive detail delineating optimal cancer care. This helps with defining what should be included in the bundles and also enumerate measures to ensure there is no stinting on the highest quality of care. Third, there are key choices in which quality can be improved and costs reduced, such as the management of predictable and preventable side effects as well as laboratory tests. Finally, bundled payments can remove perverse financial incentives, such as when oncologists prescribe very expensive chemotherapy because they then make more money even when cheaper chemotherapy is proven to be equally or more effective.

Medicare should be required to develop and implement bundled-payment pilot programs for at least 3 cancers by 2015. This would mark the first major chronic disease being moved off fee for service. It would free physicians to manage these complex patients according to their best judgment and the highest standards as defined by the profession.

As these bundled-payment approaches are being tried and implemented, other important information for additional changes in payment will be accruing. For instance, Arkansas is trying bundled payments for many conditions, from pregnancy and child birth to ADHD to congestive heart failure. If these succeed in controlling cost and improving quality, the federal government could begin implementing them as well. There are also ongoing tests of other forms of payment, especially in the private sector. As results of these efforts become available, the federal government could begin incorporating them too.

Finally, the government should implement reforms to physician and hospital payment as broadly as possible. Traditionally, when Medicare ran a demonstration project and it proved successful, it might change practices only for Medicare. Now the federal government has broader authority—and more financial incentive—to implement changes throughout the system. It could require Medicaid programs adopt these payment changes. More importantly, because the federal government now operates numerous health insurance exchanges, it could become an active purchaser and begin specifying payment policies that private insurers who want to compete on the exchanges must implement. This would be good for physicians and hospitals, as there would then be consistent payment policies from Medicare, Medicaid, and many private insurers. For instance, when Medicare expands the use of the ACE program, the part of the government that operates the exchanges could simultaneously require all the insurance companies in the exchanges to use the same ACE payment program. This would mean that more than half of payments to hospitals and physicians would change to the same type, with the same quality measures and approaches. Such consistency would be a strong incentive to transform the delivery of care for all patients and also simplify administration.

These 4 changes—higher federal excise tax on cigarettes, more competitive bidding, faster administrative simplification, and expanded payment change—are not the only changes that could further accelerate and solidify reform of the health care system. One area ripe for change is how hospitals are paid for physician training, so called graduate medical education. Each year Medicare pays $10 billion to hospitals to train physicians, with little accountability and performance reporting. Changing payment to transform medical training with more team-based and out-of-hospital training is desirable. Similarly, medical malpractice remains a topic that still needs comprehensive reform and improvement. In addition, innovative states, such as Arkansas, Maryland, Massachusetts, and Oregon, are testing out novel ideas to improve care and lower costs. The federal government could create a program to facilitate and expand such state-based innovation by making participation in such experiments easier for Medicare. But the 4 reforms above have the virtue of being "shovel ready" and would have a substantial impact on lowering prices and transforming the delivery of care. They are the place to begin health care reform 2.0.

= CHAPTER THIRTEEN =

Six Megatrends in Health Care

The Long-Term Impact of the ACA

The health care system is dynamic. The Affordable Care Act will create new institutions, such as the insurance exchanges and the Independent Payment Advisory Board (IPAB) (Chapter 8, page 231), and establish new ground rules for many activities as well as the key players in the system—insurers, hospitals, physicians, employers—and ultimately the public will respond to these new ways of delivering health care and conducting business. People will change their behavior in response to the law and then in response to what other actors in the health care system are doing. In time, various government bodies will likely also change their regulations. Even Congress will again become active and enact more health care legislation. Consequently, the system will evolve. Over the next decade or so the evolution will be quite rapid as everyone adapts to the ACA, the actual regulations, and the change in incentives and relationships. Beginning in 2020, without major additional health care reform legislation, there will continue to be change, albeit at a bit slower pace.

Making predictions is highly risky. We know how badly economists do just trying to predict basic economic data from year to year. My colleague at the University of Pennsylvania, Phil Tetlock, studied more than 28,000 predictions from 284 economists and found that economists are only slightly better than random chance. More surprisingly, the more famous the economist, on average, the worse their predictive power. And health care is more challenging than economics. There are no quantitative models that can account for all the changes the ACA is catalyzing.

Even the CBO model takes into account only parts of the system and is filled with guesses.

Nevertheless, everyone is, implicitly or explicitly, making predictions about how the system will evolve. When hospitals decide whether to expand or buy another hospital, they are making a prediction about the future. Similarly, when insurers decide to buy health systems, they are making a prediction about the future. And when venture capitalists make investments in a health care company, they too are making a prediction about the future of the health care system. For instance, many people believe big data will play an increasingly important role in the delivery of health care and improving quality. I have little to add to these predictions. But with a knowledge of the history of the system, a knowledge of the various actors' previous responses to change, and after discussions with hundreds of current actors, I will offer some thoughts about 6 megatrends for the future of health care (see Figure 13.1). I recognize the challenges—and high probability of error—in making such forecasts. Nevertheless, such predictions are necessary to inform current decisions. And unlike most forecasters, I have the courage or foolishness to write them down in order to be held accountable. So here I go.

The End of Insurance Companies as We Know Them

Americans hate health insurance companies. They are easy targets for everyone to beat up on. When premiums go up, we blame insurance companies; we do not blame the hospitals or physicians who charge high prices that help drive up insurance costs. When people with cancer, heart attacks, or other diseases are denied insurance, we blame insurance companies; we do not blame the underlying voluntary insurance market that necessitates underwriting. When our wish for a new high-priced drug is denied, we blame insurance companies; we do not blame drug companies that set the price at over $100,000. Politicians can always elicit an applause by attacking the health insurance companies, reinforcing this bad-guy image of insurance companies.

This is not to say that insurance companies are angels, but they also are also not the devil incarnate. A lot of what people consider to be their

FIGURE 13.1 Six megatrends

MEGATREND	CHANGE	EFFECTIVE DATE
End of insurance companies as we know them	Insurance companies will either become purveyors of management, analytics, and actuarial services or integrated delivery systems actually employing (or contracting with) hospitals, physicians, and other providers to render patient care.	2025
VIP care for the chronically and mentally ill	Physicians and hospitals will focus on keeping patients with chronic illnesses healthy and out of the emergency room and hospital, thereby decreasing the frequency of avoidable complications and rate of hospitalization. Then they will begin routinely screening for depression and other mental health problems and develop standardized rapid interventions.	2020
The emergence of digital medicine and closure of hospitals	Over 1,000 acute-care hospitals will close. We will see a slew of new technologies for remote monitoring, testing, and treating patients in real time outside of the hospital and physicians' offices.	2020
End of employer-sponsored health insurance	Fewer than 20% of workers in the private sector will receive traditional employer-sponsored health insurance.	2025
End of health care inflation	Health care inflation will be GDP+0%.	2020
Transformation of medical education	Medical education will be transformed in 4 fundamental ways: (1) three-year medical schools and shorter residencies; (2) half of medical school clinical training will be outside of hospitals; (3) integration of nurses, pharmacists, social workers with medical students in multi-professional team training; and (4) formal incorporation of population health and management skills in training.	2025

bad behavior is the inevitable result of the way the health care system is structured and how it incentivizes and forces certain behaviors.

The good news is you won't have insurance companies to kick around much longer. The system is changing. As a result, insurance companies as they are now will be going away. Indeed, they are already evolving.

For the next few years insurance companies will both continue to provide services to employers and, increasingly, compete against each other in the health insurance exchanges. In that role they will put together networks of physicians and hospitals and other services and set a premium. But because of health care reform, new actors will force insurance companies to evolve or become extinct.

The accountable care organizations (ACOs) (Chapter 8, page 224) and hospital systems will begin competing directly in the exchanges and for exclusive contracts with employers. These new organizations are delivery systems with networks of physicians and hospitals that provide comprehensive care. This health delivery structure is in its infancy. Today there are hundreds of these organizations being created and gaining experience within government-sponsored programs or getting contracts from private insurers. They are developing and testing ways to coordinate, standardize, and provide care more efficiently and at consistently higher quality standards. Over the next decade many of these ACOs and hospital systems will succeed at integrating all the components of care and provide efficient, coordinated care. They will have the physician and hospital networks. They will have standardized, guideline-driven care plans for most major conditions and procedures to increase efficiency. They will have figured out how to harness their electronic medical records to better identify patients who will become sick and how to intervene early as well as how to care for the well-identified chronically ill so as to reduce costs.

The key skill these ACOs and hospital systems lack—the skill insurance companies specialize in—is the actuarial capacity to predict and manage financial risk. But over the next decade this is something they will develop—or purchase. After all, actuarial science is not rocket science, even if it involves a lot of mathematical equations. Indeed, some large provider groups have already purchased insurers to acquire actuarial skills. And with that skill, ACOs and hospital systems will become integrated delivery systems like Kaiser or Group Health of Puget Sound.

Then they will cut out the insurance company middle man—and keep the insurance company profits for themselves. Therefore, increasingly these ACOs and hospital systems will transform themselves into integrated delivery systems, entering insurance exchanges and negotiating with employers, in direct competition with insurance companies.

This trend is already beginning. A recent article noted,

> More health systems are seeking to contract directly with employers with deals to bundle the price for certain services or serve as exclusive contractor for all healthcare services for a company's employees, as in a recent agreement between Intel and Presbyterian Healthcare Services in New Mexico. The direct deals have emerged as hospitals and doctors face mounting pressure to keep healthcare spending in check.

As they gain more experience in managing groups of patients, such contracts between health systems and employers—cutting out insurance companies—will become more common. At that time the health systems will make the jump to offering coverage in the exchanges.

In turn, the health insurance companies will have 3 possible responses. First, they can refuse to change, in which case they will eventually go out of business. Second, they can shift their business to focus on offering services they have expertise in, particularly analytics, actuarial modeling, risk management, and other management services. An example that foreshadows this evolutionary path is United Healthcare's Optum subsidiary, which sells management services to ACOs, hospitals, physicians, and health plans. As these customers need more help with analytics, risk management, and disease management, Optum will grow.

The third evolutionary path is that health insurance companies may transform themselves into integrated delivery systems. ACOs begin with the delivery system and will need to add the actuarial capacities to become integrated delivery systems. Insurance companies, however, start at the other end: they begin with the actuarial skills and need to add the actual providers of care. The easiest way for them to accomplish this is to buy or enter into exclusive agreements with efficient hospital systems, ACOs, or physician groups. This is just beginning to occur. A foreshadow of this future was the 2011 purchase by Wellpoint, 1 of the 5 largest for-profit insurers, of CareMore for $800 million. CareMore is a Medicare Advantage health plan headquartered in southern California with facilities in Arizona and Nevada. It delivers very high-quality care at costs that are about 20% below competitors. Presumably, in anticipation of developing efficient delivery systems, Wellpoint wanted the "secret sauce" on how to deliver high-quality, low-cost care to a sick population. Similarly, hedging its bets, Optum owns physician practices with about 5,000 primary care physicians and is on its way to developing integrated delivery systems in 75 different health care markets.

In January 2012 Jeffrey Liebman and I predicted in the *New York Times* the end of health insurance companies by 2020. We might have been a bit optimistic—or provocative. But it is certain they will end. Insurance companies will largely cease to be the middle man—taking premiums, paying providers, saying no to consumers, and making a profit—that we blame. Whether we will come to love them is another matter. That depends on how well they actually care for patients.

Some people may be concerned about the prospect of having to choose among large integrated delivery systems with selective physician and hospital networks. The worried well might wonder what happens if they contract a serious illness, such as cancer or some rare disease, will they be restricted only to the physicians in the delivery system? In the future would Erin be able to get a second opinion from the University of Colorado or M.D. Anderson? Or would she be required to go only to the oncologists in her integrated delivery system?

We should note that many people pick Kaiser or Group Health and get all of their care from those integrated systems, and they don't seem to worry that they are not getting the highest-quality care. The real issue is not whether there is a selective network of physicians and hospitals; the real issue is whether the network is of high quality. Having the assurance of a high-quality network is the key. These integrated-delivery systems will begin competing with their objectively certified, high-quality networks.

More importantly, health systems should have learned from the managed-care backlash. Just saying "no" really aggravates people, especially well-off, powerful people. Although it may be cheaper in the short run, it can be expensive, especially in terms of reputation, in the longer term. There are better ways to approach this.

I suspect these integrated delivery systems of the future will adopt 2 strategies. For rare but serious conditions they will identify recognized centers of excellence—the absolute best places in the country—and contract special arrangements for the referral and treatment of their patients. These centers of excellence may have slightly higher sticker prices, but forging these special arrangements will be worth it for integrated delivery systems because then they will be able to boast negotiated rates, better outcomes, and fewer complications. Second, richer and, thus, more expensive benefit packages, such as platinum plans in the exchanges, would cover second opinions. In addition, there will be a market for supplemental insurance that covers second opinions for serious conditions. The well-heeled and worried will be a prime target for such plans.

So be prepared to kiss your insurance company good-bye forever.

VIP Care for the Chronically and Mentally Ill

The paralyzed won't miraculously begin to walk, but patients suffering from chronic illnesses will be healthier and less prone to exacerbations and complications of their illnesses.

Use of health care resources is lumpy-bumpy (Chapter 3, page 69). About 10% of patients account for nearly two-thirds of all health care spending. To control costs and improve the quality of care, physicians and hospitals need to focus on this small fraction of patients because they account for most of the money spent in health care. Who are they? They are patients with chronic or multiple chronic conditions, such as heart failure, emphysema, diabetes, coronary artery disease, asthma, hypertension, and cancer.

A large portion of the health care spending for patients with chronic illness arises from specialists, emergency room visits and hospitalizations due to exacerbations of their illness. When I was training we frequently admitted patients who had heart failure that caused extreme difficulty breathing. We then put them on water pills and they peed out extra fluid. We tinkered with their medications to make sure their failing heart was pumping just a little bit better. After a few days of adjustments we sent them home with a fistful of prescriptions and often with a few home health visits to ensure they were staying on their medications. But a few weeks later they would show up in the emergency room, short of breath once again. The hospitalization cycle would start all over. Unkindly, we called these patients "frequent flyers."

The same kind of exacerbation cycle is common for patients with emphysema, asthma, and other chronic conditions. Patients with diabetes and poor circulation frequently have small infections on their toes and feet. If not properly cared for, these infections can become very serious, requiring hospitalization for intravenous antibiotics. And sometimes, if not caught in time, they can lead to gangrene and amputations. Cancer patients experiencing the nausea and vomiting caused by chemotherapy may become dehydrated and require hospitalization for fluids. They can also have escalating pain that requires a hospitalization for pain control.

Thus, a key to controlling costs—and improving quality of care—is prevention. Not the kind of prevention most of us think about, such as cancer screening tests or immunizations. That is *primary prevention*—preventive services for healthy people who do not have diseases. Instead, what is needed is *tertiary prevention*, or preventing people with serious illnesses from having an exacerbation of their condition or side effects of treatment that require hospitalizations or other expensive interventions. Avoiding these kinds of repeat emergency room visits and hospitalizations for preventable problems is a major area for cost control. In other words, the key to cost control and quality improvement is to keep sick patients with chronic illnesses healthy—or at least healthier. Ensure that they are managed well so that they do not have the exacerbations or amputations or that they are treated to mitigate predictable side effects.

Today, the best health care systems are focusing on this type of prevention with standardized treatment processes, and the results can be pretty remarkable. By monitoring patients who have just received chemotherapy, treating those who develop symptoms the same day in the office, a cancer group is able to reduce emergency room visits and hospitalizations of cancer patients by more than 50%. Keeping patients with chronic illnesses healthy can really pay off. Over the next decade every medical group will develop, implement, and refine care processes that keep chronically sick patients healthier so as to reduce their use of health care services, especially the emergency room and hospital.

Tertiary prevention can generate big savings, probably in the range of 10 to 20% of overall health care spending. But it can only go so far. Once preventable complications are reliably prevented, then there will be little more savings by focusing on keeping these patients with chronic illness healthy. So what comes next?

The next area to focus for cost control will be mental health. It turns out that mental health problems are actually among the leading drivers of health care costs. Mental health disorders are more widespread than we think. Approximately one-quarter of adults experience one or more disorders. More importantly, about 6% of adults suffer from seriously debilitating mental illness. Some of this relates to complex patients with schizophrenia and bipolar disorders whose care is not well coordinated, whose chronic medications are expensive, and whose institutionalizations for exacerbations can be prolonged. But a lot of this relates to patients with chronic illnesses who become depressed or anxious because of their health problems and whose depression then exacerbates their other illnesses because they fail to consistently take their medications or exercise or adhere to some other health program. In addition, patients with cancer or heart disease or other serious illnesses become anxious, and this leads them to have a low threshold for going to the emergency room for the slightest symptoms or to find reassurance in frequent check-ups or imaging tests. Isolated and depressed patients use the health care system because it offers attention and meaningful social interactions. Patients with mental health issues are expensive.

Currently, the health care system responds poorly to these patients. It is estimated that only about a third of people with mental health problems receive treatment, and only about a third of those—12% overall—are actually receiving adequate treatment. Why? Primary care physicians usually do not like dealing with mental health issues. So they refer patients to psychiatrists. But getting a new patient appointment with a psychiatrist, especially for patients who have Medicare or who have no or inadequate insurance, can take 2 or 3 months. By that time the patient may have gone to the emergency room a few times and been admitted to the hospital. Besides, these patients need more than just the care of a psychiatrist; they need to be connected to social services, engaged in social activities that replace the meaningful but expensive attention they receive from nurses.

Whereas a number of health care systems have begun to figure out how to institute preventive care for chronically ill patients—or are focused on it and will find solutions soon—only a few are beginning to attend to the mental health problems of regular patients, particularly the depression, anxiety disorders, and social isolation. The most advanced systems are experimenting with interventions. One health plan has combined routine screening of patients for depression and dementia coupled not with a referral to a psychiatrist that can take months but instead with immediate intervention by psychologists, social workers, and others. Whether this is a good intervention and will lead to better mental health care and lower costs is still uncertain. What is clear, however, is that the innovators and early adopters are experimenting now. By 2020 the mainstream of health care, what the innovation theorists call the early majority, will begin systematically tackling the mental health problems of their chronically ill patients. This early majority will have successfully built procedures and standardized care processes targeted at tertiary prevention. Their next big area for improving quality of care and reducing costs will be routinely integrating standardized mental health interventions into primary care practice. Then, over the next decade, the 2020s, patients' mental health problems will be taken seriously and seriously addressed by the mainstream. Mental health parity with physical health will finally happen—not because any legislature mandates it but because health systems find it necessary to improve quality and reduce total health care costs.

The Emergence of Digital Medicine and the Closing of Hospitals

Since the turn of the 20th century the American health care system has become ever more hospital centric (Chapter 1). In the early 1960s my father, a pediatrician in Chicago, still had a black bag and used to make house calls to remove stitches, check on an earache, rash, or fever or see whether a child was recovering well. Then, sometime in the late 1960s, he stopped, instead sending all his off-hour patients to the hospital emergency room. As a consequence, about one-third of all health care expenditures, over $900 billion (Chapter 3, Figure 3.1)—more than the nation spends on all of Social Security, all of defense, or on the federal portion of Medicare and Medicaid—now goes toward that hospital care.

This 100-year hospital habit is coming to an end. Hospitals will no longer be at the center of health care because of 2 underlying driving forces. First, in an era that focuses on cost control, when physicians are paid and incentivized to be more efficient and caring for patients in the hospital is expensive, hospitalization is a money sink to be avoided whenever possible. Second, there is a tremendous growth in the power of sensors combined with data-mining algorithms that can permit the safe remote monitoring of patients. These cost incentives are increasingly leading to at least 3 trends that will significantly reduce the use of hospitals for delivering health care.

First, if megatrend 2 occurs, sicker patients are kept healthier—that is, if tertiary prevention works—then fewer patients will be admitted to the hospital. Most of the costs saved by keeping heart failure patients from getting short of breath, preventing diabetics from getting gangrene and needing amputations, preventing cancer patients from getting serious chemotherapy side effects and uncontrolled pain comes from bypassing expensive emergency room visits and hospital stays. Better care of chronically ill patients will reduce the need for hospitalizations.

Second, the provisions in the ACA related to reducing hospital-acquired infections, medication errors, preventable readmissions, and other avoidable mistakes will also reduce the need for hospitalizations (Chapter 8, pages 224). For instance, on average, hospital-acquired infections add 7.4 to 9.4 days to a hospitalization, and millions of patients contract hospital-acquired infections each year. Under the ACA, however, hospitals are penalized for not reducing infections. Similarly, before the ACA, approximately 20% of Medicare patients discharged from the hospital were readmitted within 30 days, but the ACA penalizes hospitals for not reducing their preventable readmission rate. All hospitals are working hard to drive hospital-acquired infections, readmissions, and other mistakes down. Because of the financial penalties in the ACA, these efforts will be successful. They too will reduce the number of patients spending time in a hospital bed.

Finally and most importantly, ever more care will move outside the 4 walls of the hospital and the physician's office. There is plenty of care that once was delivered only in the hospital that now can be safely delivered anywhere, especially at home. And this trend will accelerate with the rise of digital medicine, particularly the combination of powerful sensors, wireless connections, and data mining algorithms. Digital medicine will allow physicians to monitor patients remotely anywhere they are, get labs and many imaging tests done, and perform interventions once done exclusively in the hospital.

The house call is making a comeback. Instead of sending patients to the hospital emergency room, companies are now offering to send advanced practice nurses and even physicians to patients' homes with X-ray and ultrasound machines, suture kits, IVs, medications, and other medical equipment to provide state-of-the-art treatment. Indeed, these companies are now instituting webcam-enabled "visits" instead of emergency room visits for many complaints and conditions. Imaging and surgical centers are able to do MRIs and many surgical procedures out of the hospital. Further, groups have developed a program called hospital@home in which patients who traditionally would have been admitted to the hospital for treatments like intravenous antibiotics or anticoagulants are now treated at home with a nurse visiting once or twice a day. Patients in these programs have fewer laboratory tests and recover faster with fewer hospital infections and other complications. Overall, compared to being treated in the hospital, hospital@home patients can save as much as 19%.

Digital technology will only accelerate this process, creating a positive feedback loop. As more digital medicine technologies become available, more care will be delivered out of the hospital. Greater sales, in turn, will incentivize entrepreneurs to develop more digital medicine technologies, thus enabling more care to be moved outside of the hospital.

One major consequence of the rise of digital medicine will be that about 1,000 of the approximately 5,000 acute-care hospitals in the United States will close by 2020. This may be a conservative estimate; some consultants predict that as many as 2,000 hospitals will close. Today, many hospitals are holding on by their fingernails. On average, patients occupy fewer than 67% of all hospital beds, and the more than 3,000 hospitals with 200 or fewer patient beds are operating with 40% of their beds empty. With so many beds empty, balancing the books is difficult, much less making enough margin to invest in upgrades. Even the 250 biggest hospitals, those with more than 500 beds, are running at only 75% occupancy. Simple economics means many hospitals will close over the next decade. And this will happen without any federal official or board—or "death panel"—ordering them closed. It will happen because the bond markets and others will stop lending them money. Their financial outlook and margins will not justify lending to them.

Many local populations will fight against these closures. In many communities the hospital is the biggest employer with well-paying jobs, and local luminaries sit on their boards. But fighting the closures is the wrong thing to do. Closing hospitals does not spell doom and gloom. After all, how many of us want to stay a long time in the hospital? Hospital stays are not restful, recuperative vacations; they have become almost as bad as stranded cruise ships, with constant interruptions, disrupted sleep, and risks of infection and other untoward events. Society is better off with fewer people in hospital beds.

The hospitals that close may be converted to outpatient service centers. They may serve as places for physician offices or surgical centers. More importantly, the health care personnel will continue to be employed. The shift in care out of the hospital will mean that the nurses, health aides, respiratory therapists, physical therapists, and others who once walked the wards will be employed visiting patients in their homes and at senior centers, delivering care in other settings besides the hospital. Further, the hospitals that remain open will operate much more efficiently and will be focused on only the most severely ill patients, those requiring transplants, implantation of devices, or intensive care. Indeed, hospitals of the future are likely to be intensive-care units only.

Routine use of digital medicine will become the norm. There will be extensive monitoring of patients in their real, everyday lives—monitoring of their weight, whether they take their medications, their exercise, sleep, and other health-related activities. Increasingly, patients will engage in real-time interactions with their physicians, nurses, and other health care providers, and this will create a boon in new digital medical technologies. New wireless ways of monitoring patients in real time—not only their weight and heart rhythms but also their blood counts and chemistries—will be developed and deployed, as will the software to sift through and analyze all the data so as to alert clinicians to serious abnormalities. And this will be the foundation for prompt therapeutic interventions in the 95% of chronically ill patients' lives that occur outside of the hospital or physician's office.

Long live fewer hospitals. Welcome to the new age of digital medicine.

The End of Employer-Sponsored Insurance

Before the ACA there was no employer mandate. No law required employers to provide health insurance to their workers. And yet most Americans—roughly 150 million—received their health insurance through their or their relative's employer. The large majority of employers, except for the ones with fewer than 10 employees, provided health coverage with no legal mandate. Why? To attract and retain high-quality workers. Workers demanded it because it was hard and, for some, nearly impossible to get good, reliable, and affordable health coverage on their own in the individual market. With a large pool of workers it was cheaper for employers to sponsor insurance than for individuals to buy it themselves. And the government's tax policies strongly encouraged employer-sponsored insurance (Chapter 2, page 46).

The ACA changes all of that. It created the exchanges; after the problems of healthcare.gov are resolved, these will be efficient marketplaces in which any American, even those with preexisting conditions, can get good, reliable, and affordable coverage. For many the subsidies make health care affordable. This changes the incentives for both workers and employers.

Today, most employers do not know whether they will continue to offer health insurance 5 or 10 years from now; instead, they are focused on complying with the ACA. They do not have enough information or experience to know whether continuing to sponsor health insurance or dropping coverage is the better approach. That will change. By 2025 few private-sector employers will still be providing health insurance. Some will provide defined contributions to their workers and offer them a variety of plans through the company. These are called private exchanges, in which a benefits company sets up an exchange by getting a variety of insurance plans for workers at a particular company. The workers then choose among the plans, receiving financial support from the employer. Other private-sector employers will simply increase workers' salaries to help them pay for insurance in the state-based, public exchanges.

Three things will drive the change. First, once the websites are fixed and working smoothly—certainly by 2016—the exchanges will generate positive branding. Americans need to see them as desirable places to get good health insurance. That means the websites needs to provide an engaging, "Amazon-like" shopping experience. They need to be simple to navigate, with easy-to-understand comparative information on the quality of the various plans, the physician and hospital networks, the costs, and other relevant characteristics. The problems they are having in the first year of the rollout are serious but also technical and eminently solvable. In the next few years—by 2016—people will be able to shop for health insurance on the exchange websites in a way that is similar to shopping for other common items.

Further, Americans need to have choice—but not too much choice. There needs to be a variety of good health insurance options at each price point. The more Americans use the exchanges, the more companies will enter the exchanges and offer plans. Indeed, more companies will enter as they gain experience with the number and purchasing behaviors of people in the exchange. By 2016 the insurance exchanges will provide an attractive, informative, and engaging insurance shopping experience with an adequate variety of choices.

Second, employers need to be convinced that even without offering health insurance they can attract and retain good employees. In part they will do this by shifting what they pay for health insurance to significantly higher salaries. This may be a generational issue. Younger workers who have little experience and expectation of getting health insurance from their employer and are used to shopping for books, music, shoes, clothes, smartphones, and cars on the web will probably be most amenable to now getting their health insurance on the web as well. Older workers, however, may be resistant. Using private exchanges to socialize these older workers on how exchanges work is likely a prelude to shifting them to the public, state-based exchanges.

Finally, there is a cultural element that will need to change. For decades providing health insurance was part of the "good employer" ideal. Companies will have to be convinced that they can still be viewed as good employers even if they do not offer health insurance.

Sometime before 2020—probably 2016 or 2017—these 3 factors will coalesce, and a few big, blue-chip companies will announce their intention to stop providing health insurance. Instead, they will raise salaries substantially or offer large, defined contributions to their workers. Then the floodgates will open. By 2025 almost all major employers will be out of the health insurance market, and fewer than 20% of workers in the private sector will receive their health insurance through their employer. In this regard the slowest employers to transition are likely to be city, state, and federal governments. Health benefits are part of union negotiations, and unions are very conservative on health coverage and likely to resist for a long time. Union leaders fear that without negotiations for health benefits, many workers may not appreciate the value of the union. So the leadership will be loath to permit municipalities and states to increase wages and let workers get health coverage in the exchanges.

For any company with fewer than 50 employees there is no mandate and thus no penalty for not providing health insurance. Thus, why small businesses will continue to provide health insurance is hard to fathom. Their insurance brokers may package health care with disability and life and other products to try to retain business for a few years, but, in the end, exit they will. It may be one employee getting a very costly illness that drives up premiums or the hassle of having to sift through the options that comply with the ACA that flips the switch. Or it just may be the sense that employees will get more choices and be able to get whatever they want. If companies need to convince workers that they are a good place to work, they can woo them the old-fashioned way: by offering a higher salary.

An obstacle to fulfilling this prediction is the tax exclusion: higher-income workers get a sizeable tax advantage from employer-sponsored insurance. The wealthier workers receive thousands in tax breaks when their employer sponsors health insurance. But after 2018 the Cadillac tax that employers have to pay will progressively erode the tax advantage for these workers. After all, these higher-income workers want rich health insurance plans that will have high premiums. At some point the Cadillac tax will make it undesirable for employers to continue to offer lavish health insurance.

I believe small employers will not go into the so-called SHOP exchanges for small businesses. The SHOP exchanges will have a hard time being set up. The subsidies for using them in the ACA are time limited and directed only at very low-wage workers. Workers will largely receive better subsidies if they shop in the individual exchange.

Overall this will be good for the public, state-based exchanges because large numbers of people in these exchanges stabilize them. On average, workers tend to be a relatively healthy segment of the overall population and, thus, will keep premiums in the exchange moderated.

For larger employers the employer mandate and its $2,000 penalty will alter the calculation a bit. For a company with 1,000 employees, their health insurance bill is probably between $7 and $10 million depending on how many families they cover. With the ACA, if they drop insurance, their penalty payments will be $2 million. The company can, therefore, afford to pay the employer-mandate penalty and still give each worker a big raise in cash wages to facilitate their purchase of insurance in the exchanges. For all the workers earning less than 400% of the federal poverty line, they will also get a subsidy to purchase insurance. At the time of the switch this may be revenue neutral, but over time the company will not have to worry about a component of compensation that grows much faster than increases in productivity or the GDP.

Alternatively, the company could comply with the ACA by giving each worker a defined contribution for their purchase of insurance in the exchanges. This would allow the company to avoid the employer-mandate penalty. But it would also mean their workers would get that tax exclusion but would not get the exchange subsidy.

Over time the employer-based market is likely to look a lot less like the current system, with employers covering much of the employees' health insurance. Increasingly, it will look like a voucher system. Individuals rather than employers will be choosing from a variety of health insurance options in a marketplace, the exchanges. Their purchases will be subsidized by vouchers that will come either as income-linked subsidies from the government or as employer-defined contributions.

The important point is that with the voucher, the consumers will have a strong incentive to be frugal in their purchase of insurance, thus providing downward price pressure on premiums.

Some people may be worried that if employers are out of the health insurance business, they will stop caring about their workers' health and will terminate their wellness programs and efforts to improve the nutrition of their food services. After all, currently many employers are establishing wellness programs on the promise of lowering health care costs. However, most of the available evidence suggests that the impact of wellness and nutrition programs on health insurance premiums takes a long time to occur if at all; instead, the real impact of these programs is on lowering disability payments and absenteeism and increasing workers' engagement and productivity on the job. Even without any financial interest in health insurance, employers will be interested in developing wellness and nutrition programs for these other benefits.

The End of Health Care Inflation

For the last 5 decades health care costs have increased much faster than the overall growth in the economy. If the economy grows at GDP, according to the Congressional Budget Office health care expenditures have grown at GDP+2% since 1975 (Chapter 4). This means that each year health care takes increasingly more of all economic output. This is why health care has grown from 8% of the GDP in 1975 to just under 18% today. This growth in health care costs is a financial cancer that undermines state support for education, wage increases, and the nation's long-term fiscal health. A central rationale for health care reform was to control health care costs—in the jargon, to "bend the cost curve," to reduce health care cost growth from GDP+2% to something less.

There was a small window in the 1990s when health care inflation was low. Indeed, during those years health care costs remained, as the CBO put it, "relatively stable as a share of the economy"—about 13.7%. This was the managed-care era. It had a downward effect on costs by reducing both excess hospital beds and prices paid to physicians and hospitals. But with the managed-care backlash came the return of the growth in health care costs, building to their near-historic levels from 2001 onward. This growth, however, has moderated over the last few years, partly because physicians and hospitals have changed how they care for patients, partly because of the Great Recession, partly because of increases in patients' deductible and co-pays, and partly in response to the ACA.

The ACA will succeed at controlling the growth in health care costs. It is important to be very clear here. This does not mean total national health care expenditures will go from $2.87 trillion per year *down* to $2.6 trillion, much less $2.4 trillion per year. Instead, it means health care expenditures will rise from $2.8 trillion to $3.5 and $4 trillion more slowly. The important point is that the *growth* in health care costs as a proportion of the GDP will slow down.

Five important factors arising from the ACA reforms will lower the growth of health care costs. One is that high prices paid for health care goods and services will decline. There are high and variable prices for many health care products (Chapter 3, page 90), but a variety of reforms will lower input prices, especially for devices and other items. For instance, competitive bidding for durable medical equipment, prosthetics, and other items is part of the ACA. In the regions of the country it has been implemented, competitive bidding has already significantly lowered prices, by about 40%. The ACA requires this to spread nationwide by 2016. And competitive bidding is likely to expand to other medical items that are really commodities and have been highly automated, such as laboratory tests and imaging. In addition, the push for transparency in medical prices has just begun and is gaining momentum. This will lead to increasing public awareness of prices and, thus, a downward price pressure. Finally, as more physicians and hospitals are paid a fixed rate and learn to change their business model from revenue to margin generation, they will seek lower prices from their various suppliers as well as from other physicians and providers to whom they refer patients. Thus, we are likely to see lower prices on a wide range of medical goods and services.

Second, consumers really will care about the price of insurance in the exchanges. Consumers have not really shopped for health insurance with their own money. Their employer has made a contract with one or more insurance companies, and they have selected among those. Increasingly, with the exchanges and as more employers place their workers in the exchanges, the majority of consumers will shop primarily based on price. In turn, insurance companies—and, then increasingly, ACOs and integrated delivery systems, when they enter the exchanges—will be forced to develop health plans that lower costs in order to lower premiums and attract more customers. This will put pressure on physicians and hospitals to cut out unnecessary services and deliver quality care more efficiently.

Third, the focus on tertiary prevention will lead to lower health care utilization. As this focus on keeping chronically ill patients healthy spreads to more medical organizations, it will generate savings and control costs throughout the system. And as digital medicine and the focus on prevention develop and expand into the home, there will be other areas for additional savings.

Fourth, moving care out of the high-cost hospital setting to the home will also generate additional savings. In early efforts hospital@home programs can save 20% when caring for patients in their own homes instead of admitting them to the hospital. This too will spread to more institutions and to more conditions, again lowering the cost that comes with more complex interventions.

Most importantly, there will be a change in incentives because of a change in the payment structure to physicians and hospitals. As the payment structure moves away from fee for service toward more bundled payment or capitation, physicians and hospitals will have a strong incentive to focus on delivering high-value care efficiently. They will focus on interventions that make a big health impact and those that cost less when there are equivalent therapeutic choices. This will catalyze each of the previous trends, as physicians decrease the use of unnecessary services and search for lower prices. They will identify interventions that preempt more expensive ones, and they will provide care in lower-priced settings. Ultimately this payment change will incentivize a mentality that strives to do more—with higher quality—at lower costs.

This change in incentives will have an additional benefit in terms of cost: it will change the kinds of medical technologies being developed. Instead of companies developing interventions heedless of their cost,

FIGURE 13.2 National health expenditures

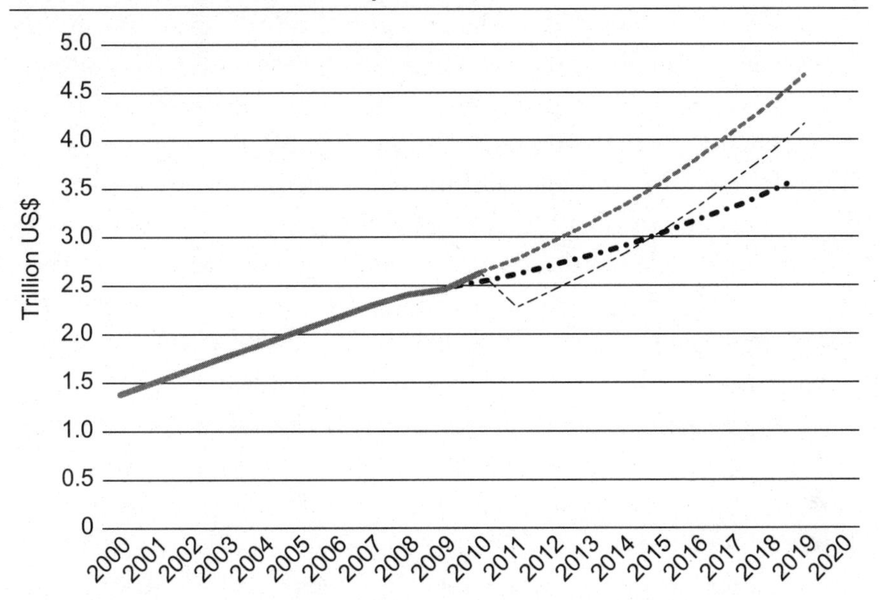

companies will increasingly develop technologies that can lead to better health care at lower costs. Their selling point will no longer be just the clinical benefits they offer but, instead, the value they offer—their benefits per dollar. The change in payment structure will not undermine medical innovation but rather change its direction for the better.

Some of these changes, such as competitive bidding, will be one-time decreases in the level of health care spending. Although necessary and helpful, it does not lead to lower growth over time (see Figure 13.2). But some of these changes, such as those related to technology and prevention, will lead to a bending of the cost curve.

How much? GDP+0%. My prediction is that by 2020 per capita health care spending will grow at GDP+0%. This will mean that a relatively stable amount of the GDP will be going to health care. Health care spending will grow only because of the increase in the population.

Health care costs will not go down; they will still be growing. But they will not be growing faster than the economy can afford. We will repeat the period from 1993 to 2000. Remember, that was a great economic time. The economy was growing, employment was growing, wages were growing, and investment was booming. In addition, the federal deficit declined, and by the end of the period the budget was actually in surplus. Clearly, not all of this booming economic activity is attributable to lower increases in health care costs; many factors, from higher taxes on the wealthy to the Internet to changes in production, contributed to the economic boom. But a substantial portion was related to lower health care inflation.

GDP+0% per capital health care growth is a bold, maybe unbelievable, maybe even reckless prediction. After all, it has occurred exactly only one time in the last 40 years. But the confluence of these 5 trends has never occurred before. Already there is some evidence that health care inflation has slowed over the last few years, and not just because of the Great Recession. My own discussions with hospitals, physician groups, insurers, venture capitalists, and others indicate a real seriousness in focusing on cost control that was absent prior to the ACA. Seriousness and effective cost control are different things, however. Nonetheless, there are real changes in financial incentives that are translating into changes in how care is delivered and, therefore, what technologies will be adopted that are going to permanently make health care more efficient and, thus, lower the growth rate.

GDP+0%! If this occurs—or even comes close—we will not become Switzerland or Norway, much less Japan and Singapore in terms of our health care spending. We will still be the highest-spending country in the world. But at GDP+0%, the American economy will be significantly transformed, and the federal budget and long-term debt situation will look much healthier.

The Transformation of Medical Schools

For the last 100 years medical education has largely been unchanged. Despite all the advances in biomedical research and technological transformations in the delivery of medical care, despite the growth and complexity of hospitals, despite all the new types of medical interventions, the training of physicians remains firmly in 1910. That was when the Flexner Report recommended collegiate science education and a college degree for prospective physicians, with the first 2 years of medical school devoted to preclinical study of physiology, microbiology, anatomy, and other basic sciences, followed by 2 years of clinical training in hospital wards (Chapter 1, page 24).

Recently, medical education has changed formats from lectures in the preclinical years to more small-group discussions and study. It has also introduced students to a patient or 2 in the first week of medical school. But fundamentally, this 4-year training, with 2 preclinical years focused on the basic sciences and 2 clinical years occurring in large teaching hospitals, has hardly changed in the past century.

Today's medical graduates are lacking the skills they need to practice in the coming era of digital medicine, and they are not getting those skills during their postgraduate training as interns, residents, and fellows. Medical education is probably the slowest-evolving institution in society. This will need to change.

In what ways? In every way—how long it takes, where it occurs, who is in the classroom, and, most importantly, what subjects are taught. Over the next 15 years there will be 5 major transformations in medical education. First, the duration of medical school will go from 4 years to 3 years, and the years of residencies and specialty fellowship training will also be shortened. The drive for efficiency in medical delivery will likewise force medical schools to be more efficient. At my current medical school, the University of Pennsylvania, preclinical work is already down from 2 to 1½ years, and at Yale and Duke it is 1 year, proving that top medical schools do not need to waste 2 years on preclinical work, much of which has little to no relevance to the actual care of patients. At Penn the required clinical rotations in medicine, surgery, pediatrics, obstetrics and gynecology, and other core clinical courses last just 1 year. Students then spend 1½ years doing electives, taking time at other hospitals to audition for internship and residency, and vacationing. This extended elective time could easily be shortened to just a half year. This would make medical school 3 years. Yale and Duke have 2 years of clinical work, and their 4th year of training is a required year of research. But why all medical students even at the top medical schools should engage in research when few will pursue it as a career is not clear. Already, some major institutions are experimenting with 3-year programs. For instance, recently NYU admitted 10% of its class for a 3-year medical degree. As pressure builds on the health care system to be more efficient, medical education will not escape this push. Further, the need to do something about ever-increasing medical student educational debt, which averaged over $160,000 for the class of 2013, will place additional pressure on shortening the training time. The transformation will occur when the first major medical school—one of the top 25 schools—shifts to a 3-year program. Then the dominoes will fall.

Similarly, many residencies and fellowships require trainees to spend one or more years conducting research, even though few will ever be researchers. This added training is very expensive and not a terribly productive use of some of the best minds in society. For instance, many surgical and specialty training programs, such as urology and cardiology, add 2 years of research separate from learning clinical skills. Much of this is done not for the benefit of the trainees but rather for the convenience of the faculty, so that there are sufficient residents to take night call. This exploitation of trainees for no improvement in clinical skills will end.

It is not just the length of medical education that will change; so will where it occurs. Today, most clinical medical education is still hospital based. Medical students may visit a patient in a nursing home or at their own homes, but this is the exception; most training is still in the hospital's emergency room, intensive-care units, radiology departments, surgical suites, and patient wards. But with digital medicine, care is moving out of the hospital, and medical training will too.

By the middle of the next decade half of clinical training during medical school, internship, and residencies will occur out of the hospital, and a good portion of that will be where patients live, not where physicians have their offices. This is where care is migrating to, and physicians need to learn how to care for patients where the vast majority live, not where only a few of the sickest go.

Since at least 1910 medical educators have perfected how to integrate students into the fabric of hospitals, with time for rounding on patients, teaching, and then ordering tests and changing care plans. Increasingly, only the very sickest patients will be cared for this way. Medical educators have had a hard time developing nonhospital training sites that have appropriate activities for medical students and time carved out for teaching. Educators will need to devote more time and resources to cultivating training sites outside of the hospital for students as well as interns and residents, including doing house calls and working in other facilities. In addition, they will need to develop more formalized curricula for training at these sites so as to ensure students learn the full range of lessons. They will also need to develop appropriate faculty who can teach in these new training sites. This may seem easy, but it is not. Office and clinic time is heavily booked, without set periods for student learning. Educators will need to work with physician practices to make them teaching practices.

A third change will be who is in the medical school classroom. Medical education will become multi-professional training. When I was in medical school we did not train with nursing, dental, pharmacy, social work, or respiratory therapy students; indeed, we were implicitly taught to look down on them as people we would eventually give assignments to with our all-powerful physicians' orders.

Over the next decade the delivery of health care will become much more integrated and team-based. Medical care will evolve away from the traditional physician-patient relationship toward a much more effective but complex health care team-patient-caregiver relationship. This will require a change in how we train not just medical students but all health professional students.

To prepare for team-based care, medical students—indeed, all health professional students—will need to learn with other members of their future care teams. This means there will need to be more training of medical students, interns, and residents with health care professionals from other schools. Part of this multi-professional training will involve learning about how to assemble well-functioning teams, the appropriate roles of each member of the team, and how to manage teams effectively.

As medical training transforms to include other health professionals, the faculty teaching medical students will also change. There will be a role for experts from business and management schools to assist in medical education to help teach medical students about team building and other topics. This multiprofessional evolution of medical education will integrate training across professional schools.

Finally, the content of medical education will need to change. One important omission in current medical training is population health—how to take care of not just the patient in the office but also the patient who fails to show up with a complaint but is sick or the patient who doesn't even know he or she has risk factor(s) for a serious illness. Medical schools as well as internships and residency training will increasingly include population health training.

Management styles must change too. One of the most important things physicians do is manage—their patients, their offices, their colleagues, and their time. As megatrend 2 shows, another important thing they need to do is change how they practice. So they will need to manage change. They also negotiate with patients and families as well as with other physicians, nurses, and hospitals. And yet medical school leaves medical students and physicians totally unprepared to manage effectively. It is as though medical schools think management skills are either innate or irrelevant. Similarly, over the next few years hospitals and other medical facilities, from physician offices to neighborhood clinics to nursing facilities, will need to subject their practices to the LEAN production process based on the Toyota production philosophy of eliminating waste that does not add value to the customer. Future physicians will need to understand and know how to implement LEAN or a similar standardized production process that is focused on value.

Not too long ago there was absolutely no formal training in communication skills at medical schools or during internships and residencies. That ended when medical educators realized communication skills are important to being a good physician and can be formally taught and improved. Similarly, management training is absolutely necessary for future physicians. Because of this, increasingly it will not be seen as something a select few students pursue by combining their M.D. with an MBA, but instead it will become a standard constituent of medical education for all future physicians. This management training will probably be introduced during students' last year of clinical training and then reemphasized in various ways throughout their internship and residency. This change in curriculum will mean that medical schools will need to affiliate more closely with their sister business and management schools. Between changing who is in the classroom and adding management training, medical schools will be a major force in breaking down the silos between university schools.

Finally, medical education will need to implement training in digital medicine. The future is digital medicine, including using electronic health records, integrating more real-time data on patients, knowing how to use analytics as well as decision supports, delivering tests and treatments outside of the hospital and the physician's office, engaging in electronic communications with patients and their caregivers, and constant monitoring of quality.

To educate students and young physicians in the ways of digital medicine there will need to be training in new sensors and digital monitoring devices, telemedicine, and how to integrate them effectively and efficiently into the care of patients. Students will also need training in how to use all the data that they have to better care for their patients.

The big problem with putting more emphasis on digital medicine in medical schools is the paucity of well-trained faculty. Few medical school–affiliated physicians do house calls or practice using continuous at-home monitoring devices. How, then, can they teach those techniques? Not only will medical schools need to change their curricula; they will also need to add nontraditional faculty to address this gap.

These changes for medical schools are a tall order, especially considering these schools have changed so little since the 1910 Flexner Report. But the rapid changes in the practice of medicine will necessitate medical schools' adaptation.

Conclusion

Clearly these 6 megatrends interrelate. Instituting tertiary prevention and keeping chronically ill patients healthier requires greater use of digital medicine and is essential to achieving lower health care inflation. Similarly, having physicians use digital medicine more effectively requires a change in medical education. Having more integrated care through digital medicine and other transformations will be key to having accountable care organizations that can compete with traditional insurance companies.

These 6 are not the only megatrends. For instance, there will be a shift in medical innovation. Significant investment is already moving away from new pills and devices for the surgical suites or intensive-care units. Increasingly we will see investments that emphasize interventions to keep patients healthy, increase patient compliance with physician orders, monitor patients remotely and noninvasively, and improve processes of care.

Finally, the realization of these trends on the time scale I have suggested depends on other trends. The end of insurance companies as we know them and employer-sponsored insurance depends on the health insurance exchanges working effectively and being attractive marketplaces for many Americans to shop in. Similarly, the focus on tertiary prevention and the end of hospital-centric care as well as the rise of digital medicine requires changes that move physician payment away from fee-for-service to alternative payment methods that incentivize a health care system, not a sick care system.

But given all the provisions of the ACA along with the responses from insurers, employers, hospitals, and physicians, I am fairly confident these are likely to occur. I may be aggressive in my timelines, but I am certainly not shy, cautious, or fearful of writing down my predictions—or the future.

CODA

A Final Thought

In the short term the ACA has been a political disaster for President Obama and the Democrats. Its enactment produced a strident conservative backlash, which led to one of the largest electoral landslides in recent memory when the Democrats lost control of the House and their filibuster-proof majority in the Senate during the 2010 midterm elections. And it has left the Obama administration in a perpetually defensive stance, depleted of the political capital needed to achieve progress in other important policy areas such as immigration and the federal budget.

Prospects have not exactly improved with time. The disastrous rollout of the federal exchange website along with the postponement of various ACA provisions, such as the employer mandate, the small business exchange, and regulations for menu labeling, have added to the public's negative view of the ACA, the Democrats, and the president. Indeed, it has even led some to question whether the very idea of liberal governance is viable in 21st-century America. As one conservative columnist mused, "We have not just Obamacare unraveling, not just the Obama administration unraveling, not just the Democratic majority of the Senate [unraveling], but we could be looking at the collapse of American liberalism."

It did not have to be this way. The ACA did not have to lead to such political bloodshed for the Democrats. The Democrats fumbled in 2 fundamental ways: communication and execution. Leading up to the summer of 2009 and the angry August that gave birth to the Tea Party, the Obama administration did not have an effective communications strategy to explain health care reform to the public. As the president showed during his impassioned September 9, 2009, speech to a joint session of

Congress, galvanizing the nation to reform health care is not impossible. However, although deploying the president's rhetorical skills in support of the ACA was necessary, it was not sufficient. Rousing presidential speeches can certainly spur momentum, but they cannot by themselves sustain a campaign to enact legislation. The administration never empowered surrogates to constantly carry the message nor did it develop a coherent and persuasive narrative that others could repeat when explaining reform.

The administration had to do 2 things from the start. First, it needed to keep opinion leaders in medicine, such as leading physicians, nurses, hospital executives, and others, regularly coming to the White House for briefings and brainstorming sessions. With this constant engagement the health care leaders would have been more invested in reform's success and more inclined to positively influence organized medicine, frontline physicians, and the rest of the health system, and through the health care providers influence patients and the public. The administration actually did convene such a meeting in early March 2009 and supportive editorials in medical journals ensued, unfortunately, they did not follow up with monthly engagements. It was a one-off meeting. As a result, an opportunity to engage medicine's leaders as strategic partners was lost.

On health care the American public trusts physicians and nurses (nurses more than physicians). The administration should have appointed 10 or 20 physicians and 10 or 20 nurses as public ambassadors for health care reform and armed them with a PowerPoint presentation that explained the need for reform, the contents of the ACA, and the positive impact it would have on the average American. These ambassadors could have been sent out to the American people, clad in white coats and stethoscopes, to explain the ACA and persuade people of its virtues.

Would these communications strategies have mitigated the 2010 political disaster? Who knows. At least they are likely to have blunted the talk of death panels and socialized medicine more effectively than the administration's actual communications strategy.

As I noted, the second major fumble was when the administration did not properly manage the implementation effort once the ACA was enacted. Senior administration officials never placed ACA implementation at the very top of the postpassage agenda. Passing the legislation was exhausting and hard enough, but implementation was going to be harder. Nonetheless, senior leadership had moved on to other issues, such as the depressed housing market, continued unemployment, and the persistently distressed economy. And they did not empower anyone with well-honed managerial skills to run the implementation day-to-day. We have experienced the results of this absence of focus on execution.

The poor communication and management of the ACA may yet cause even more political damage for President Obama and Democrats in Congress. Technological fixes will be ongoing. It is unclear how much more political impact the ACA will have in the 2014 and 2016 elections, but it is safe to say that the law's opponents are not ready to give in and will continue to highlight the problems of health care reform unless the American public begins to find it beneficial.

Regardless of the short-term political costs, in the longer sweep of history, beginning in 2020 or so, the ACA will increasingly be seen as a world historical achievement, even more important for the United States than Social Security and Medicare had been. And Barack Obama will be viewed more like Harry Truman—judged with increasing respect over time. Why?

The ACA is stimulating a transformation of the entire American health care system—that is, 18% of the economy. Before the ACA, the American health care system was literally killing the country. Government estimates were that the population of uninsured Americans would rise from 45 million in 2009 to 54 million in 2019. For more than 4 decades health care costs were rising much faster than the growth in the economy, sucking off tremendous amounts of money. Not all of this spending was bad, however. It built tremendous academic health centers and modern community hospitals, spurred development of many new medical technologies, and filled medicine cabinets with groundbreaking new pills that were more potent with fewer side effects. But it also diverted resources away from many other vitally important social programs, from education to infrastructure to middle-class wage increases. Bridges were aging and crumbling as adjacent hospitals were brand new and stuffed with amazing technology. And, even worse, over this 4-decade period cash wages for private-sector workers stagnated—and health care was a major contributing factor. As the Congressional Budget Office put it in 2009:

> The high and rising costs of health care impose an increasing burden on the federal government as well as state governments and the private sector. Under current policies, CBO projects, federal spending on Medicare and Medicaid will increase from about 5 percent of gross domestic product (GDP) in 2009 to more than 6 percent in 2019 and about 12 percent by 2050. [For context, all federal spending amounts to about 21% of GDP.] In the private sector, the growth of health care costs has contributed to slow growth in wages.

Probably most abstract but worrisome was the impact of health care costs on the United States' long-term fiscal stability. As numerous economic and financial commentators noted, the inexorable rise in the nation's debt was fueled not by defense spending or Social Security but rather by Medicare and Medicaid spending. And if nothing was done, Medicare and Medicaid would drown the country in a bowl of red ink.

But something was done, and that was the ACA. Although the ACA is far from perfect and could have done more, especially in regard to changing the way physicians and hospitals are paid, it has stimulated change in a way nothing had done before. The talk of efficiency and value as well as cost control and accountability for quality, not just by health policy experts but increasingly by hospital executives and medical societies and associations representing practicing physicians, signals a sea change. If this change in perspective and psychology takes hold, it will fundamentally transform all physicians' and hospitals' practices. And the ACA will have done nothing short of save the United States from fiscal calamity. If the ACA does transform the practice of medicine and control per capita costs at GDP+0%, although health care spending will still be at 18% of GDP, its growth will slow, generating a tremendous economic boom and transforming a significant federal budget deficit into a significant surplus. This in turn will free up governmental resources and allow the country to invest again in the many things that have been starved for funds: rebuilding roads, bridges, and other infrastructure and investing in early childhood education, scientific research and development, and the like.

Yes, the initial growing pains of ACA implementation are reigniting Americans' inherent skepticism of government. The botched implementation of the federal exchange website, even if fixed over the next year, could feed the suspicion that government cannot get anything right, that it cannot be trusted. This is a credibility issue: once lost, trust can take generations to regain. And perhaps it will fuel even more antigovernment feeling and set back American liberalism a generation.

Although the short-term political costs of the ACA have been enormous and enormously damaging to Democrats, the judgment of history is likely to be much kinder to the ACA. Because of the size and reach of the American health care system, it will take a decade to truly take stock of the system-wide changes. By 2020 the transformative impact of the ACA will be clear through the change in how patients are cared for. The ACA revealed a classic tension between politicians fighting for the next election and policy makers looking over the horizon to the next generation. In the case of the ACA President Obama, Speaker Pelosi, Majority Leader Reid, and the Democrats had their eyes fixed on the next generation. And all Americans will be better off for it.

Further Readings

Introduction: Erin's Disease

Cohn, Jonathan. *Sick: The Untold Story of America's Health Care Crisis—and the People Who Pay the Price*. New York: HarperCollins, 2009.

Part I: The American Health Care System

Chapter 1: How Did We Get Here?

Cunningham, Robert, and Robert M. Cunningham. *The Blues: A History of the Blue Cross and Blue Shield System*. De Kalb: Northern Illinois University Press, 1997.

Fein, Rashi. *Medical Care, Medical Costs: The Search for a Health Insurance Policy*. Cambridge: Harvard University Press, 1986.

Hacker, Jacob S. "Part III: The Politics of Public and Private Health Insurance." *The Divided Welfare State: The Battle over Public and Private Social Benefits in the United States*. Cambridge: Cambridge University Press, 2002.

Roberts, Jeffrey A. "A History of Health Insurance in the U.S. and Colorado." University of Denver, Center for Colorado's Economic Future, November 2009. www.du.edu/economicfuture/documents/HistoryOfHealthInsurance_CCEF.pdf.

Rosenberg, Charles E. *The Care of Strangers: The Rise of America's Hospital System*. Baltimore: Johns Hopkins University Press, 1995.

Starr, Paul. *The Social Transformation of American Medicine*. New York: Basic Books, 1982.

Stevens, Rosemary. *In Sickness and Wealth: American Hospitals in the Twentieth Century*. Baltimore: Johns Hopkins University Press, 1999.

Chapter 2: Financing Health Care

Aaron, Henry J., and Jeanne M. Lambrew. *Reforming Medicare: Options, Tradeoffs, and Opportunities*. Washington, D.C.: Brookings Institution, 2008.

Cutler, David M., and Richard J. Zeckhauser. "The Anatomy of Health Insurance." In *Handbook of Health Economics*, ed. Anthony J. Culyer and Joseph P. Newhouse, 563–643. Amsterdam: Elsevier North-Holland, 2000.

Henry J. Kaiser Family Foundation. "Medicare: A Primer." April 1, 2010. www.kff.org/medicare/upload/7615–03.pdf.

Henry J. Kaiser Family Foundation. "State-by-State Estimates of the Number of People Eligible for Premium Tax Credits Under the Affordable Care Act." November 5, 2013. www.kaiseredu.org/Tutorials-and-Presentations/Private-Health-Insurance.aspx.

Kaiser Commission on Medicaid and the Uninsured. "Medicaid 101. Kaiser-EDU." Henry J. Kaiser Family Foundation. March 1, 2013. www.kaiseredu.org/Tutorials-and-Presentations/Medicaid-101.aspx.

Kaiser Family Foundation and Health Research and Educational Trust. "Employer Health Benefits: 2013 Annual Survey." 2013. http://kaiserfamilyfoundation.files.wordpress.com/2013/08/8465-employer-health-benefits-20132.pdf.

Chapter 3: How Americans Get Their Health Care

American Hospital Association. "AHA Hospital Statistics." 2013. www.ahadataviewer.com/overview/Hospital-Statistics/.

Shi, Leiyu, and Douglas A. Singh. *Delivering Health Care in America: A Systems Approach*. Sudbury, Mass.: Jones and Bartlett Publishers, 2009.

Chapter 4: Five Problems with the American Health Care System

Brill, Steven. "Bitter Pill: Why Medical Bills Are Killing Us." *Time*. March 4, 2013. http://content.time.com/time/magazine/article/0,9171,2136864,00.html.

Chernew, Michael, David M. Cutler, and Patricia Seliger Keenan. "Increasing Health Insurance Costs and the Decline in Insurance Coverage." Health Services Research 40, no. 4 (August 2005): 1021–1039. www.ncbi.nlm.nih.gov/pmc/articles/PMC1361195/.

Congressional Budget Office. "The 2013 Long-Term Budget Outlook." September 17, 2013. www.cbo.gov/publication/44521.

Elhauge, Einer. *The Fragmentation of U.S. Health Care: Causes and Solutions*. Oxford University Press, 2010.

Elmendorf, Douglas W. "Federal Health Care Spending: Why Is It Growing? What Could Be Done About It?" Congressional Budget Office. November 13, 2013. www.cbo.gov/sites/default/files/cbofiles/attachments/44761-Wharton.pdf.

Lee, Thomas H., and James J. Mongan. *Chaos and Organization in Health Care*. Cambridge: Massachusetts Institute of Technology Press, 2009.

Organisation for Economic Co-operation and Development. "Health at a Glance 2013." November 21, 2013. www.oecd.org/els/health-systems/health-at-a-glance.htm.

Part II: Reforming the American Health Care System

Chapter 5: The Surprising History of Health Care Reform in the United States

Altman, Stuart A., and Shactman, David. *Power, Politics, and Universal Health Care: The Inside Story of a Century-Long Battle.* Amherst, N.Y.: Prometheus Books, 2011.

Blumenthal, David, and James A. Morone. *The Heart of Power: Health and Politics in the Oval Office.* Berkeley: University of California Press, 2009.

Falkson, Joseph L. *HMOs and the Politics of Health System Reform.* Chicago: American Hospital Association, 1980.

Johnson, Haynes, and Broder, David S. *The System: The American Way of Politics at the Breaking Point.* Boston: Little, Brown, 1996.

Marmor, Theodore R. *The Politics of Medicare.* Piscataway, N.J.: Transaction Books, 2000.

Oberlander, Jonathan. *The Political Life of Medicare.* Chicago: University of Chicago Press, 2003.

Starr, Paul. *Remedy and Reaction: The Peculiar American Struggle over Health Care Reform.* New Haven: Yale University Press, 2011.

Starr, Paul. *The Social Transformation of American Medicine.* New York: Basic Books, 1982.

Chapter 6: Enacting the Affordable Care Act

Cohn, Jonathan. "How They Did It: An Inside Account of Health Care Reform's Triumph." *The New Republic.* May 2010. www.tnr.com/article/politics/75062/how-they-did-it-part-one.

Daschle, Thomas. *Getting It Done: How Obama and Congress Finally Broke the Stalemate to Make Way for Health Care Reform.* New York: Thomas Dune Books, 2010.

Jacobs, Lawrence R., and Skocpol, Theda. *Health Care Reform and American Politics: What Everyone Needs to Know.* New York: Oxford University Press, 2010.

Washington Post. *Landmark: The Inside Story of America's New Health-Care Law and What It Means for Us All.* New York: PublicAffairs, 2010.

Chapter 7: What the Supreme Court Said

Blackman, Josh. *Unprecedented: The Constitutional Challenge to Obamacare.* New York: PublicAffairs, 2013.

Elhauge, Einer. *ObamaCare on Trial.* CreateSpace Independent Publishing Platform, 2012.

Persily, Nathaniel, Gillian E. Metzger, and Trevor W. Morrison, eds. *The Health Care Case: The Supreme Court's Decision and Its Implications.* Oxford University Press on Demand, 2013.

Rosen, Jeffrey. "Big Chief." *New Republic.* July 13, 2012. www.newrepublic.com/article/politics/magazine/104898/john-roberts-supreme-court-aca.

Supreme Court of the United States. National Federation of Independent Businesses et al. v. Sebelius, Secretary of Health and Human Services, et al. N. 11–393. June 28, 2012. www.supremecourt.gov/opinions/11pdf/11–393c3a2.pdf.

Chapter 8: What Is in the Affordable Care Act?

Gruber, Jonathan. *Health Care Reform: What It Is, Why It's Necessary, How It Works.* New York: Hill and Wang, 2011.

Kaiser Family Foundation. "Health Reform Implementation Timeline." 2013. http://kff.org/interactive/implementation-timeline/.

Kaiser Family Foundation. "Summary of the New Health Reform Law." March 2010. www.kff.org/healthreform/upload/8061.pdf.

McDonough, John E. *Inside National Health Reform.* Berkeley: University of California Press, 2011.

Chapter 9: What Does the ACA Mean for Me?

Newhouse, J. P. "Assessing Health Reform's Impact on Four Key Groups of Americans." *Health Affairs* 29, no. 9 (September 2010): 1714–1724.

Part III: The Future of American Health Care

Chapter 12: Health Care Reform 2.0

Antos J., et al. "Bending the Curve." Engelberg Center for Health Care Reform. 2013.

Center for American Progress. "The Senior Protection Plan." November 2012. www.americanprogress.org/wp-content/uploads/2012/11/SeniorProtectionPlan.pdf.

Emanuel, Ezekiel, Neera Tanden, Stuart Altman, Scott Armstrong, Donald Berwick, François de Brantes, Maura Calsyn, et al. "A Systemic Approach to

Containing Health Care Spending." *New England Journal of Medicine* 367, no. 10 (September 2012): 949–954.

Chapter 13: Six Megatrends in Health Care

Christensen, Clayton M., Jerome H. Grossman, and Jason Hwang. *The Innovator's Prescription: A Disruptive Solution for Health Care.* New York: McGraw-Hill, 2009.

Dishman, Eric. "Health Care Should Be a Team Sport." TED Talk. March 2013. www.ted.com/talks/eric_dishman_health_care_should_be_a_team_sport.html.

Scoble, Robert, and Shel Israel. *Age of Context: Mobile, Sensors, Data and the Future of Privacy.* Patrick Brewster Press, 2013.

Topol, Eric J. *The Creative Destruction of Medicine: How the Digital Revolution Will Create Better Health Care.* New York: Basic Books, 2012.

Index

About the Author

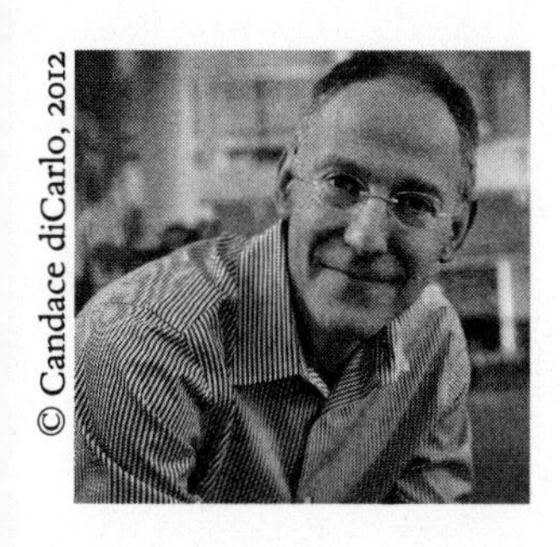
© Candace diCarlo, 2012

Ezekiel J. Emanuel is Vice Provost for Global Initiatives and chair of the Department of Medical Ethics and Health Policy at the University of Pennsylvania. He is a breast oncologist. From January 2009 to January 2011, he served as special adviser for health policy to the director of the White House Office of Management and Budget. Since 1997, he has been chair of the Department of Bioethics at The Clinical Center of the National Institutes of Health, a position he left in the summer of 2011. Dr. Emanuel has written and edited 10 books and over 250 scientific articles. He is currently a columnist for *The New York Times* and a senior fellow at the Center for American Progress. He appears regularly on television including *Morning Joe, Real Time with Bill Maher,* and *Hardball* with Chris Matthews.

Dr. Emanuel received his M.D. from Harvard Medical School and his Ph.D. in political philosophy from Harvard University. He has been on the faculty at the Dana-Farber Cancer Institute and Harvard Medical School, and was a visiting professor at the University of Pittsburgh School of Medicine, UCLA, the Brin Professor at Johns Hopkins Medical School, the Kovitz Professor at Stanford Medical School and New York University Law School. Raised in Chicago, Dr. Emanuel has three grown daughters, and now splits his time between Washington, D.C., and Philadelphia.

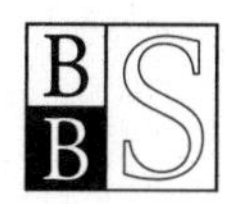

PUBLICAFFAIRS is a publishing house founded in 1997. It is a tribute to the standards, values, and flair of three persons who have served as mentors to countless reporters, writers, editors, and book people of all kinds, including me.

I. F. STONE, proprietor of *I. F. Stone's Weekly,* combined a commitment to the First Amendment with entrepreneurial zeal and reporting skill and became one of the great independent journalists in American history. At the age of eighty, Izzy published *The Trial of Socrates,* which was a national bestseller. He wrote the book after he taught himself ancient Greek.

BENJAMIN C. BRADLEE was for nearly thirty years the charismatic editorial leader of the *Washington Post*. It was Ben who gave the *Post* the range and courage to pursue such historic issues as Watergate. He supported his reporters with a tenacity that made them fearless, and it is no accident that so many became authors of influential, best-selling books.

ROBERT L. BERNSTEIN, the chief executive of Random House for more than a quarter century, guided one of the nation's premier publishing houses. Bob was personally responsible for many books of political dissent and argument that challenged tyranny around the globe. He is also the founder and was the longtime chair of Human Rights Watch, one of the most respected human rights organizations in the world.

· · ·

For fifty years, the banner of Public Affairs Press was carried by its owner, Morris B. Schnapper, who published Gandhi, Nasser, Toynbee, Truman, and about 1,500 other authors. In 1983 Schnapper was described by *The Washington Post* as "a redoubtable gadfly." His legacy will endure in the books to come.

Peter Osnos, *Founder and Editor-at-Large*

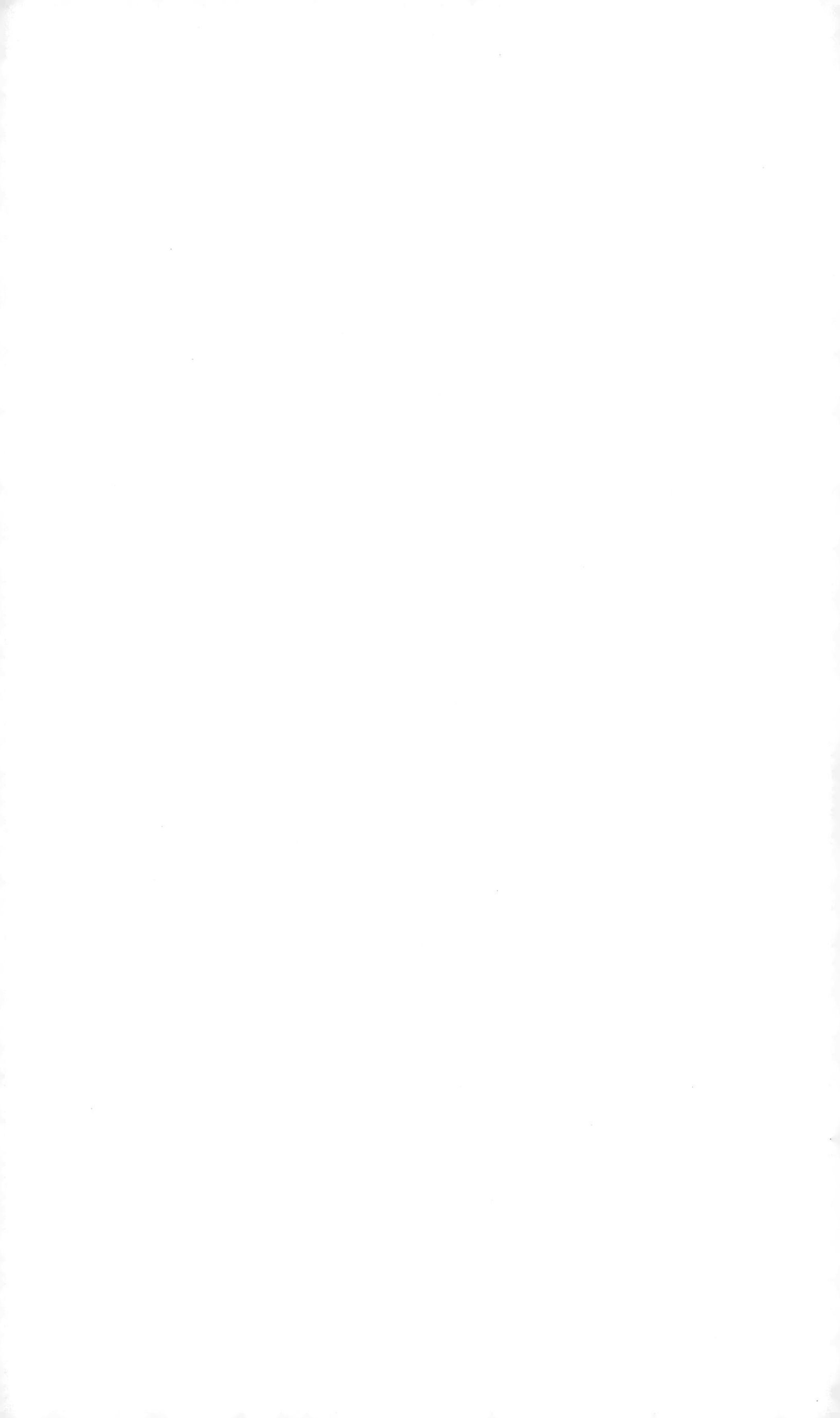